ISSELS

The Biography of a Doctor

ISSELS

The Biography of a Doctor

---

by

GORDON THOMAS

HODDER AND STOUGHTON
LONDON SYDNEY AUCKLAND TORONTO

For Edith

Science is the tool and the reinforcement of the spirit, and the spirit will find its salvation, not in turning back upon itself, which is the pursuit of a shadow, but in seeking out the object and grappling with it.

ALAIN

Contents

Illustrations

Key to acknowledgments:

1 Foto-Schäfer, Berchtesgaden, Bavaria
2 Quick-Foto: Th. Martens & Co., G.M.B.H.
3 Georg Schödl
4 Mac Slee
5 Ernst Grasser

Introduction

IF CONTROVERSY WAS SYNONYMOUS WITH ACCEPTANCE DR. Josef Issels long ago would have assured himself of a place in that elite of all establishments, the medical establishment. Few other doctors this century have so consistently aroused the medical profession to anger as he has with his approach to the treatment of cancer—cancer often beyond further surgery, irradiation and the conventional use of cytotoxic drugs which inhibit or kill malignant cells. For cancer is not just a biological and medical problem calling for a solution. It is also a human situation often presenting a crisis of suffering.

Cancer—or more precisely malignant growth caused by a disorder in which some cell type in the organism begins to grow in an apparently unchecked way—is an emotive word. Most doctors assume a quite proper hard disbelief towards claims of recovery for the disease which is said to have happened outside the accepted use of surgery and radiotherapy. Cancer, more than any other serious illness, attracts the charlatans, the quack doctors and the mystical healers. In the last twenty-five years alone dozens of 'cures' have been claimed by such people. All were scientifically proven cruelly false.

His harshest critics say that Issels belongs among those pedlars of bogus remedies.

It is a charge his advocates refute. They argue that Issels is a properly qualified doctor and that the Ringberg Klinik in

Rottach-Egern, Bavaria, meets the strict requirements of the West German Government who license it annually; they stress that doctors from all over the world, many of them recognised cancer specialists, continue to send patients to the clinic for treatment; finally they point to the astonishing record of success for his treatment: almost a 17 per cent remission rate for those termed 'incurable'.

Nevertheless the attacks continue. They gained impetus in 1968 when the American Cancer Society Incorporated—the largest voluntary agency of its kind in the world with donations of over sixty million dollars a year—placed Issels in its 'Index of Unproven Methods', a slim paperback, which it circulated to other cancer societies in the world through the offices of the International Union Against Cancer in Geneva. The American Cancer Society Incorporated did not spend one dollar to send an observer to investigate the claims made by Issels before black-listing him.

The British Cancer Council, through its secretary, Dr. Graham Bennette, expressed this opinion in 1970: 'Issels has little to offer except the potential to raise false hope.' Bennette admitted that no member of the British Cancer Council had up to then ever actually been to the Ringberg Klinik to establish if in fact such a statement was true.

Professor Karl Bauer, *der Altvater* of German cancer specialists, in 1970 said of Issels: 'He is a dangerously misguided man who does no good at his clinic.' Bauer, professor of surgery at Heidelberg University, has never visited the clinic.

In 1970 the B.B.C. invited Professor Michael Shimkin to visit the Ringberg Klinik as part of a television enquiry it was conducting into Issels. Shimkin, of the University of California in San Diego, is one of the world's most eminent cancerologists. At first he was enthusiastic. Then he talked to the American Cancer Society Incorporated. What was said is not known. But Shimkin cancelled the first-class return air ticket which the B.B.C. had bought him. He told the Corporation: 'It would be inappropriate for an American to go to Germany to look at German work in this field just as it would be wrong for a German to come to America under these circumstances.'

Issels was baffled; every year there is a steady exchange of cancer specialists between Germany and America. But he was accustomed to such behaviour, though he was surprised that Shimkin, traditionally so open-minded, should have refused in such a manner.

Bitter experience had, however, taught Issels that nowhere was opposition to his ideas more strident, more ill-informed, than among those members of the medical establishment, unable for many reasons, to become divorced from an orthodox approach to treating cancer.

Yet, he could never give up trying to persuade them. He was one of those whom the Russian philosopher, Chernshevsky, described as 'the movers of the movers'; the shout which one day let loose the avalanche. Issels believed his shout had been finally heard when Sir David Smithers, cancer adviser to the British Government's Department of Health, visited the Ringberg Klinik with five other cancer experts after an unprecedented public call in Britain for an 'impartial inquiry' into the methods practised by Issels. The team spent five days at the clinic, charged with examining over 6,000 case histories in a foreign language. Their verdict was Issels had little new to offer in the treatment of cancer.

Following the furore created by the report's publication, Josef Issels drew comfort from what other distinguished cancer scientists had earlier told him. One of them was Mr. Denis Burkitt of the Medical Research Council, London, a scientist whose place in medical annals is forever assured through his discovery of one of the most significant of cancer diseases, cancer of the lymphatic tissues. In 1970 he had met Issels in London and told him how much he admired Issels' approach to managing cancer patients. It was a view shared by another respected physician, John Anderson.

Professor John Anderson, professor of physical medicine at one of Britain's better teaching hospitals, King's College Hospital, London, spent a considerable period of time, spread over two years, on behalf of the B.B.C., and for his own interest, conducting a detailed scientific investigation into Issels' claims. Anderson later gave me permission to quote from his assessment of Issels:

I advise that Dr. Issels has a new approach of interest to

doctors and patients. Looking at the data which is available I accept his findings of a long remission rate of nearly 17 per cent in terminal cases. I am of the considered opinion that this is a new approach to cancer treatment and appears to be a considerable improvement on what is usually offered. My overall opinion is that the Issels approach to the treatment of cancer is an unique and pioneering solution to a very difficult problem. He is undoubtedly producing clinical remission in patients who have been regarded as hopeless and left to fall back on their own resources. From the clinical, scientific point of view an independent trial is essential if his treatment ideas are to be accepted more widely and further research must be undertaken to evaluate what he has started.

When Anderson's views became public, an event he regarded as significant happened: his research grants from some of Britain's cancer societies were threatened. Such a move has often proved an effective way of disciplining a recalcitrant member of the medical establishment. Anderson found himself a victim of the fierce emotions, and sometimes near hysteria, that the medical establishment displays when Issels and his work is discussed.

It is an established fact that his opponents sincerely believe they are right to reject Issels and his belief that cancer, even in the imprecisely defined 'terminal stage', can still be successfully treated after all other conventional methods have failed. It is also equally true that some of his influential critics have failed to keep the scientist's open mind. Denis Burkitt wrote of their attitude towards Issels: 'It is quite unscientific to say, "it can't happen: therefore it didn't happen".'

Issels' approach to his work is synthesised in what he wrote when he first treated cancer patients:

Even when it is obvious that a patient has reached the terminal phase of a cancer, it is impossible for me to give up treatment, believing, as I do, that the treatment I prescribe often offers a positive alternative to just quietly bringing comfort to the dying. Distress must be relieved;

> no patient should be faced with a burden of suspended dying where only a truncated semblance of life is maintained. Equally, I believe more can, and should be done to offer the chronic and incurable a real extension of valuable living.

The words are a private litany of rejection of the universally held scientific belief that beyond surgery, radiotherapy and drugs little else is practical in treating cancer. When still young Issels decided to make his life his argument; to show that his methods offered a genuine alternative to merely prescribing pain-killing drugs in the final stages of the illness. By the time he reached middle-age he developed and lived for ideas which were both revolutionary and greatly misunderstood. Always orthodoxy found him to be a total opponent. In refusing to accept the conventional hypothesis on how cancer should be treated, Issels found himself changing public attitudes towards the disease; he brought it into the headlines, often in a manner he would not have wished.

Though pilloried in the courts, and the centre of wrangling in the legislature, comfort came from his belief that some of the mystery, superstitious fear and dread surrounding the disease was removed under such scrutiny. Despite the attacks, and possibly because of them, Issels sees his clinic as a kind of oasis where patients from Europe, America, Africa and Asia experience a rare peace.

To the outside world he has become in recent years almost an unbelievable figure; so often has legend and fantasy become entwined with the controversy and bitterness that any real judgment on his work is lost. Rumour reached a fantastic level in 1971 when it was seriously put about that the Ringberg Klinik was under surveillance by West German intelligence agents who suspected patients from behind the Iron Curtain were somehow using it as a 'dead letter-box' for Soviet espionage. It took some weeks for the story to die.

Sometimes those he has helped, his patients, have added to the confusion. In publicly parading their recovery in the press—done so without the approval of Issels—they conferred on him what one critic savagely likened to 'sainthood by acclamation'. At one stage the rush of embarrassing paeans threatened to reduce Issels to the status of a mere 'celebrity' and allowed his detractors ample room to attack.

Men like Josef Issels will always attract critics, both great and small. For his part he has never avoided them. Often he has found himself alone, but never lonely, for he enjoys a real fellowship with those who share the beliefs he has pursued with single-minded determination and incredible resources of energy for so many years.

His long working life spans much of the period when modern research, management and control of various types of cancer were expanding.

Roentgen discovered X-rays in 1895; a year later the first case of radiation-induced dermatitis was reported. Undoubtedly the seminal period for cancer research were the early years of this century. First came a redefinition of the cause of coal-tar cancer. Then came the discovery of the first cancer-producing virus. Since then the progress of cancer research has been one of generally painstaking advances with success in a number of areas. Skin and breast cancer are not the scourge they used to be, especially if treated early on.

Even so surgery and radiotherapy still represent the main treatments generally available; hormone therapy and drugs play supportive roles. Though surgical techniques are more sophisticated, operations are still only locally effective and virtually useless when dissemination of malignant cells has occurred; while irradiation now allows X-rays to be accurately focussed upon a cancer it does not always achieve permanent inhibition of malignant growths.

Meanwhile unprecedented sums of money are spent to find that elusive of all the answers: the actual *cause* of cancer. Many of the cancer-producing influences are known; possibly complete understanding will come only with full realisation of the vital processes of normal cell growth. But these are days of high expectancy in the field of cancer therapy; while effective control of the illness is still a hope of the future, much has been accomplished today.

For Issels, achievement, and possibly even fame, could have been attained by working alongside those engaged on such orthodox lines of inquiry. He had the qualifications and potential to be an outstanding surgeon; with it went the rarer gift of a mind capable of genuine original thought that, properly channelled, could have been an asset to any research institute.

Quite deliberately he chose a different course. From the outset it brought him into conflict with colleagues in Germany, and later in Great Britain, the United States of America and numerous other countries. Over the years his opponents—whom Issels castigates as exponents of *medi-politik*—have remained consistent in their efforts not only to discredit him, but also those members of the medical profession who support Issels. In spite of their campaigning—the attacks reach into his personal and political as well as his professional life—Issels has managed to attract continuing support for his methods.

Today, there are many men, women and children who say they owe their lives to the treatment he has given them. They were designated as 'terminal cases' by their own physicians and surgeons. A growing number are still free of detectable cancer after the arbitrary five-year interval customarily used to express effective remission. Some of this success came at a time when immunotherapy agents were still the exclusive province of the microbiologist and chemotherapy was a relative newcomer to the fight. Available treatment was summed up in that crude slogan of *stahl und strahl*—steel and radiotherapy.

Issels maintains that is not enough.

Without the support of the State, or the full thrust that funding by an appropriate foundation brings, he refined an idea fallen from favour as medical science became more specialised. Put at its simplest, he argues that cancer is not a local affliction, but a general disease which places the whole body at risk from the outset; success lies he says, in the use of a treatment devised to ensure effective distribution throughout the whole body.

Embracing Einstein's concept—'imagination is more important than knowledge; knowledge is limited, imagination embraces the world, stimulating progress, giving birth to evolution'—Issels has devoted a lifetime to popularising his theory. Over the years he has exercised a flair for public relations; he must be one of the most travelled medical men in Europe. His readiness, unusual among scientists of any discipline, to offer his ideas to a lay audience increased professional opposition.

He has attracted powerful lay interest. Pope Pius XII blessed his work during a private audience. Lord Snowdon showed Issels royal interest by attending a short public debate on his methods which the B.B.C. sponsored. It was held at the Royal Institution in London. Members of the medical profession were outraged that this bastion of their establishment should have been used for such a purpose.

An increasing number of the components of what has become known as Issels' 'whole body treatment', or *ganzheitstherapie,* are now regularly used in all parts of the world. On learning in 1970 that New York's Sloan Kettering Institute for Cancer Research had carried out trials on the 'fever treatment' he used many years previously, Issels observed:

> For so long I have felt like a voice in the wilderness that it is still almost a shock, though a pleasant one, to see such a pillar of the medical establishment coming round to my way of thinking. I am not unique in this reaction; the innovator, especially in medicine, has always been looked upon with suspicion, especially if he uses techniques that have not been tried before.

His implacable belief that he is right, earns him a secure place among the private hates of the medical establishment. He is the embodiment of the truism that a man is known as much by his enemies as by the friends he keeps.

Issels remains an excellent example of the medical establishment's institutional memory being far longer than the careers of individual members. It neither forgives nor forgets. It has also been said, and with some truth, that Josef Issels early on in his career obliterated any chance of receiving the benediction of his peers by his obstinacy, habitual arrogance and a damning self-assurance. To this charge, Issels answers that kid gloves are no use when handling barbed wire.

As his work became more widely known—his daily postbag can come from up to thirty-two countries—there were repeated demands for his co-operation in telling his story. He refused all such requests, believing that however well-meaning were the writers they still failed to grasp the fundamentals upon which he lays such store.

A study of the voluminous newspaper coverage, founded on casual, short-term interviews he has granted over the years, tends to support his doubts. The phrases recurring most frequently are 'miracle doctor' and 'medical maverick'; much is made of his dictatorial approach, his life style, his willingness, as one American newspaper put it, 'to try anything'. Those closer to him regard this widely-held view as a serious misrepresentation of the man and his methods. Little understanding has been shown of the unique patient-doctor relationship he has developed over many years; nor has there been any rational understanding of his treatment by the media. Issels long ago shrugged such things aside, though he was momentarily shaken when the *Times of India* announced his death in November, 1971.

If it achieves nothing else, this biography would hope for a clearer picture of the methods, and the man, to emerge than has hitherto appeared. It is not a book about cancer; though the word appears on many pages, such a book could only be written by an expert. Neither is it a history of cancer research or a treatise about a highly unusual treatment. Nor is it a story about a total cure for all cancer.

I first met Josef Issels on behalf of the B.B.C. at the outset of the Corporation's marathon investigation into his claims. I was one of the two producers in charge of the project, with special responsibility for research. The production team found itself at loggerheads with some executives within the B.B.C. who were alarmed, as the investigation deepened, in case we became protagonists for Issels. Those executives saw their role as one of making sure that the B.B.C.'s traditional 'balance' was in no way threatened. At times they felt the production team, in its enthusiasm, showed too strong a committment to Issels.

Both my co-producer and myself had in fact from the outset made it clear to all concerned with the inquiries that particular care must be taken to remain impartial. In turn, this produced problems with Issels; the relationship between the doctor and the production team was frequently strained. On at least two occasions Issels told me during our investigation that he was 'tired and upset' with what he regarded as our excessive probing. In the end he was persuaded that an uncritical assessment of his claims would be useless to him and that we would be failing in our duty to adopt such an approach.

From a beginning of wariness on both sides I began to grasp the complexity of his own story and also the wider picture of how powerful pressure can be in the medical profession. Further and deeper investigation continued to destroy the neatness of our original interpretation, and as material accumulated, it became clear to me that no matter how the massive, though at times fragmentary, evidence was marshalled and selected, there was an overwhelming case for screening the results. Looking back now I honestly believe that all of us concerned with researching and making the film were acutely aware that such a study is fraught with the temptation of uttering premature personal judgments—and that we took good care not to do so.

Of the many impressions I gained, one constantly returned: Issels had never lost the enthusiasm for the rebellion he proclaimed long ago against many of the hallowed concepts of his profession. As a student he had little patience with rote and example. For him the value of original discovery rode rough-shod over all else. This heuristic attitude remained constant all his life, providing stimulus for the tumbling with practical experience. It became clear he had made mistakes, many of them. Equally, he had also made a contribution to the *awareness* of cancer.

In his mature years when he already had treated some 6,000 cases of what he regarded as chronic cancer, two events projected him again into the headlines. In November, 1970, B.B.C. television screened the results of our investigation; the Olympic athlete, Lillian Board became a patient of Issels—and died in the full glare of the mass media. Both events profoundly affected him. He found himself having to defend to an audience far greater than almost any doctor had faced not only his immediate medical decisions, but also his whole philosophy. It was then that the possibility of my writing his biography was seriously raised. Issels hesitated. He doubted whether the project was viable. He felt a biography should not be published while he was alive. But I knew the nature of the problems he had faced probably better than anybody outside his immediate family, and in the end a promise was made that his huge library of private papers would be made available. This source would enable a direct and first-hand presentation of the evidence; occasionally there was an uneven wealth to the material and in places it contained an apocalyptic note by Issels. I was initially uncertain about my ability to explain many of his actions and attitudes without falling into that pitfall of all biography—rationalising them at the expense of contemporaries and predecessors. Any such biography would be misleading. Again the weighing of oral evidence—the recall of patients, doctors, the Issels family—in such an enterprise could be imprecise and even risky, and perhaps its only justification is that it might provide a vital fragment or two. Finally, the character of Issels, an explosive and dedicated man, would be difficult to portray. But difficulty is itself a challenge, and in the end I accepted it.

In the only editorial guidance he ever offered me Josef Issels said:

> Not just my own story, but also the story of how the medical establishment closes its ranks and its collective mind when cherished opinions, however wrong, are brought into question. In an age when science is changing human life for better or for worse, it is natural to take an interest in the scientist, in his attitudes, the way his mind works, the nature of his investigations. What needs to be stated also is that unless the scientist, or clinician, works within the strict confines of what is acceptable to orthodox thinking at the time, he will engender doubtful curiosity. I have suffered a lifetime of it.

He asked no more. Neither of us knew that when I began to write this book it would be only a matter of months before Issels would find himself with no alternative but to close his clinic and find himself in a desperate personal battle to survive. He survived both closure and near bankruptcy, and, when these words were written in 1974, he was planning a new life, evaluating offers from various medical centres around the world which had offered him posts. One thing is clear: the last has not been heard of Josef Issels or his ideas.

Gordon Thomas,
Ashford,
Co. Wicklow,
Ireland.

I

Early Years

ON A DULL NOVEMBER 21, 1907 JOSEF MARIA LEONHARD Issels was born in the textile town of Mönchen-Gladbach in the Rhineland of Germany. His middle names came from a family tradition of naming children after a paternal grandmother and a favourite uncle. On the evidence of photographs he was a solemn-faced baby with startlingly clear eyes, the first son of a marriage of convenience. The knowledge later had a marked effect on his life.

He was born into circumstances far different from those the first recorded Issels faced in 1750: nothing is really known about him except that he was the son of a land worker in Holland. For nearly another hundred years successive Issels tilled the fertile Dutch soil, untroubled by the cultural tides of the time. Around them individual fortunes rose and fell, princes died, kingdoms were redefined, mercenary armies advanced and retreated, but the range of success or failure for the antecedents of Josef Issels was strictly measured by the rotation of a crop.

In 1866 another Josef Issels sold his plough and plodded out of Holland eastward into Germany. In the month he crossed the border, May, the *Bruderkrieg* between Austria and Prussia began; in seven swift weeks Prussia had absorbed Austrian Silesia and all of north Germany. The roots of a world power had been planted.

That nineteenth-century Issels also set about laying a proper foundation for his family. With money he husbanded from peddling goods in the streets of Mönchen-Gladbach he bought three properties in a prized position in the town's market place; within a short time 1–3 Alter Markt had established a wide reputation for good quality linen and household goods. The family lived over the store: five of the nine children born in the house died in infancy. For the survivors life became increasingly good.

By the time Hermann Josef Issels was born in September 1869, the family was one of the wealthiest of the town's merchant class. As the full hammer-blow of industrialisation came to the Rhineland and changed its face with shattering impact that wealth increased. No. 4 Alter Markt was brought into the Issels fief. The four houses with their elegant façades offered a marked contrast to the surrounding Brueghel dreams of towers, spires and gabled roofs.

In 1888 Hermann Josef Issels took over the family store on the death of his father. Only nineteen years old, he firmly established that efficiency was his religion. Under his frugal and canny direction business prospered; soon customers were travelling the fifty kilometres from Holland to buy his goods. By the age of thirty-six Hermann Issels was a key figure in the town's business oligarchy, that controlled trading hours, ran the fairs, appointed public officials and saw to it that Jewry knew its proper place. Apart from work—'the best relaxation'—his only hobby was a schoolboy passion for stamp collecting. There is nothing to show he ever had a serious romantic entanglement until 1905, when he was approaching middle-age. In January of that year, the traditional carnival month in the Catholic Rhineland, he was persuaded to temporarily put away his stamps and go to a *fasching* ball.

It was his good fortune to be partnered early on in the evening by Adelheid Heinen in those endless waltzes and polkas characteristic of *fasching*. She was one of the belles of the town—a slim, vivacious twenty-three-year-old with a fine-boned face and a winning smile. She captivated the inexperienced Hermann Issels.

Both families were delighted. *Mutti* Issels saw in Adelheid the prospect of a wife she had almost given up hoping Hermann Josef would ever take. For Frau Heinen, Issels was a catch she, too, had desired for her daughter. For years the Heinen family had spent a brave, though unsuccessful, time trying to maintain their place in the community's business life; their investments had foundered and by 1905 they lived in genteel poverty.

The romance was actively encouraged by both families, even though Adelheid expressed no great enthusiasm for it. She was in love with a law student. But by April 1905, her mother had persuaded Adelheid to put that young man aside and prepare for a formal proposal of marriage from Hermann Josef Issels. A month later they became engaged and they were married in the September of that year, securing for at least one child the assured future Frau Heinen so desperately wanted for all of her six children.

If passion was absent Adelheid brought other qualities to the marriage. Her lively mind pursued first one and then another avenue of intellectual exploration. She encouraged her husband to look beyond his stamp collection; she read poetry to him and revealed a real interest in nature study on their Sunday rambles into the countryside around Mönchen-Gladbach. From the comfort of middle-class security she tried to comprehend the new socialism that was emerging in Germany: she found it beyond her capacity to sympathise or understand it. But she knew her duty: every week she called on a number of poor families in the Hogarthian alleys around the store and brought them food and clothes.

Hermann Josef Issels still maintained a public self-defending reserve, but to the marriage he brought a sense of duty, of dedicating the present entirely to the future. Soon this sense of duty became the central factor in both lives; in many ways it replaced the true intimacy to be found in other marriages. A daughter, Maria, was born on 8th August, 1906. The event kindled, briefly, an ecstatic relationship between Hermann and Adelheid, who wrote of:

> The great happiness she has brought me, brought both of us. This is a great chance to have the perfection of family life which is so important. Hermann Josef is a new man. He cannot do enough for the baby. Pray that it is always like this.

The first months following the birth were probably the happiest the couple experienced. But gradually a pattern which was to be familiar established itself: for Hermann Josef the shop took precedence in his life; he minded it for thirteen hours a day and meal times were given over to discussing new lines to be offered, outstanding accounts to be settled. What little leisure he had, he spent with his stamps.

Adelheid accepted it as a part of the price she had to pay for the security her mother had deemed so necessary. While the gaieties and frivolities of a still new marriage were noticeably not there, there was a burning determination to expand in business on Hermann Josef's part and a recognition within Adelheid that in future she must be the hub and guardian of the family. She embraced fervently the four great 'K's' of German womanhood—*kirche, kemenate, küche, kinder:* church, bedroom, kitchen, children.

It was in that frame of mind that she looked forward to the birth of her next child: Josef Maria Leonhard.

A number of incidents occurred in Josef Issels' childhood which helped to mould his character.

His parents now shared 1–4 Alter Markt with his uncle Otto's family—Otto Issels worked in the shop—and all told there were eighteen adults and children in the house. Appearances were carefully maintained. Hermann Josef Issels believed a merchant had to present a prosperous front if he was to hold the confidence of his customers: there was a cook, a daily help, and a parlour maid who received one pound a month and her keep. When she asked for a shilling increase on her salary, it needed several family conferences before it was agreed. Money, and how it should be spent, was a recurring theme in the household. One of Josef's early memories is of his father returning home with a considerable purchase of valuable stamps and his mother quietly reproaching: 'But the money could have been used on the children.' The cost of stamps was to be a matter of some contention on several occasions, even though the money was there to pay for them.

If the house had its moments of emotional struggles, care was taken that the electricity of conflict was kept from the children who were born at regular intervals. In October,

1909, Charlotte arrived; Margot came in February, 1912; Adele in July, 1913; Helmut in July, 1916 and Reinold in November, 1922.

Josef was undoubtedly a favourite not only with his mother, but also among his brothers and sisters. From early on his mother concentrated upon him the love, hopes and ambitions she herself had never fulfilled, and that she accepted her husband would never satisfy.

She taught Josef to read and say his bed-time prayers. In those devotions he learnt not only to include his immediate family and relations, but also the creatures of the earth. It helped to develop in him a compassion and sensitivity for all life, and was the first important watershed in his normal and intellectual development.

There were also other factors shaping the life of Josef Issels.

Mönchen-Gladbach, like most Rhineland towns had its Jewish ghetto. The Jews would daily venture forth from their quarter about their business. They were sufficiently few in number to be an oddity. The town's children, reared on lurid tales, often regarded Jews as enemies of Christ, and they would catcall and jeer at any passing Jew. One day a Jewish pedlar trundled his cart over the cobblestones outside the store. Behind, at a safe distance, came a group of youths chanting insults. Josef Issels was forcibly struck by the forbearance and patience the pedlar showed towards his tormentors. In years to come he recalled: 'His behaviour offered me a valuable lesson in how to behave under persecution.'

It also instilled in Issels a freedom from religious prejudice which became a hallmark of his mature life.

The early years were blissfully happy ones for Josef and the other children, with the highspot coming on those warm summer Sundays when the entire family would pile into a farm cart pulled by two horses and picnic in the fields outside the town. But even on the sunniest of days the sky to the north appeared overcast: the Ruhr, with its priceless lode of coal, threw up a great pall of greasy smoke that never lifted.

From the age of eight until his fifteenth birthday he spent his school holidays on a farm, tending animals, sowing and reaping crops. Like his mother Josef had an abiding interest in nature and frequently returned home with a specimen to add to the growing collection of bugs and insects he kept in a box-room at the top of the house. His sister Margot recalled:

> Over the years he spent hours up there. He had an endless curiosity about anything that moved. He simply had to know why and how. But he was gentle with everything. His interest didn't extend to pulling off wings or doing any of the other nasty things little boys do when they want to find what an insect is made up of.

By the age of twelve his interest widened to include human physiology. An entry in the family diary for May, 1920, reveals:

> Jupp [the family nickname for Josef] has again spent hours being a doctor. Maria is his nurse. The other children are the patients. He takes it all very seriously. He can take an accurate pulse and thermometer reading. He is very thorough in his examination. The patients are laid out on a table in the scullery and examined most carefully. Frequently Jupp diagnoses that only surgery is helpful; he is quite keen on operations and goes through all the motions. First he and Maria wash their hands, then Jupp inspects again the area to be operated upon . . . in the last few weeks Charlotte has had both her legs and arms removed by this tyro surgeon among us! But he does it with such gentleness that she is willing to undergo further 'surgery'. When he is not operating he is busy prescribing pills for all sorts of ailments: his patients don't mind this as he dispenses peppermints. He says he still wants to be a doctor when he leaves school, but he will have to concentrate more on his studies if he is to achieve his wish.

Those last words reaffirmed a view his teachers held almost from the outset of his schooldays. He had entered the Mönchen-Gladbach Gymnasium at the age of six, a thin and rather sickly-looking boy who became the occasional victim of bullying. He solved that problem by conscientiously building up his physical strength, until, in his teenage years, he was the school's outstanding athlete. By then he was also engaged in a hard race to catch up on the academic side. Issels had the misfortune early on to have been placed in a class run by an old-style pedagogue who showed no interest in his pupils—'a great part of the day was spent catching flies', Issels later wrote. When he moved up to the senior school he discovered how poor the basic grounding in his education had been.

Encouraged by his mother—to whom he had confessed the sorry story of those wasted early years in class—Josef Issels set about seeking academic respectability. He was helped in his task by his new master, Dr. Hoven; while the teacher remained constant to the adage that for boys the road to success was paved with Latin declensions and French verse, Hoven had a rare skill of making lessons both stimulating and informative.

Under his guidance Issels discovered that learning was both a knack and a pleasure; he was not brilliant, but his natural ability was supported by a new determination to do well. In many ways he was coming to accept the responsibility of satisfying his mother's expectations for him.

There was a tradition in the family that every weekday afternoon the children gathered in the drawing room around a sofa on which their mother rested and gave faithful and detached reports of the school day: in his last years at the Gymnasium Josef Issels undoubtedly found the reports easier to give because they were, for the most part, accounts of modest success.

If academic brilliance at school had been blighted by a poor start, there can be no doubting his athletic prowess: it was little short of phenomenal. The puny six-year-old had, by the age of ten, developed skills more in keeping with a circus acrobat. He could handspring around the dining room or walk upstairs on his hands, supporting a smaller child on his upturned feet. Tipped into the school swimming pool by a group of older boys, and nearly drowning because he could not swim, Issels mastered the crawl and breast stroke in three punishing days. He brought the same dedication to his tennis and other ball games.

In August, 1914 the streets of Mönchen-Gladbach, as in all German towns, were filled with great columns of men marching for the Fatherland to war, singing *Deutschland, Deutschland über alles* and:

Lieb Vaterland, kannst ruhig sein,
Fest steht und treu die Wacht,
Die Wacht am Rhein . . .

Hermann Josef Issels did not go: the nation felt no need to call upon a forty-six-year-old shopkeeper to answer the *Hoch* 'For Kaiser, people and country'.

For the next four years, by the junk heap of no-man's land the opposing armies squatted opposite each other in France, living troglodytic lives in dugouts and trenches; there in the chalk of Friscourt, or the clay of La Bassée, or the mud swamp of Flanders a whole generation of idealistic young men bled to death. Raised to valour, taught loyalty to the tribalism of *Gott* or *God* or *Dieu,* they sacrificed themselves to a civilisation that died with them.

By 1918 in Germany talk of *Siegessturm* (stroke of victory) had given way to a succession of *der schwarze tag,* with each day becoming blacker. Finally, in the cold of that year's November, a few days short of his eleventh birthday, Josef Issels saw an age reach Journey's End: the door of history closed forever on the princes and potentates and their toy-soldier armies. Inside Germany, the taste was bitter, and for millions, unbearable. In the Issels household, the Armistice did little to raise the gloom. Prophetically Hermann Josef Issels told his wife that it was no more than a truce; true peace, as they knew it, had gone forever.

That morning of November 11, 1918, the bells tolling for peace were also a definite omen to Adelheid Issels; the belfries calling joyously to each other seemed to represent a divine warning. After breakfast she called the children together and told them to prepare themselves for difficult times ahead.

The war years had already produced a marked decline in the fortune of the family store; only Hermann Josef's relentless drive kept the business going. The strain affected his health. Early in 1919 the family doctor diagnosed diabetes and became a regular caller at the house to carry out treatment.

Over the years Josef found the housecalls offered an opportunity to satisfy his increasing interest in medicine. The family diary for April, 1921, shows:

> Jupp again asking Dr. all sorts of questions. 'How much blood in the body?' 'Why does hair grow again when it is cut?' 'Why must we close our eyes to sleep?' Poor Dr. He will need an extra fee for all his answers! Jupp gives only one answer now about his future: he will study to be a doctor.

At school Issels took extra pains with chemistry and biology; his work in those subjects became clear and acceptable to his teachers.

Outside school he became more aware of the worsening political situation within Germany. On January 24, 1920, the Versailles *Diktat,* as most Germans had come to regard the Armistice Treaty, was ratified by Germany. Two months later right-wing elements tried to topple the fledgling Weimar Republic. The move was thwarted by a general strike called by the Social Democratic Party. The streets of the Ruhr became battlefields for the militant workers, the *Rote Soldatenbund,* and the Rightists.

In Mönchen-Gladbach the demands of the workers filled the air with that deep-voiced north German accent that, say the Bavarians, 'makes the ears bleed'. Finally those demands erupted in the late summer of 1923.

Issels had just completed a term in which he continued to make progress for the crucial examination he must eventually pass to go on to university and study medicine. Physically, he had already reached manhood: he was tall, muscular and incredibly fair. He had begun to have a roving eye for the girls. His sister Charlotte recalled:

> He was very grown up with the girls. They loved his charm and the way he could talk on all sorts of things. And he was very good about ending a relationship. He would not just drop a girl, but he would do it slowly

and gently until she was left with the feeling that it was her decision to end the relationship.

The first weeks of the summer holiday were idyllic for Issels: an endless round of tennis, swimming, country hikes and dances. The troubled world outside was temporarily forgotten.

Then, late in September, 1923, the bottom finally dropped out of the money market: 5,000,000 RM were equal to one American dollar. The German bank rate was raised to a meaningless 90 per cent. The long summer had already been one continuous eruption of sniper shots and grenade explosions. Now events became hopelessly out of control as a fresh series of strikes swept Germany.

For days gangs roamed Mönchen-Gladbach, looting and burning shops and factories. Business came to a standstill. The streets were filled with charging riot police and insurgents.

In 1–4 Alter Markt, the Issels family waited impassively behind shuttered windows. From time to time grave news was brought by fellow merchants: the looters were becoming more senseless in their reactions. The spectre which had haunted Adelheid Issels since Armistice Day was assuming an ominous form. Yet to flee meant losing everything. To her husband and children she calmly said: 'Here we stay to see what happens.'

They had not long to wait. Lunch was over on the last day of September when a gang gathered at the far end of the street. In minutes their number had grown close to a hundred—unkempt men with clubs and some jubilantly waving red flags. There was a shouted command and the band swept down the Alter Markt. Above the babble of shouts one word clearly reached the family: *Issels*.

Adelheid Issels did not hesitate. She ordered her husband and children away from the windows. Then turning to Josef she said: '*Komm!*'

Smoothing down her apron she walked briskly down the stairs.

What followed Josef Issels committed to a private diary:

> From the foot of the stairs we could hear the rioters. They were preparing to charge down the door. Mother did not falter. She unbolted the door and opened it. Beyond, the street seemed filled with men. She stepped out of the door and faced them. I stood behind her, ready to pull her to safety if there was trouble. For a moment the crowd was muttering. Then they fell silent as Mother continued to look calmly at them. She waited until they were totally quiet for almost a full minute. Then she said, very clearly 'What is it you want?' From the front of the crowd a man shouted that they wanted something for their family, that they were starving. Mother nodded. 'Very well. Then you must have something. All of you. But there will be no looting. Understand? There will be strict order.' Mother turned and walked back into the shop. For a moment nothing happened. Then, one by one, the gang filed in, took whatever Mother handed over, and walked out quietly again.

In the coming days several neighbourhood shops were plundered, but 1–4 Alter Markt remained untouched.

> What Mother did [Issels diary continues] is to make me realise that I must never run away from a situation, however difficult it may seem. She taught me to always face up to a situation and try to see it from the other side as well.

Summer faded into an autumn of growing violence. Chancellor Wilhelm Cuno's government fell; his successor, Gustav Stresemann, fared little better. In Munich, yet another political factor flexed its muscles: the new *Nationalsozialistische Deutsche Arbeiterpartei* tried, and failed, in a putsche. For the first time the name of its leader, Adolf Hitler, was heard outside Bavaria. By Christmas the deeds of the party forced newspapers to shorten its title to Nazi Party.

Silvester, the celebration of a new year, 1924, was marked by the family gathering together for a carp dinner and to sing *Grosser Gott wir loben Dich*. Afterwards the children played party pieces on the piano—Josef was a poor musician—and at midnight exploded the traditional fireworks and shared a toast of champagne.

The new school term meant extra studies for Issels to ensure he moved up a class at Easter, and so stayed among the aspiring university entrants. His school report shows he made it—just.

There was a tradition of scholastic integrity higher up in the Gymnasium, of pure rationalism in the classroom that did not allow for emotion. Strangely, it suited Issels remarkably well, and his progress for a time was steady, though unspectacular. More than one teacher echoed his senior master's observation: 'The boy has a lively mind. He does not always accept something because it is there. Often his thinking is more intuitive than logical.'

But intuition was no substitute for the sheer hard work the curriculum demanded. Issels did not help matters by skimping homework to devote more time to sport. In Easter, 1924, he paid the supreme penalty: he was the only boy in his class who failed to move up. The shock was salutory. Little was said at home, but the warning was clear in his mother's words: 'This must never happen again, never.'

Throughout 1924 the shop on Alter Markt slowly regained lost ground though the nation was still gripped by serious dissension. Hermann Josef Issels hoped his eldest son would take over the business, but Adelheid firmly vetoed the idea. In the family diary for October, 1924, she recorded: 'Jupp, if he successfully finishes his present studies, will go on to be a doctor. Of that I am now sure.'

His interest in things medical was becoming mildly obsessive. At school, when there was a playground accident or fight, Issels was always on hand to help with the bandaging or stop a nose-bleed. He read avidly contemporary popular medical magazines; Pasteur and Lister became heroes. And the continual visits by the family doctor to attend his father offered fresh chances to widen his knowledge. To his brothers and sisters he was, quite simply, a hero. Margot remembered years later:

> Anything he suggested we followed. But he took great care never to lead us into trouble. And he was always

passing on extraordinary bits of information that he read or heard, such as the first man who invented a special stitch to make it easier to sow up the stomach after an operation. Jupp had a wonderful way of finding out things. He would pursue a problem until he ran up against a brick wall. Then, when he was quite sure there was no way through the wall, he would retreat and approach the problem from another angle. In that way he nearly always solved it. It was something Mother taught him to do.

Adelheid Issels continued to play an important role in her son's development. She taught him respect for freedom by allowing him as much freedom as he wished. She showed him what tolerance really was by her own example; only once did she forget herself to confess to him that her life might have been far different if she had followed the dictates of her heart all those years ago. His mother's attitude towards life had much to do with determining the one Issels was visibly beginning to reveal in himself. He had a religious perspective that rose above stifling sectarian walls. There was a depth of mind that allowed him to pursue a problem long after others would have given up. There were his loyalties that never became corroded by nationalism. But he never absorbed his mother's grasp of diplomacy; it would be a serious drawback all his life.

By the end of the autumn term of 1926, it was almost certain that Issels would pass the *abitur* examination to take him on to university.

Then, close to his nineteenth birthday, Josef Issels fell in love. There had been girl friends before. Some had come home to the big house on Alter Markt for tea with the family. But things never went much further than holding hands under the table or a brief kiss while the girl was being escorted home.

Rita Kümmel was different. She was the popular image of a Rhine *mädchen*: blonde, busty and shapely. She was seventeen years old, in her final year at school, and a contemporary photograph shows a face remarkably mature for her age. For Issels: 'This is love, real love. I cannot bear to be away from her. I adore her. I love her.'

Before long the whole family was aware of his feelings. Hermann Josef Issels left his wife to handle the situation. She recognised the dangers of intervention; such a move could drive the affections of the couple underground with potentially disastrous consequences. She fell back on a well-tried strategy by encouraging Rita to visit the house. She explained to the girl that Josef hoped to become a doctor and that there would be years of study ahead before he qualified and was in a position to support a wife, leave alone a family. Adelheid said no more, but sat back to await developments.

The romance progressed through long country walks, an exchange of small books of poems and the Saturday dances. Issels would frequently return home at dawn on Sunday, and, still in evening dress, hurry to join his brothers and sisters at 6 a.m. mass. But time, as it will, brought a leavening: passions cooled; no more was heard of the talk of marriage—which had sent a shudder through Adelheid with its prospect of a bleak end to her dreams. By Easter, 1927, Josef Issels was back on course, passing his entrance examination to university, and at the same time gently disengaging himself from the eager arms of Rita Kümmel.

He ended his schooldays as one of the few who achieve the paradoxical glories that makes a boy memorable to his fellows: he was an outstanding sportsman and at the same time he managed to avoid arousing the enmity of anybody.

It was a distinction he would never again repeat.

2

Medical Student

Josef Issels had been accepted as a medical student by the Albert-Ludwig University at Freiburg, the first member of his family to achieve such status. Something of the pride everybody felt in Alter Markt comes through in the family diary for August, 1927. His mother wrote:

> The tailor has delivered Jupp's new wardrobe. There are three new suits, sports clothes, a dozen shirts etc. He looks very fine in them. We all agree he looks very grown-up and will be a credit to us. Though he says he is very calm, if the truth were known he is as excited as we all are. It has been settled, after almost no discussion, that he will receive a monthly allowance to start with of RM 400. More will be found if he needs it.

Later that month Issels said farewell to his family. The emotionalism of the occasion survives in his private diary:

> Father was very brief. Just a quick handshake, and 'do it well'. No more. I had expected nothing else. As I was leaving Mother took me into her bedroom. She cried a little. Then she said: 'School is over. All your childhood problems are at an end. There will be new problems. But work hard. It is your future that matters now'.
> I took Mother in my arms and told her I would always remember the words. She looked at me very directly and

said: 'I don't want to say very much. But I want to tell you that I expect more from you than anybody else. It is not easy for us, sending you to university. We have seven children. Don't forget that. It costs money. Do something with your life, and for us.'

The train journey to Freiburg was broken overnight for a stay with an old schoolfriend. The two youths went out and got drunk to celebrate their maturity. The high spirits splash on to Issels' diary entry: 'I am Free!! Free!! Must not ask Anybody! I can do all things. I feel like a King! I am King! Nothing is impossible.'

Freiburg did not dispel this euphoria. Set in the Black Forest it is one of the old university towns of Germany. Issels took a room near the town walls: it was little more than a box at the top of the house, and stuffed with heavy furniture that bore the marks of generations of students. Issels gloried in the cubby-hole, just as he did in the sense of history all around him.

The city and the deep woods beyond reflected something of Germany's heritage. In the Thirty Years War—that national calamity between 1618 and 1648—the town served as a bloody doormat for the Swedes and their dreams of conquest. After the Swedes came the French. Finally they went and the castellated walls were never again breached. Behind those walls a great cultural explosion burgeoned; the atmosphere was rich with the judgments of such revered German philosophers as Hegel and Kant, and the *grossen* men of German theology, Troeltsch and Harnack.

While the university medical faculty had imposing traditions of subject matter, rules and regulations, Issels did not find it stifling. All signs of the slackness he had sometimes displayed at the Gymnasium disappeared and he developed the habit of driving himself hard in all his studies. Anatomy, physiology, botany, histology—to each subject he applied an astonishing recall and a tempered intelligence, which, like a surgeon's knife, pared away the essentials of any argument. He was fortunate in his choice of tutors: anatomy was taught by Professor von Müllendorf; physiology by Professor Hoffmann. Both had national reputations. He also developed a natural gift for expressing himself both verbally and on paper. There was a particular elegance and clarity about his writing from now on, as a note he wrote to his parents in the spring of 1928 shows:

> Every day I realise a little more that medicine is more than just textbooks. It is people and human nature. Even at this stage, when I have done no clinical work, it is very obvious that to be a *good* doctor, and there is no point in being anything else, I must never forget that fact.

Just as his tiny academic triumphs at school had been a source of deep happiness for his mother, his success at university gave her more open pleasure: the family diary for 1928 is filled with such entries as:

> Jupp wrote a clear account of an afternoon spent dissecting the leg he has been given for his anatomy classes. He writes that it is a man's leg, and that he is now becoming quite good at exposing the muscle . . .

or:

> . . . he is spending time now dissecting an Asian. Says she is very fat and came to the class, he believes, from the local hospital. He thinks she may have been the victim of a street accident. When he began to dissect, all the fat tissue was liquid. He says it must be the diet Orientals live on. He is sounding very matter-of-fact about it all . . .

As a boy he had watched the hearses bringing the dead for burial in the church behind Alter Markt. Death, and awareness of death, came to be natural and acceptable. Death was an abstract; he had yet to face the disturbing personal issues it brings.

Socially his life widened enormously under the campus influences. Early on he joined the *Ripwaria*, one of the best Catholic Students' Union—whose motto was 'religion, science and Fatherland'—and made his mark as a swordsman. He had girl friends in plenty among the 3,000 students, but they were casual relationships with the minimum of emotional involvement.

His stay at Freiburg ended in the autumn of 1928 when he went north, to Bonn, to continue his studies at the university by the Rhine. Freiburg had provided the basics in his medical education; in Bonn he would widen his knowledge further before moving on to the medical school at the University of Munich to gain clinical experience. This chopping-and-changing is common practice at university level in the German educational system; it is said to give students a broader academic perspective.

Bonn, on the Rhine's left bank, was Caesar's outpost when the land to the east was trackless forest. Tacitus, the Roman historian, had been depressed by its hard winters, the fog and the rain: the first altar raised by Caesar's legionaries on the Rhine bank was to Nemesis, the goddess of retribution. Issels revelled in the timelessness of it all.

He was drawn to Bonn by the reputation of three men at the university: Professor Johannes Sobotta, professor of anatomy and author of a standard work on the subject; Professor Ulrich Ebbeke, professor of physiology, and also author of a definitive textbook on his subject; Professor Peter Junkersdorf, who taught physical chemistry, and had not managed to get a textbook published. Maybe that was the underlying cause of his dislike of Ebbeke. Where Sobotta was a remote exalted figure—he appeared punctually for a class, delivered a lecture and walked out again; personal relationship between teacher and student did not exist for him—Ebbeke and Junkersdorf carried on an open war of attrition that embraced all those they taught. Issels noted:

> To survive one has to accept totally their private codes, quarrels and customs. They have the authority in a world where authority is what counts. If one of them likes you and gives you a good mark, the other is duty bound to give you a harder time. Sometimes I have the odd feeling that they seem to exist largely for their feuds.

Issels followed with careful attention their lectures, taking copious notes of what was said. That, however, was only part of his success. He came to the perfectly good conclusion that, with sound common sense, and a proper grounding in a subject, it was possible to improvise the right answer to any question. On those Sunday rambles in the countryside around Mönchen-Gladbach he had learnt how to use his eyes. He applied the knowledge to work; no important detail ever escaped him.

In Bonn Issels faced his first major examination in medicine; he approached it with a thoroughness few other students equalled. Relying on his memory, he literally stored away whole textbooks in his mind. Nights passed without sleep as he assimilated vast quantities of information for his oral, the *Physikum*, that stern examination in the natural sciences which comes at the half-way point in German medical training.

It was in two parts. The first was an examination by Junkersdorf. At the end of a rapid-fire, twenty-minute question and answer session, the professor gave Issels a coveted First. Next he faced Ebbeke. Noting the high mark for physical chemistry, Ebbeke subjected Issels to a hard line of questioning about human physiology. At the end he also gave Issels a grudging First. Rarely had the two professors shown such agreement over a student. At the end of his time in Bonn, in the autumn of 1929, Issels wrote to his parents: 'Bonn has been the preparation for meeting the patient. That is the real reason, the only reason for being a doctor.'

But his thoughts were moving in a direction in which contact with patients would be largely confined to the operation theatre. He wanted to be a surgeon. In a dissertation home in October, 1929, he explained:

> Surgery is attractive to me because the surgeon faces a constant battle. The long history of the art itself is really a story of battle. There have been four great conflicts. Each one happened at widely spaced intervals. But without them surgery as we know it today would be impossible. There was the battle to control haemorrhage, the battle against pain, the battle to master infection and the battle to overcome shock. Each victory allowed surgery

to progress. What fascinates me most is that in each instance the main, *decisive* battle, was fought by one or two, or at the most a few, men with the ability to see, as their colleagues could not, that further progress was impossible until the decisive battle was won. It is clear to me that advances in surgery have largely come because of the ability and the character, and often the obsessions of a few great men. They were the ones who made the new discoveries, who developed the new techniques. These are the men of vision and the daring to face up to the unknown. And, apart from their great achievements, they are also exciting people in their own right. All of them are linked with more than just a common vitality, though that they had in plenty. They are pioneers of surgery. Their characters are complex and even startling. And, they have dedicated themselves to medicine. That is not a bad epitaph to be remembered by. From my own reading, it appears that these men believed that winning a battle was even more important than their own personal happiness; they all had the strength to sacrifice the happiness of even others when it might conflict with their own expectations. To carry on working, however modestly, in the footsteps of such men must be the most exciting and stimulating thing in medicine.

In the course of his voracious reading of all things medical, Issels came across cancer. He paid no great interest to the disease. In a note-book he jotted some general observations: 'Afflicts all living things. Old disease. Hippocrates said to have 'cured' cancer of neck by cautery and taught disease must be treated early.'

Regularly Issels took stock of the world outside and by 1929 he had grown more perplexed by it. Intensely non-political—he would remain so all his life—he failed totally to understand the machinations which brought the Great Depression to America, and in Europe, especially in France and Germany, the real possibility of the international Communist movement overthrowing shaky capitalist systems. Nor did he grasp why George Bernard Shaw and H. G. Wells influenced millions with their panacea of Utopian Socialism and rejection of middle-class morality.

Nearer to home, the words of Sigmund Freud were equally hard to comprehend, let alone accept.

Easier to understand, and reject, were the speeches of Adolf Hitler, forging the new German sword. His words offended everything Issels believed in. But in 1929 he did not take the fanatic of Bavaria seriously; at most he looked upon Hitler as no more than a passing phenomenon. Nevertheless Issels was depressed on regular visits home to find increasingly the unemployed of Mönchen-Gladbach eagerly taking up the jingoism of the Nazis.

Bonn University was free of such crudity. Socially, it was also a completely self-contained community. There were clubs catering for every interest, and Issels belonged to many of them. He fenced, went riding, and was an enthusiastic member of the gymnastic club. In the evenings he played chess or sat in a *weinstube* endlessly talking out the future. Outwardly, he developed an easy manner towards women, and consequently they sought out his company. He displayed an old-fashioned courtliness which always aroused in some women something approaching adoration. By the end of his stay in Bonn more than one girl was infatuated with Josef Issels. He cheerfully accepted the situation, loving them and leaving them. His *traumfrau* was always tall, blonde, clear-skinned and lissom. Curiously, Issels never saw her as German but rather as Swedish. In reality, she was a figure to be turned to in moments of great stress, to provide a measure of solace; her role was no more than an emotional safety valve in which love had no part.

Early in his student days Issels began to recognise there was also a 'dark side' to his personality that periodically produced a tug-of-war within him. Only in 1972 could he express what he felt but could not yet describe in 1929:

> My friends thought I was the most cheerful person they knew. They didn't know the effort it sometimes cost me. For instance I would be faced with a situation which I could resolve sensibly or put myself at risk. It could be a girl, work, no matter. Some part of my mind would urge me to take the risky course, while the rest of my brain was warning of the dangers. This inner struggle

would go on until I would win the battle and do the right thing. But it was often exhausting.

He discovered other things about himself. He needed the security, the comfort, the feeling of *belonging* to a group. He surrounded himself with small pockets of friends he could always turn to. With them he was expansive and generous; his substantial monthly allowance often went on entertaining them. Left to his own resources, Josef Issels found it hard to make the first move with strangers: a basic shyness, inherited from his father, took over. He was poor at small talk, becoming almost tongue-tied in its presence.

Yet he hid all this from the outside world. In his youth only his mother really recognised and understood the torment that periodically wracked him. The separation of university life had not lessened the very real influence she had on Issels. Her expectations of him in many ways made her the focal point of his existence. In turn, she made it repeatedly clear he was the mainspring of her life. On his visits home she questioned him endlessly about his studies, his tutors, his progress. When he was back on the campus she dreamt about him and regularly prayed for him. Her letters to him were full of ambition that he would make his way in medicine. She appeared not to mind whether he chose to be a surgeon or a general physician. What mattered to Adelheid Issels was that her eldest son should be successful.

Towards his father Issels expressed filial duty. Nothing of the intimacy or sympathy was ever present on either side of their relationship that brought such a profound contentment to his contact with his mother. In time he judged all women by the qualities he saw in her. No woman could hope to have more than a passing connection with him unless she had the intrinsic qualities of intelligence, charm, courage and the devotion his mother so clearly expressed for him. On his last day at Bonn he penned a note in which he expressed his recognition of her desires: 'I am very conscious that the next step in my career is a critical one. But be assured I will not disappoint you through lack of application. I, too, long for the day when I will be a doctor.'

Then he travelled south to Munich, to the splendidly endowed Ludwig-Maximilian University which was the pride of Bavaria.

Issels approached Munich University with something between high excitement and reverence. It rated with Berlin as a seat of learning. He wrote home: 'There is a unique atmosphere. For a start the place is so *big*. And my professors have reputations respected in all of medicine. It will all take some getting used to.'

His tutors included four men with international reputations. Physical medicine was taught by Professor Friedrich Müller; the professor of surgery was Erich Lexer. Pathology was in the hands of Professor Max Borst. The professor of gynaecology was Albert Döderlein. Issels settled in quickly. The theory of general medicine, pathology, gynaecology and surgery was supplemented by teaching rounds in the university hospital. He saw that medical treatment was a blend of science and routine, and that it was all part of a new world in which the hospital professors were exalted figures:

> They rule us, and their patients with, on the whole, kindly autocracy. Each reproduces in miniature the structure of the hospital hierarchy as a whole. Always the students are around the bottom of the ladder, below the new housemen and just above the nurses.

At night there were lively student discussions in *bierkellers* to sit in on. Issels developed the rewarding, though often embarrassing, gift of isolating the weakness in any argument and ruthlessly destroying it. He could deflate a glowing oratorical performance with an irrefutable: 'why?'

Munich offered more than animated talk. At weekends through the winter of 1929–30 Issels put away his books, locked the door of the garret he rented near the station and escaped to the ski slopes outside the city. As the weeks passed those excursions held an increasing importance for Josef Issels. Munich University, for all its excellence, was too impersonal. A diary entry for February 1930 conveys his growing dismay: 'I am a number. Every student here is a number as far as the teaching faculty goes. It is not the fault of the teachers. It is the system they work in.'

He continued to study; to answer precisely such professorial booby traps as 'what defence can the organism under natural conditions offer against pathogenic germs?' The exact nature of pus—that complicated cellular process when phagocytes digest microbes—was observed along with other clinical phenomena. His note-book filled with observations on what was then available to combat bacteria: surgery, 'if the focal point of the infection can be reached'; antiseptics; increasing the 'general resistance' of a patient; specific products for specific bacteria—'for malaria, quinine', 'in the case of syphilis, mercury'.

But the social life of Munich held an increasing fascination for Issels. He became a familiar figure at the theatre, opera and in the city's artistic colony, where he impressed the painters and sculptors with his handsome body and gymnastic agility. That winter, the famous Krone Circus returned to Munich. Issels was attracted to the circus atmosphere and soon became deeply drawn to the special discipline of the performers; his circle of friends widened to include a knife thrower, a lion tamer, trapeze artistes and a team of bare-back riders. Finally, perhaps inevitably, he was offered a job as a clown. He felt it possible to combine at least temporarily an academic and circus life.

> It's not the money [he wrote], though that is always useful. It's the chance of a new experience. And that is very important. It is life! I know there are some people who firmly argue that a medical student should spend every moment just learning medicine to the exclusion of all else. But that does not necessarily make for a better doctor at the end of it all. Contact with people, all kinds of people, is also what matters.

Face rouged and whitened with flour paste, Issels tumbled and did prat falls in the circus ring as if he was born to the sawdust life. When the circus moved on, he was invited to travel with it.

Instead he went back to the lecture halls and the world

Adelheid Issels
with (*left to right*)
Maria, Josef
and Charlotte

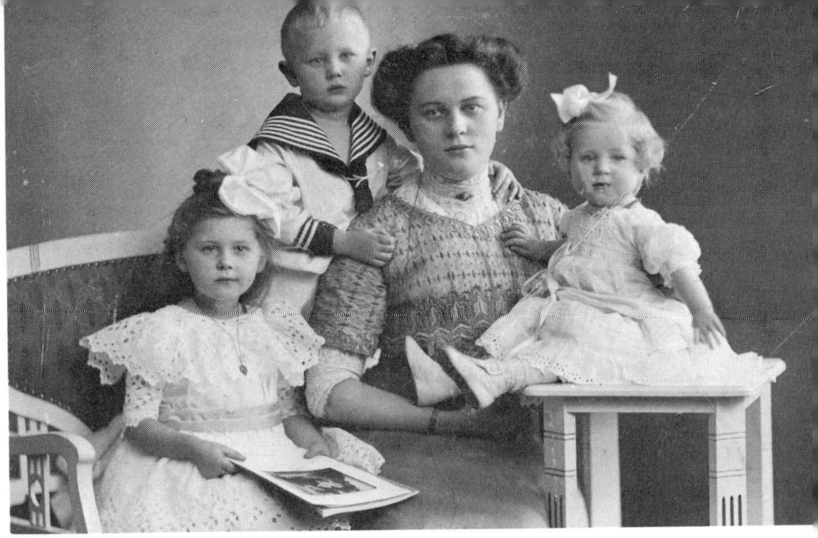

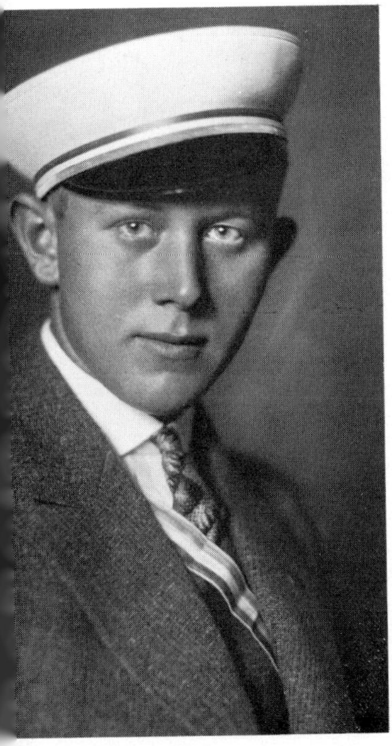

Josef Issels,
rst-year medical student

Issels modelling for 'body beautiful' pictures
during his days as a medical student in Rostock.

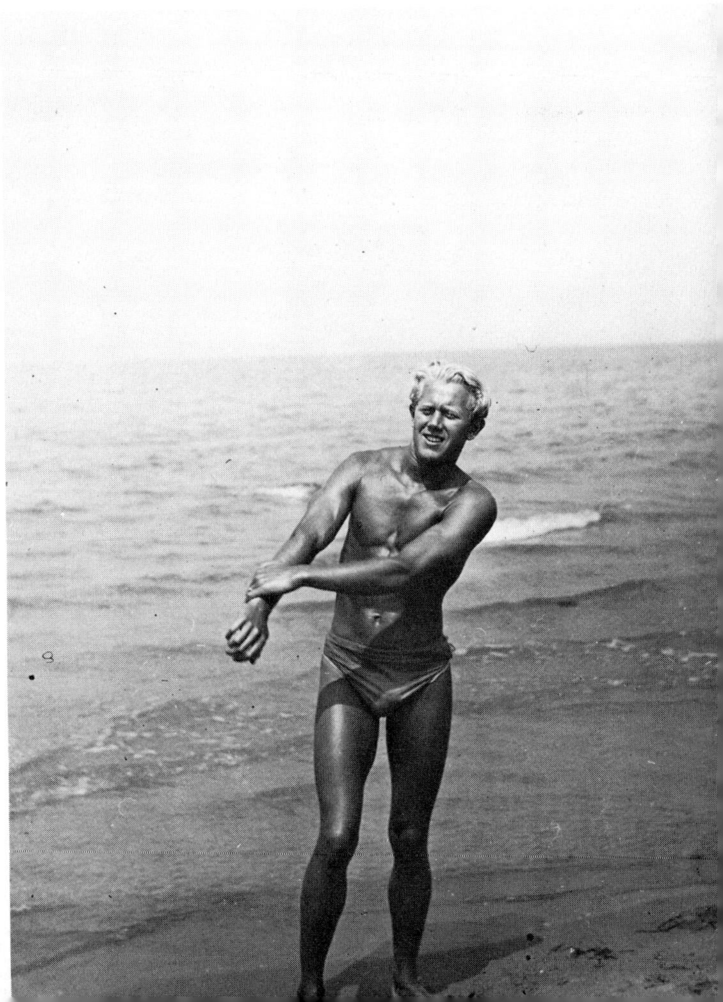

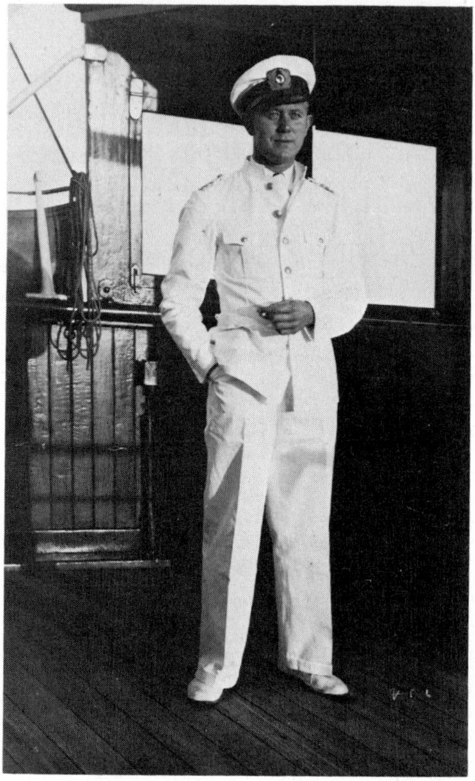

Issels: ship's doctor

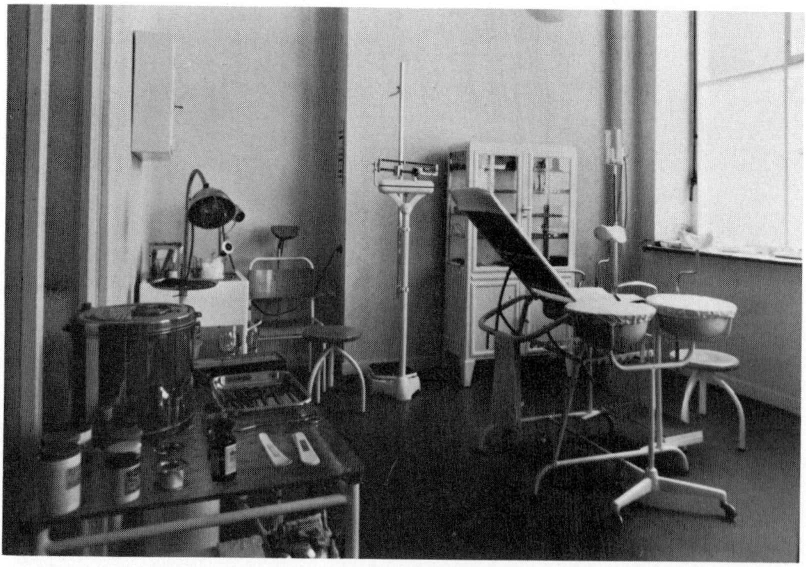

His first surgery in Bismarkstrasse, Munich

of clinical observation. There were ample opportunities to examine and diagnose a wide variety of patients. From such contact came a deeply-ingrained lesson:

> It's surprising how many doctors, and students, when they meet a patient, put on a special professional manner. It makes it difficult to have a good relationship with a patient if he feels he is in the presence of some Special Person. And the students often copy this attitude, so that in later life they will probably forget the patient is a human being. It is a tragic error, and one that I will try never to make.

Munich, for all its pleasures, finally palled. Issels applied to enrol in the University of Rostock, far in the north of Germany. It had a good academic reputation for a small university, but it must also be stated that Issels was attracted there by tales of fine beaches, beautiful girls; it was a place for *viel spass,* much fun.

While waiting to enter Rostock he worked in his home town general hospital, the five-hundred-bed Maria Hilf Hospital. Apart from furthering his clinical experience, Issels found that a doctor's manner was often what mattered: it was a show of confidence, as well as drugs, that helped.

At home the intense and exclusive relationship with his mother continued. He found himself reliving his hospital day for her benefit. With the other children his closest relationship was with his sister, Margot, grown into a pert eighteen-year-old: towards her he displayed brotherly protectiveness that remained all their lives.

The move to Rostock indeed turned out to be an excuse for *viel spass.* Issels hardly saw the inside of a lecture hall, but spent the days sunning himself with his friends on the beach. In between came a chance to earn some extra pocket money posing for 'body beautiful' pictures on the sands at twenty marks a session. The money went towards drinks for the endless parties.

Summer over, Rostock lost its appeal. The fun moved elsewhere. Issels decided the most exciting place would be Vienna, famed as a seat of learning. He applied, and was accepted by the university, for the winter semester of 1930.

He arrived in Vienna on a wet September morning in 1930: even grey overcast could not dampen his sense of history. Vienna was a cross-roads of Europe. A score, and more, of armies had marched over its cobbled streets. The Romans garrisoned it. The French held it for four years during the Napoleonic War of 1805–9; a century later a Gaelic aroma was still there. In his imagination Issels detected another pervading influence: he sensed the music of Beethoven, Schubert, and above all, Johann Strauss, whose waltzes turned Vienna into a musical confection known throughout the world.

It was not just the ambience of the café society which stirred him, but also the knowledge that here he could learn something of Freud and Adler. He plunged into the world of the *id and libido* with the same furious energy he displayed before taking the *Physikum* at Bonn. It was, in fact, his exceptionally high marks in the *Physikum* that gained him easy entry into Vienna University.

Issels found for all the 'good manners and gentle smiles' of his professors he was expected to work hard, and not just at his psychology lectures. There was a rigorous discipline where intense study and accurate information was the very minimum accepted by the professors of surgery, gynaecology, bacteriology, pathological anatomy, pharmacology and general medicine. To his parents Issels wrote towards the end of term:

> . . . every fact and every statement must be justified. I really believe this sort of pressure has helped my general intellectual development. And I have also learnt a most valuable lesson. In medicine you can have more than one opinion, and that they can both be right . . . but this is also a wonderful place to relax in, though there is not much time for that. When there is I go to the Opera (very formal in my cloak and silk hat: the custom here is to keep the hat under your seat during the performance). But for the most part it is hard work, and very exciting to see at first hand what the 'Viennese school of medicine' really represents. At this moment I feel that I could stay here for my final examination.

By return post came a note from his mother saying that his father had been taken seriously ill with a lung infection. Issels took the overnight train to Mönchen-Gladbach.

Hermann Josef Issels had pneumonia. Adelheid took over the shop and the elder children rallied around. But a sense of crisis greeted Josef as he arrived home, and he was the cause of it. There was a family feeling that he should give up studying and assume the traditional role for the eldest son: minding the store. Adelheid Issels firmly rejected the idea. Over dinner she told the family that Josef would remain at university and that 'somehow we will all manage'. Issels enshrined those words all his life—and no more was ever heard of the proposition that he should enter commerce.

But he felt he could not return to Vienna; it was too far away should his father grow worse. Issels looked around, and settled on the Academy of Medicine at nearby Düsseldorf, one of the fifteen cities of the Inner Ruhr.

The Academy was dwarfed by the true majesty of the city: the giant mills sent great gouts of flame skywards heating the air to an uncomfortable degree in pressing out steel and other products. Düsseldorf reminded Issels of the old Ruhr joke about the steel baron who arrived in Hell and shouted, '*Verdammt!* I forgot my winter coat.'

The Academy numbered under two hundred students; the teaching faculty included two of Germany's outstanding men: Professor Frey, professor of surgery, and heart specialist, Professor Eden. Issels worked hard in and out of the lecture rooms. In the short train journeys home he read and filled note-books with such thoughts as:

> Amusing reference to homoeopathic medicine. Professor called it folk medicine. Says it is impossible to understand how anybody can take it seriously who claims to have a scientific training. One thing is very clear: it will have no place in the teaching curriculum here.

and:

> Cellular theory replaced humoral theory. But why reject action of body fluid substances, especially blood serum?

A Russian scientist, Metchanikoff, popularised the cellular theory at the Pasteur Institute in Paris in the 1880s. He observed that certain specialised cells offered a vital defence for the body against intruders, dissolving them by a process similar to that of the digestive ferments of saliva. German medical schools adopted the theory with the same enthusiasm they once taught the humoral concept.

Issels felt increasing pangs of dissatisfaction over the way he was taught orthodox medicine. Unformed though his doubts were, they emerge in such note-book jottings as:

> The rigidity of thinking can be stifling at times . . . there is too much a feeling that if it is in a textbook then it must be absolutely accepted . . . some of the professors give the impression that they have given the same lecture for forty years. . .

He began to question the supremacy of rote and example; he by no means rejected it entirely, but doubted its value in all cases as a substitute for original thinking. His own thoughts ranged far and wide. He pursued the early researches of the German, Pollender, who played a large part in opening up new medical territory with his work on micro-organisms. Issels became fascinated with the ways the body's defences could be mobilised by vaccines to fight illness. He wrote: 'In 1888 Vidal and Chantenesse proved conclusively that even a vaccine of dead germs could develop in the blood the potency to destroy the microbes of typhoid fever.'

He was attracted to such nineteenth-century innovators as Robert Koch in Germany and Louis Pasteur in France; intrigued not just by their discoveries but also the way they rejected the conventional thinking of the day to plunge down new and unexplored avenues.

As his own *leitmotiv* Issels copied into a note-book the words of Lister in 1898: 'I regard all worldly distinctions as nothing in comparison with the hope that I may have been the means of reducing, in however small a degree, the sum total of human misery.'

By Christmas 1931 Hermann Josef Issels was about his business again and his son made yet another move, this time to the Julio-Maximilian University at Würzburg to sit his final state examination. It was the sixth medical school Josef Issels attended. Again he was lucky in his choice of teachers. Surgery was taught by Professor Fritz König; physical medicine was the province of Professor Erich Grafe and Professor Ernst Magnus-Alsleben; Professor Karl Josef Gauss taught gynaecology.

The university had a long history of liberal tradition and Issels felt immediately at home. He failed however to register the changes occurring outside the campus. In the Reichstag elections of November 14, 1930, the Nazis emerged with 107 seats, second only to the Social Democrats; the Weimar Republic increasingly looked like a *Zwischenreich*, a temporary regime. As the storm gathered, Issels remained still unaware of the mounting resentment towards Jewish students and staff at the university.

He roomed in a house owned by a Jewish butcher, Stern, who provided 'good food, a clean room, all very pleasing'. Stern supplemented a decent income from kosher killing by offering similar terms to nine other students, He paid them all the compliment by addressing them as 'Herr Doktor'.

One day Stern knocked on Issels' door, who recorded the somewhat bizarre sequence of events which followed:

> S. said his wife was ill and that the professor of gynaecology recommended an operation. Did I agree? For one moment I wondered what S. would have said if I had not approved. Refused the operation? I said I was sure the professor was right. S. was relieved at my 'second opinion'. Later Frau S. had the operation—and died. S. came to me and said it was all my fault because I had agreed to the operation! I tried to explain I was not even a doctor, but he would not have it, repeating the reason he consulted me was because he wasn't sure of the professor!
>
> All the students in the house agreed to send a joint wreath. But who would take it to the funeral? One said we should draw lots. I looked surprised, and they asked me if I was not aware of the hostility towards the Jews. I shook my head, saying 'just because they come early to class and take the best seats is no reason to dislike them'.

The others looked strangely at me. One said: 'it's not just the Jewish students; it's Jews everywhere who are hated.'

I drew the lot to carry the wreath. I arrived at the cemetery just as a funeral procession moved away. I tagged on at the end. I recognised nobody, so I started to move up through the long file of mourners. I was sure S. would be at the head. When I reached the coffin it was to hear the rabbi reciting final prayers for a *man*. I was at the wrong funeral. Everybody looked very oddly at me, an obvious stranger, clutching a huge wreath. All I could do was leave it at the graveside and make as dignified a retreat as possible.

His friends did not accept his story. They believed he avoided the Stern funeral because of the political situation. He was angered and hurt by the charge. His whole attitude towards religion was one of tolerance.

Issels worked hard for several months, eschewing parties, girls, relaxation of any kind. Then, in the summer of 1932, he was invited to a weekend tennis tournament in the Tegernsee valley of Bavaria:

There are two of us and we picked up the prizes in the singles and doubles. We booked into the best hotel, and found we couldn't afford it. So we took back the prizes and asked for cash. Even that didn't cover us for more than one night! We ended up next day sleeping in a hut behind the local chemist shop; it was filled with bottles of vile concoctions.

The weekend stretched into a week, a fortnight, a month. Two more students joined them, and the four had a giddy whirl which they helped pay for by giving tennis and swimming lessons. One day Issels walked around the lake to a small village: it was Rottach-Egern: twenty years passed before he returned and made the village world famous with his clinic.

But in those balmy days of 1932 common sense finally prevailed. Issels returned to Würzburg, and devoted his time to the *paukverband*, cramming sessions in which he revised and memorised everything he would need for the Finals.

In December, 1932, he collected a First in twelve of fourteen subjects; his overall position in the examination was fourth out of 136 students.

For his thesis he chose a dissertation on leukaemia. In forty pages he showed that the disease, unlike other forms of malignancy, has no primary focus and growth; the quality of the malignancy is only determined by the virulence of the cells themselves. It was a workmanlike piece of work with only occasionally a glimpse of his usual lively prose to brighten a depressing clinical picture of invasive cancer ending in swift death.

To this day Josef Issels does not know why he wrote a paper on that particular subject. Cancer still held no real interest for him.

3

Herr Doktor

ON JANUARY 15, 1933, ISSELS JOINED THE STAFF OF THE Maria Hilf Hospital in Mönchen-Gladbach as a houseman. His salary was RM 97 a month: as a student he had frequently spent more in a week's good living. He joined the firm of Dr. Sickmann, the hospital's senior surgeon. Sickmann was an excellent surgeon and teacher. He taught Issels all he needed to know of practical surgery. He had a demonstrative and highly original way of imparting knowledge. When Issels made a mistake, he patiently corrected him. Sickmann had established a local reputation as a surgeon of daring by performing complicated operations. The only feature that enlivened his rather mousy appearance was a glass left eye that often caused him problems when operating on the right-hand side of a patient. The surgeon tended to miss the incision area, and on one memorable occasion he removed the wrong digit entirely—cutting off the right toe when he should have removed the left one. Sickmann sportingly did a second operation at no extra charge. It was, he said, a fact of life that anybody could make a mistake.

Issels discovered that other medical facts of life could only be acquired by perseverance. Successful treatment depended not only on exact knowledge, but also on understanding the patient and recognising the significance of all kinds of factors not directly related to immediate symptoms. He found it was not enough for him to simply assess the degree of cardiac stress in an old man, or prescribe the right quantities of drugs to a young mother with a failing circulation system. He began to look beyond the visible signs of distress, to see, and comprehend, underlying factors. In becoming so involved he discovered an important thing some doctors never learn: a patient was always a person, that a seemingly trivial complaint sometimes masked a more serious problem, that vagueness over symptoms was not always a sign of malingering. He had spent five years learning about the body; he knew how to treat a mechanical failure or one arising from infection. He now set about learning something the textbooks did not teach: while it was possible to save time by a firm assertion and no explanation, nothing was ever lost by letting a patient feel reassured. To a classmate in Würzburg he wrote:

> Some of our colleagues forget a simple but important truth. A patient cannot be expected to be calm and totally coherent when he lies naked on an examination couch being prodded and jabbed with no proper reason given for it. I think you must take the patient along with you as far as possible.

Issels also developed skills as a surgeon. His mornings passed, first assisting, and then actually performing, simple operations in the hospital's operating theatre; an appendix followed a hernia, to be followed by another appendix: a steady cycle of scrubbing, cutting and stitching. Sometimes the list contained a case of cancer and the relatively cheerful atmosphere in the theatre was dispelled. Even with full vision there was little Sickmann could have done. Issels' diary for May 10, 1933, recreated a typical situation:

> The patient was a man with rectum cancer. Sickmann took a look at the case notes again and became gloomy. We proceeded with the first part of the operation. After minutes Sickmann said, 'too late, too late, too late'. The man was sewn up and returned to the ward as inoperable, and now incurable. In the changing room Sickmann leafed through the case notes. The patient has suffered much pain with his cancer before coming into hospital. Sickmann said, 'always if there is pain it is a symptom of a

progressive cancer for which surgery is no use'. What a very depressing situation.

After every possible cancer operation Sickmann had a fixed routine. The tumour he removed was placed in a specimen pot. He took it to the laboratory, cut the tumour, extracted the fluid and examined it under a microscope. Issels was surprised to find a surgeon in a laboratory. His colleagues told him Sickmann had a fixation about finding the cause of cancer. They looked upon it as one more eccentricity on the part of the surgeon. Issels was impressed that at least Sickmann tried to do something more than just operate. While Issels slowly discovered that surgery was not a magic bullet for all cancer—nor was it intended to be—he took the first steps towards mastering a problem many doctors find difficult: having a meaningful relationship with the dying.

In June, 1933 a workman was admitted with an acute infection of the arm. Sickmann decided amputation was impossible: without penicillin or other antibiotics of a later age nothing could be done except make the patient comfortable as death approached.

Issels refused to believe the patient would die. He spent all his free time either thinking about, or tending, the workman. But after a few days he saw the prognosis taking an inevitable course. Still Issels refused to give up. Then, one night, when he was alone with the patient, the man rallied enough to whisper: 'I know I'm dying.'

Issels did not reply.

'Doctor, I *know* I am dying. Just as I know you doctors can't tell me. It's your job to save lives.'

The workman sank back on his pillow relieved in the knowledge he was right. In the remaining days of his life he derived an emotional reward from the fact that Issels knew of his acceptance of death. It was a bond they shared to the end.

The death greatly distressed Issels. He was shocked that medicine had no life-saver in such a case. His teaching professors had not dwelt on the limitations of treatment; rather an impression was given that the armoury of available drugs could meet any challenge. Nor had the semesters offered any preparation for simply coping with the dying. The patients selected for teaching purposes were interesting specimens. But they were not at death's door. Nothing he saw or read in the past five years offered a hint in handling somebody who knew he was dying. Nor had the senior doctors at the hospital followed any fixed approach to the situation. Aware of the impending tragedy, and accepting nothing more could be done, they retreated, leaving the final scene to the nurses and Josef Issels.

When the immediate trauma of the death receded Issels reflected on the disturbing ignorance he had experienced in not only *what* to say but *how* to say it. He thought seriously for the first time over the vastly complicated doctor-dying patient relationship. His search for information soon revealed that well-established knowledge was scanty. The impersonal aspects of death—the statistics, the details of the average number of deaths over years in particular fatal diseases could be dug out. But there was no systematic study in 1933 on what people experienced at the point of dying, and what lessons those concerned with their welfare could draw from that experience.

Issels' mind filled with questions orthodox sources could not answer. Did people know when death approached? And if they did, did they wish independent confirmation from their doctor? Should the whole question of incurable illness be discussed openly with them? And at death's point: was it fear or sadness they experienced most? What were they frightened of: an increase in suffering or death itself?

There were no ready answers. He recognised his psychological knowledge was inadequate to quantify suffering, even though his semester at Vienna University gave him an insight into fear, courage and depression, all of which he associated with dying. In the end he recognised that to have any worthwhile, and proper, relationship with the dying meant creating his own rules. Once more the questions spilled out. How much of a fight should he make, *should* any doctor make, in the face of inevitable death? Or, in the final stages, should the main emphasis be on comfort? Again, his experience was too limited to provide solutions for such problems. Many years, and deaths, passed before he developed a workable philosophy for managing patients suffering from incurable illnesses. Recognition that many accepted death rationally, neither ignoring it nor denying its finality, was a slow process in which he increasingly saw that death was often ennobling for those facing it; the dying did all they possibly could to spare the feelings of loved ones, and towards their doctors and nurses they displayed similar consideration. Eventually, Josef Issels believed such courage deserved only one answer—a total honesty on his part when faced with a similar situation he met in the Maria Hilf Hospital in June, 1933.

Socially the summer was a full one for Issels of tennis tournaments, country walks at weekends and dances. He lived at home, but enjoyed all the freedoms of a young bachelor. On Sundays, after midday mass, twenty or so worshippers, business friends of Hermann Josef Issels, joined the family for wine in the drawing room of the house on Alter Markt. Josef found himself in a situation familiar to all doctors at a social gathering: more than one matron or burgher sidled up for a few words of advice. He was flattered by their attentions and answered their questions gladly.

In turn he listened to the talk of *Götterdämmerung*. Hitler had become Chancellor and the Third Reich, in the jargon of Goebbels, the 'Thousand Year Reich', was a reality that was epitomised in the words composed by Horst Wessel:

Die Fahne hoch! Die Reihen dicht geschlossen,
S.A. marschiert mit ruhig festem Schritt. . .

There were some guests at the Sunday morning gatherings who still believed that the country was only temporarily occupied by a gang of ruffians; that eventually Hitler would be forced from office by public pressure. They failed to see the reality of the situation.

In the welter of Nazi decrees and orders changing the lives of everybody in Germany, one affected Josef Issels. From April 1, 1933, it became compulsory for all doctors working in hospitals run by religious orders to join the *Schutzstaffel*, the S.S., or the *Sturmabteilung*, the S.A. The law became known as the 'April butterfly' order—trapping all those who until then had hesitated at becoming actively involved with the Nazis. Issels was bluntly told by the hospital administration that he could not continue working there unless he joined one of the organisations immediately. That night an old family friend, a priest, advised him to join the up to then more moderate S.S. Next day he enrolled with no great enthusiasm and was ordered to instruct other members once a week in first aid. He attended compulsory parades, wore the familiar black shirt and pants with the S.S. insignia over the heart and gave the *Heil Hitler* salute like the rule book said. He did no more, or less, than thousands of young men did.

His work settled into a definite pattern: operating theatre in the mornings, ward rounds in the afternoons, night duty at regular intervals. It was a life of solid application rather than any memorable incidents. Then, in the first week of August a young married woman was admitted to the surgical ward with cancer of the left breast. After careful examination and tests, Dr. Sickmann pronounced there was every chance of success with a radical mastectomy, removal of the entire breast by surgery. It was the first time Issels assisted in such an operation: the experience changed his whole outlook as his later account showed:

> By the time we scrubbed up and gowned, the patient was on the table. There was a heightened atmosphere in the theatre. An outsider might have thought it all part of the ritual that gives every operating theatre its own style: the way the trolleys and instruments are positioned. But the sense of atmosphere, or drama, came from the patient. Even though she was anaesthetised, she looked so peaceful and vulnerable. The operation area had been clearly marked out. The breast rose and fell with the patient's breathing. It was large and firm. The only blemish was a small neat cut, a few centimetres long where Sickmann had performed a biopsy a few days earlier which confirmed the presence of a malignant tumour about the size of a large pea. He had removed the growth intact so that there was no risk of metastases occurring. Laboratory tests confirmed the tumour was malignant. Yet it was clear, at least to me, that the patient was no longer at risk once

the growth was safely removed. But the procedure to be followed in such a case was clearly laid down in the text-books: the breast must still be totally removed.

I looked again at the operation area. The breast was truly a thing of beauty, perfectly formed with the nipple glistening from swabbing with antiseptic. Satisfied that everything was positioned properly, Sickmann started to cut. A line of spurting blood marked the progress of his knife. He kept on staring intently at the incision area. I wiped the area clean with surgical sponges and pinched shut the main bleeding points with blood-vessel clamps. Then Sickmann went on cutting.

Nobody spoke. The only sounds were the rustling of a nurse's gown as they passed over instruments, or the click of one instrument following another into the discard tray.

In ten minutes it was all over. Ten minutes to destroy what had taken twenty years or so to form. With a last snip, the breast was cut away like a piece of meat and thrown into the waste bucket. I kept on saying to myself, 'My God. How terrible. Was this really necessary? Has anybody thought of the after-effects for this poor woman? The psychological problems she faces?'

The whole operation stunned me. I was nearly sick at the way it ended. One minute she was a complete woman—then she was disfigured forever. That was all I could think of: the hideous disfigurement she had experienced at the hands of surgery.

The psychological after-effects for her were indeed severe. She was shocked into almost a total breakdown by the loss of her breast. Her husband also failed to understand, and within a year he had divorced her. None of that I could foresee as she was wheeled out of the theatre. All I felt was a sense of outrage that such a thing had been necessary.

I hated the disease which had caused it.

He turned to the one person for comfort and understanding he trusted implicitly: His mother listened quietly as he poured out his anguish about such surgery. She asked him if he knew of any alternative. He shook his head. Even in his anger he knew of nothing that could change a situation where the surgeon's knife dominated cancer treatment.

In spite of his experience Issels still wanted to be a surgeon—though he knew he could never again face another breast operation. Shortly after it, in fact, he went to work as an internist on the hospital's medical wards. There was nothing significant in the move: it was all part of his compulsory first year of hospital work. On the wards he found new challenges to throw himself into and new relationships to establish with patients and colleagues. The months passed swiftly and by December, 1933, Issels eagerly scanned the medical press for a suitable vacancy that would take him further along in his career. He soon found one—an opening for a senior surgical assistant to Professor Victor Orator, one of the most respected abdominal surgeons in Germany. Issels applied, was interviewed and got the job in a few hectic days. He had taken not just a step, but a sizeable leap up the medical ladder.

In January 1934 Issels began operating with Orator in the general hospital in Duisburg-Hochfeld, a dark, concrete jumble of a city broken by a network of polluted canals feeding coal barges to the bottle-shaped furnaces. Duisburg had a milieu all its own: a by-product of the air thick with dust, the regular blinding flash of molten metal being tipped from giant furnaces, the constant cherry-red glow in the sky that gave even the newest of buildings an aura of age.

The hospital was an old building, caked with grime which only the theatre remained free from. Orator ran a fast-moving operating room, lecturing, as he cut and cauterised, to all those around the table. Small and sturdy, with piercing brown eyes, he had stubby arms and hands tapering to surprisingly long fingers. Nothing escaped his notice during an operation: his eyes constantly monitored the reading on the scale of the blood-pressure cuff—an essential gadget for detecting shock—and the level of anaesthesia. When he was not lecturing, Orator kept up a monologue about a previous night's visit to the opera or theatre.

Apart from the abdominal operations Orator's reputation was built on, the surgical team dealt with emergency cases from the surrounding factories. An average week brought a crushed leg or two, a severed arm, and on one horrific occasion a man with a steel rod driven clean through his chest: he lived.

Sometimes death came unexpectedly. Anaesthesia was in its infancy, and nitrous oxide, ether and chloroform were still used for general anaesthetics in many theatres. A newcomer was the barbiturate anaesthetic, Penthothal Sodium. It was marketed in 1932 following a search, pioneered in Germany, for a drug to put patients to sleep without the unpleasantness of a chloroform mask or the threshing that often accompanied the first moments of ether anaesthesia. Penthothal was quick and easy. Issels had the responsibility of administering it, or another anaesthetic, such as the new drug, Evipan, whose main advantage was holding a patient at a shallower level of sleep than was before possible.

Orator was impressed by the claims made for Evipan, and tried it on the first suitable patient. It was his twenty-five-year-old nephew who needed an exploratory operation. The man was cheerful as he was wheeled into an ante-room beside the main theatre where Issels administered anaesthetics. He had developed a knack of slipping the needle into a fold of skin while bantering with the patient.

He was about to prick the boy's arm when Orator came into the ante-room.

'Might as well keep it in the family,' he said, reaching for the syringe in Issels' hand.

The professor of surgery turned and looked down at his nephew, nodded reassurance, and injected the measured dose of Evipan. For a moment a surprised look came into the boy's eyes and was gone. Other moments passed while Orator stood there. Suddenly he dropped the syringe and felt the boy's pulse. His nephew was dead—killed by an unforeseen side reaction to the drug. 'All deeply distressed [Issels wrote to his mother]. Another practical lesson that science is not the clear-cut thing that the textbooks tell you.'

But there was little time to dwell on the limitations of textbooks. In that first year Issels assisted in over two hundred stomach operations and almost as many accident cases.

Orator, for all his skills, was a specialist. He knew his way around the abdomen, but constantly needed to refresh himself from manuals when it came to amputating a leg or

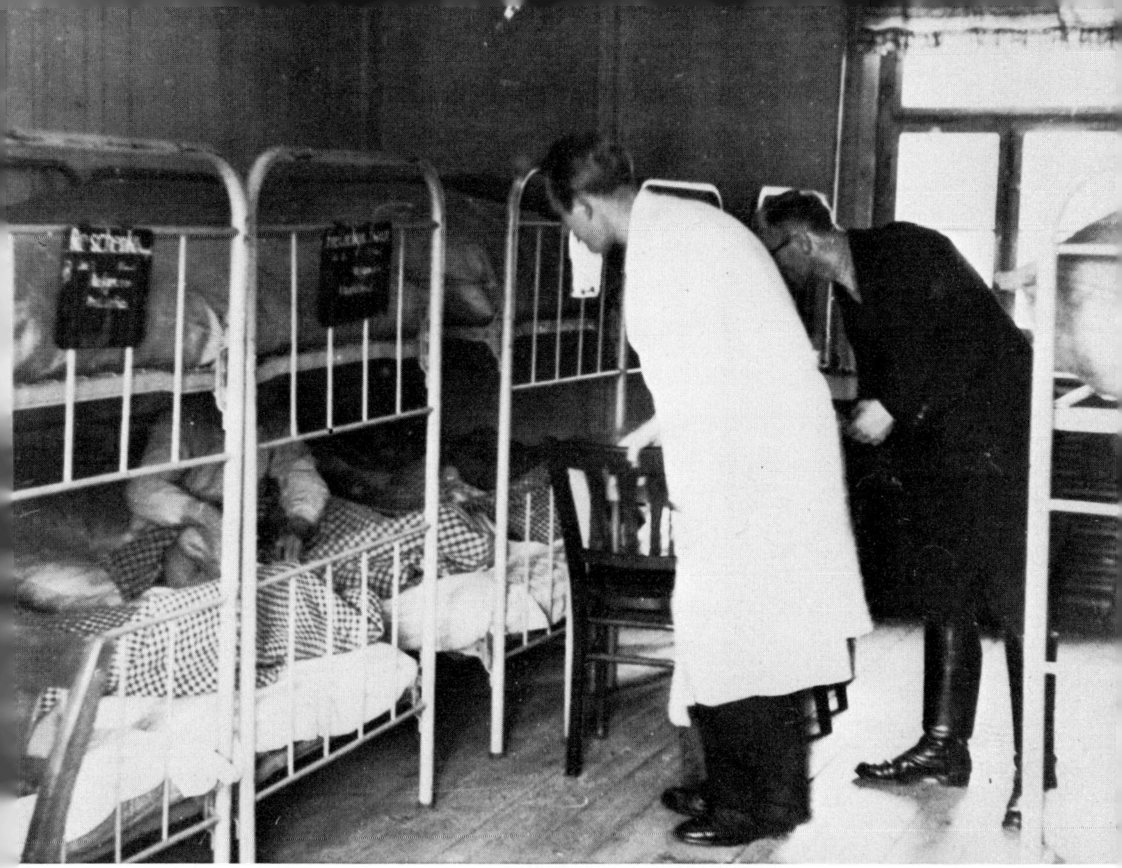

Issels (in white coat)
working in a field hospital

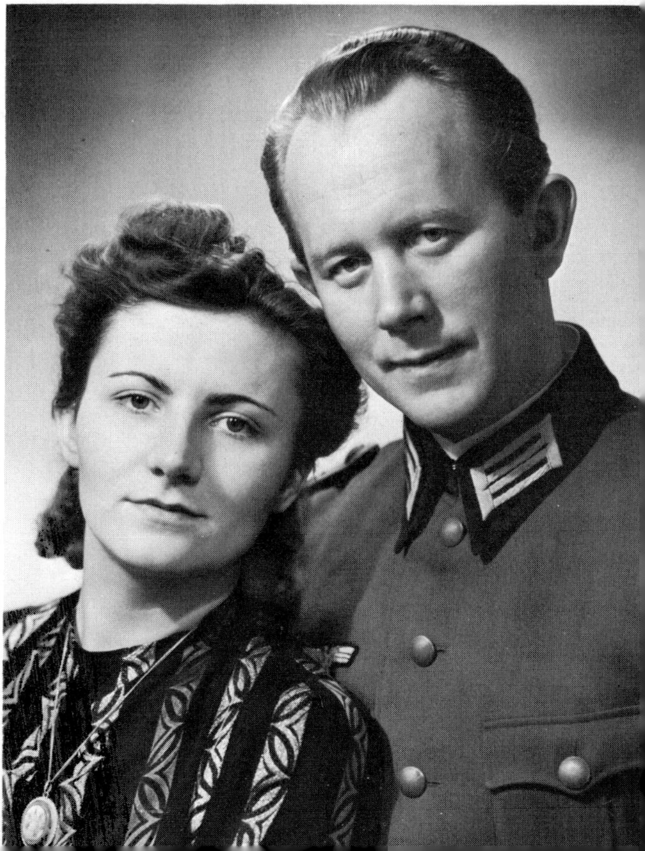

Issels' engagement portrait
with his first wife, Irmengard

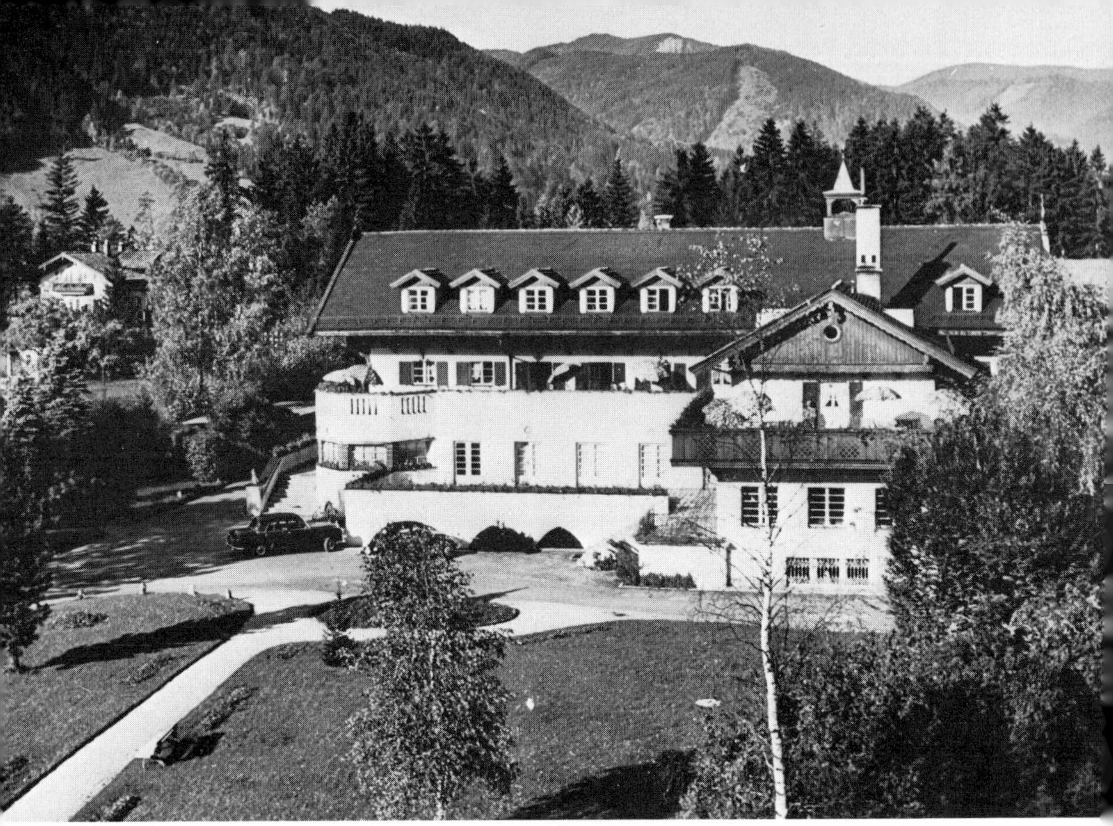

The Ringberg Klinik in 1951

The first patients at the clinic, 1952

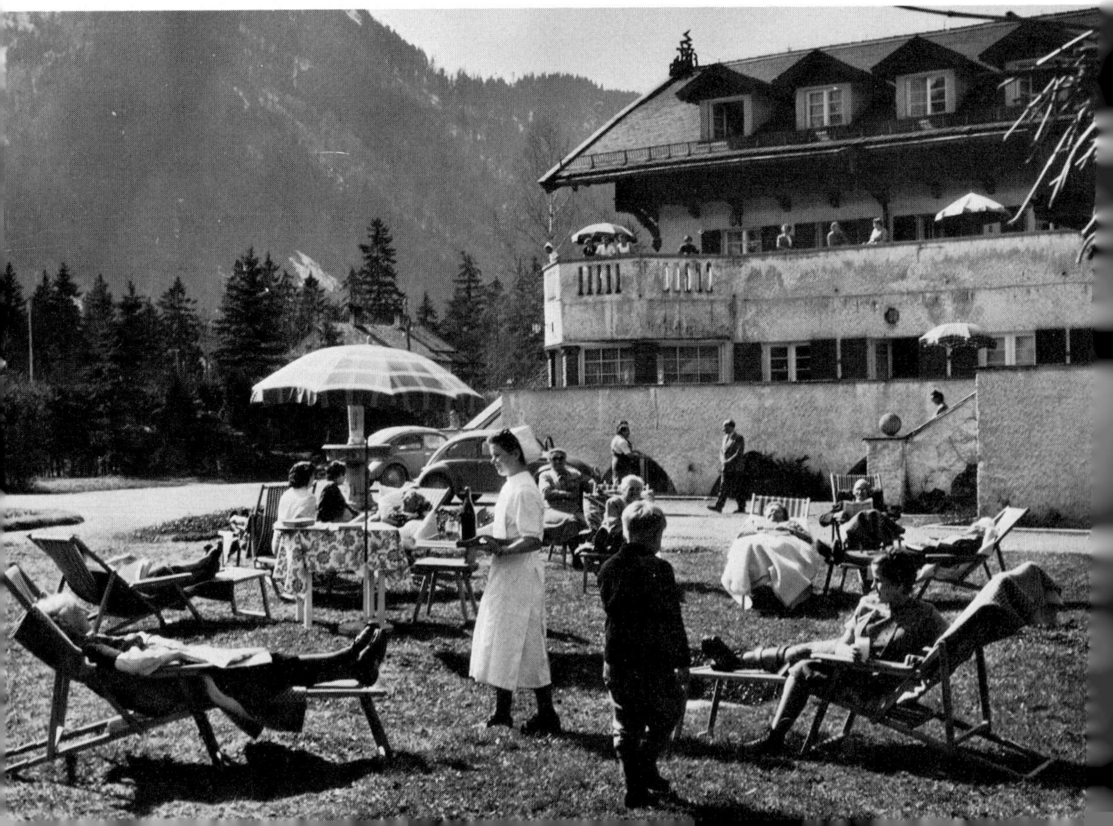

arm: a routine established itself where the surgical team poured over reference books in Orator's office before rushing to the theatre to cope with a compound leg fracture or a crushed rib-cage.

The sudden occasion, the unexpected emergency, played havoc with the best of private plans Issels entertained and made chaos of the most orderly of his days. He found his social life constantly dislocated; only compulsory attendance at the local S.S. lodge remained a regular part of his life. The S.S. men of Duisburg were far different from those he had met in Mönchen-Gladbach. The Duisburg black-shirts were stokers and welders, ham-fisted men who relished the part they played in the local solution of the *Judenfrage*, the Jewish problem. They looked on Issels with little favour: they disliked his good manners, superior knowledge, and, above all, that his Party number showed he remained aloof from the Nazis until the 'April Butterfly' act. In turn, Issels confined to his diary in June 1934: 'They are crude beyond belief. Towards me, and towards each other. There is an unpleasantness about them hard to describe. They are always seeking out trouble, for somebody to get their hands on.'

From time to time a cancer patient turned up for surgery, and Issels marvelled at the skill Orator displayed when cutting out a malignancy. But the operation still did not usually result in permanent healing. Within a year, and often less, the patient returned for a new growth to be removed. Finally, when no more surgery was possible, the man or woman was sent home to die, usually unaware of their condition, or even misled about it. Some were told they were not suffering from cancer.

> It is very hard for the doctors. We know it may be inhuman to lie. But what else can we do? We know no other way. Many of my colleagues believe that to tell a patient the truth brings a loss of hope. And there are some patients who simply do not wish to know the harsh facts of their fate. For them it is probably enough to live from day to day. Yet we would all like to establish an honest relationship if it was possible. But we are taught never to use the word *incurable* in front of a patient. If he

is inoperable, he must be told. Yet there are avenues open to such a patient when surgery is no longer a possibility. There are many examples where spiritual healing has worked. The teachings of the Church show that a Greater Power than surgical skill can prevail. We should never forget that God is the greatest instrument of healing that we have.

Those words, written on a hot summer evening in July, 1934, mark a step forward in the development of Josef Issels as a doctor and a man of strong religious convictions.

From early childhood—when his mother taught him to pray for the animals of the earth as well as its people—his Christianity developed into a deeply private faith. He was baptised and raised in the tradition of the Roman Catholic Church. Early in manhood he felt no need to provide continuing proof of his beliefs by regular attendance at Church. Rather, he set off on his own search for God. It was not an easy journey to make. Issels approached religion in much the way Peer Gynt regarded the onion in Ibsen's play: if it was stripped of all its outer layers, nothing might remain in the centre—or, there might be a hard core upon which he could build a meaningful spiritual life.

The search for truth, as for so many people, was a slow and pensive inner probing that continued all his life. The basic elements of his belief were childlike in their simplicity: God and Heaven were real images; at death there was a pause and then a moving on to Eternal Life; Hell was a torment inside a person here on earth. He built on that foundation a structure rejecting the parochial limitations of religion: God intended no doctrinal boundaries; a Jew or Moslem had just as much right in his beliefs as a Christian.

His religious thinking received a new clarity from two events occurring in middle-age: a long private audience with Pope Pius XII and the support of Albert Schweitzer. The Papal Audience gave Issels renewed strength and purpose not only in his professional standards but also in his religious beliefs. Schweitzer had a similar effect. The two men had common bonds. Orthodox beliefs were not enough for either. The philosopher constantly offered himself the deeds of his life: 'I am only a person living his religion,' he said; and again, often: 'My life is my argument.' Issels adopted an identical stand. Both recognised the importance of rational thought in their attitudes towards God. Schweitzer, possibly the last of the great minds of the Enlightenment—though he was born over a century later—embodied for Issels the true principles of reasoned thought and naturalism. For Schweitzer those ideals formed the bases of his religious life. In time they did the same for Josef Issels.

That summer, in his holidays, Issels took a job as a locum near the small Rhineland country town of Grevenbroich. The rural life proved a welcome respite from the Ruhr and the work brought its own satisfaction. There was time to develop a genuine relationship with a patient. Issels came to recognise which one of two basic approaches to call into play. Some patients wanted him to be authoritarian; for them the doctor's word held the same reverence as religious dogma. Others preferred Issels to be fraternal, sensitively feeling his way to the root of a problem. For these patients the biggest asset Josef Issels offered was a sympathetic ear: he listened patiently and never condemned. He gave the impression the problem was a mutual one, to be solved by the joint efforts of doctor and patient. Over the weeks he came to understand the family life of the community as he tasted the home-made wines or joked over a bowl of thick country soup. The knowledge he gained gave him a new approach to diagnosing: the patient was not isolated in a hospital bed, but could be reviewed against his normal family background and environment; Issels found that the inter-relationships inside a family often added another dimension to be taken into account when diagnosing. Searching for the causal effects of an illness—as distinct from treating the immediate symptoms—often meant knowing the family history for several previous generations. He looked at a patient as a whole; cause became as important as effect. In that way he laid down another foundation stone for the system that eventually started him upon a heterodox career.

In the autumn of 1934 Issels divided his time at Duisburg Hospital operating under Professor Orator and learning something of the specialised craft of Dr. Schmitt, who handled all the hospital's bladder, kidney and prostrate operations. Schmitt was a good technician, but Issels noted in a diary entry for September 1934:

> We can take away the stone in a gall-bladder, but the cause is still there. The stone is a symptom of a sickness of the whole kidney. It is no good removing the stone if the whole kidney is left untreated. I put my idea to Schmitt. He listened politely enough, but said it was impossible to do anything like I suggested. '*Kindchen.* You will find nothing in any textbook to confirm your idea,' Schmitt said kindly enough, making it very clear that he worked only from textbook principles. It wasn't very convincing, and I still believe it is simply not enough to take away the stone and say that is the end of the matter.

Issels' reputation as a competent surgical registrar increased: he was firmly balanced on the medical ladder that so many young hopefuls constantly fell off. He was ambitious to widen his experience in such areas as gynaecology, and early in 1935 he travelled a few miles along the Rhine, returning to Düsseldorf to work at the Marien Hospital as senior registrar under Professor Franz Kudlek, professor of surgery and gynaecology. The unit's case load was heavy and Kudlek, though into his sixtieth year, was tireless, shuttling between ward rounds and operating room with brisk strides.

Düsseldorf faced Issels with the full reality of how limiting surgery could be in cases of progressive cancer. Over half the operations carried out on women patients were for cancer. Kudlek was a courageous surgeon, operating on cases other surgeons considered inoperable. But his knife proved, too often, a mere delaying tactic: the cancer returned, sometimes in sites where even Kudlek could not cut with impunity. Death followed.

If there was any one turning point in the life of Josef Issels it was that day in Düsseldorf, February 17, 1935, when he wrote:

> Surgery offers no hope of getting to the *cause* of cancer. We concentrate on the actual tumour, at the expense of all else. It is clear removing the growth does not remove the *cause*. Getting to the *cause* is as important as dealing with the tumour itself. Take just one recent case that explains the point too well. Kudlek did a good, clean job on a woman with a tumour in the breast. Within six months she was back with metastases in the liver and abdomen. There was nothing more to be done. She was sent home to die. But her case shows the dilemma. In the case of that woman, cancer of the breast meant her whole body was at risk, even from the outset. The cancer would still have spread. So it seems there is a good cause for believing the whole basic attitude we have towards the disease is not the perfect one by any means. Surgery concentrates on the local area of the tumour. It seldom looks beyond that. It is the same, I understand, with irradiation. The local area is attacked and no more. But there would also seem to be a real need to examine the wider effect of the disease on the body as a whole.

He combed the orthodox textbooks for support for this view. He found none.

But his experience at Düsseldorf finally crystallised his ideas about a surgical career. It had lost all appeal in spite of the assured future it offered him. Professor Orator had once extended the graph of professional progress that was indicated for Issels: at thirty he would be a fully-fledged surgeon; ten years later he could head a surgical team in some middle-sized State hospital; around the age of fifty he would move to a large hospital as chief surgeon, finally retiring to live in the country on his sixty-fifth birthday.

Having decided against that sort of future, Issels cast about for a new branch of medicine; in a moment of sheer escapism he decided to become a ship's doctor. He wrote to the Medical Registry in Hamburg, who replied there was already a list of 248 doctors waiting to go to sea; it would be two years before he could expect to get a ship. Undaunted, Issels packed his bags and took a fast train to Hamburg on April 1, 1935.

He haunted the shipping offices by day and the waterfront at night looking for a berth. In between he fitted in a crash course in tropical medicine. Within a fortnight he talked himself aboard the s.s. *Ingrid Horn* as its medical officer for a voyage to South America and the West Indies.

The next months were idyllic. He learned to speak English and French. There were pleasant dalliances with some of the comely matrons on the passenger list, thought it was not until the ship reached Caracas that he found himself caught up in a really torrid affair with the dusky daughter of the Venezuelan President's lawyer. With her black hair and dark eyes Conchita Lopez was far different to his usual *traumfrau*, but they made a handsome couple in local high society. Nevertheless, when the family offered Issels his own hospital as a wedding present, he recognised the danger signals, and only finally breathed a sigh of relief when sailing time came. Those weeks at sea also helped dim the memories of cancer operations which had failed and the limitations of surgery for incurable diseases.

After a brief stop-over in Hamburg, Issels shipped out as a doctor on the s.s. *Ussukuma*, on a voyage around Africa. The outward journey passed uneventfully; the small sick bay in the ship's stern remained unopened for days on end, and then it was mostly to dispense sun-burn lotions or tablets for upset stomachs. Issels and the ship's nurse had ample time to acquire magnificent tans.

Then, four hours after the *Ussukuma* sailed out of Port Elizabeth in June, 1935, the nurse reported that one of the passengers, an Englishwoman, was suddenly seriously ill. The high drama that followed was preserved in an account Issels wrote immediately after the event:

> I found a woman of forty collapsed in her cabin. She had a high temperature, weak pulse, drawn face and an abdomen as hard as a plank. It was a classic case of peritonitis, an acute inflammation of the lining of the abdominal cavity. She would die without surgery. Leaving the nurse to watch her, I ran to the bridge and told the captain of my findings, adding that he must return at once to Port Elizabeth for the woman to undergo emergency surgery.

'Impossible! The company would never sanction the loss of a whole day!'

I told him I was not concerned with the balance sheet of the line—only whether a patient lived or died. I said he left me with no alternative except to carry out the operation on board. 'I forbid you! I am the Captain! You will obey me! And when we reach Hamburg you will be dismissed ship!' I ignored his threat. As calmly as possible I told him that when it came to a patient's life he had no authority over me. Momentarily baulked, he sought the backing of the line to curb me. He cabled them—and received a swift reply that the ship was to maintain course and I simply must not operate. I refused the order.

'Listen, Dr. Issels, these are difficult times. If the woman dies during the operation there will be much bad publicity for you, for the line, even for Germany!' I told him I was not interested in the finer points of image building. I was going to operate—and that was the end of the matter. I hurried to the sick-bay, and the situation there did nothing to reassure me. The instruments locker contained a poor selection of scalpels, clamps, needles. The line had not equipped the locker in anticipation of any major operation. Though I had checked the locker on joining the ship, I too had not anticipated the situation I now faced. The nurse arrived, white-faced and nervous. The patient's condition was worsening. I asked if she could give an anaesthetic for the operation. She shook her head. 'Then find somebody who can assist me—and quick!'

She returned with a first-class passenger. He was a young sea captain on a busman's holiday. He had taken a course in basic first aid at sea. Together we prepared the room for surgery. A dining table was plonked in the middle; the pitiful selection of instruments positioned on a breakfast tray. Then, gowned and wearing tablecloths around our waist to afford some measure of asepsis, we awaited the arrival of the patient.

'I've never done an operation before,' said the captain brightly. 'I fancy a drink!'

I nodded. I knew the feeling. He rummaged around and found a half-bottle of cognac. He took a generous mouthful and said he was ready for anything. The patient arrived on a stretcher carried by two sailors who dumped her on the table and then took up positions of interested spectators in a corner of the room. 'Nervous, doctor?' one of them asked cheerfully. I shook my head, hoping to give the impression that I had faced this situation many times before. I inducted the woman. A silence came over the room. The sense of impending drama seemed to have reached the bridge. The ship had slowed down; possibly her captain was trying to make it easier for me to operate. I picked up a surgical knife. My two assistants stood on either side of the exposed abdomen. I made the first firm stroke with the knife. Nothing happened. I pressed harder with the scalpel. It was so blunt it simply would not cut. One of the sailors volunteered that my predecessor was in the habit of sharpening his pencils with a scalpel. I took another knife, uncomfortably aware that the captain was bent over the incision area to have a closer look. The skin parted—and a fountain of pus spurted into his face. He promptly fainted. One of the sailors revived him with another large swig of cognac, washed his face and hands and guided him back to the table.

In the meantime I scooped out the pus with a handy coffee cup. In a cupboard the nurse found some clean handkerchiefs and I soaked these in a bottle of sterile water and washed out the stomach. The site of the infection was a huge cyst near the right ovary. I cut it away and prepared to sew up. The nurse had threaded gut through the handful of needles and held them in her hands. The first needle broke on contact with the skin. So did the second. Salt air must have corroded them. Then the patient started to wake up. I snatched a fresh needle and slipped in a few stitches. 'Quick!', I shouted to the sailors. 'Grab her hands and legs and keep her still!' To the captain I said: 'Put her under.' He sprinkled ether on her nose and she started to drop off again.

The line had been right! It was too much! Too big an operation! But I simply had to go on now! The woman was still restless. I told one of the sailors to bring me all the sticky plaster he could find. Then I lay across the exposed abdomen, in case she managed to get a hand into the still open cavity. I was soaked in sweat. In that position the wallowing of the ship made the floor rise and fall alarmingly.

The sailor returned with the sticky plaster and I slowly plastered up the abdomen until only one piece of intestine remained exposed. Before I could stop him the sailor popped it inside with his dirty, meaty fingers. I put in a drain.

It was over. I went to the bridge to report that my patient was still alive—if only just. The captain looked bemused. Then, without a word, he fetched a bottle of champagne and we drank a toast. There was still more to do. I spent the next twelve hours at her bedside until she opened her eyes. After two days she showed marked improvement. I spent most of that time listening to her abdomen, to see if the intestines were working. On the third day there was a satisfying rumble—and I knew she was on the road to recovery—which she fully made.

The operation brought Issels his first taste of international publicity as newspapers and radio stations in a dozen countries recounted the story. The shipping line cabled him congratulations. When the *Ussukuma* reached Zanzibar, he was invited to the Sultan's birthday party. In every port local doctors came on board to discuss the operation. His eventual return to Hamburg in the autumn of 1935 had all the trappings of an instant celebrity. He accepted his status graciously, rejected further offers to go to sea, and returned to Düsseldorf.

4

New Methods

In his absence the Marien Hospital had not changed apart from acquiring further coats of grime from the Düsseldorf chimneys. But the world around the building assumed a new and menacing aspect. Germany was tooling-up for war, and the Ruhr disgorged a vast flow of weaponry. The hospital's casualty department handled a growing number of workmen injured while turning out gun barrels and tank tracks.

There was a law from 1935 that all German men working abroad, on returning to the Fatherland, must report to the local Party headquarters to be assigned some role in the unfolding Wagnerian tragedy. Issels ignored it. The hospital's administration assumed he had complied with the law. He let them believe that. But nothing escaped forever the efficient Party machine. Issels was finally confronted by an S.S. officer, berated for his disloyalty, and forced to re-enlist in the *Schutzstaffel.* He had no stomach for the mood of violence that gripped the S.S. or the general need to purge everything that did not meet the strict requirements of National Socialism. He grew skilled at finding work within the hospital which kept him from marching to the tune of *Heil Hitler* or debating *Mein Kampf.*

His work in the months following his return left him little time for any outside activity. There were a few brief, and unsatisfactory, affairs, only remembered later because they were so empty. His thinking otherwise seldom ranged beyond the hospital's medical wards and clinics. Issels had returned to Düsseldorf to complete his medical education in physical medicine—and he set about the task with characteristic drive. He was filled with a sense of the importance of his work. In January, 1936, he wrote to his mother:

> Internal medicine is so important for my fuller understanding of the patient. Surgery was often only the end of the story. It failed to reveal the *cause*. Yet *cause* is the factor that matters most—and that is what my life here now is concerned with.

He might have added that the twists in the path were numerous and surprising, but that in the end it was the winding road that reached the top of the hill. Along that journey he worked in the ears-and-throat, skin and paediatric clinics. To a variety of clinical problems he applied the same basic rule: the root of a disease must be fully exposed. He became an observer without preconceived ideas as he followed the trail of illness in all parts of the body. Heavily underlined is a diary entry for March, 1936, which he regarded as:

> Very important. Most hospital patients are in a progressive state of illness. Therefore, hospital is not the stage to get to the *cause*. Here we are concerned primarily with the treatment of the presenting symptoms. If a man has an ulcer it is treated locally, but generally the *cause* is not sought. That seems to me to be very wrong.

He discussed his feelings with colleagues at every opportunity. For the most part they remained unconvinced by his thinking; for them it was enough that the immediate illness was successfully treated.

To complete his training in general medicine he moved, in January, 1937, to the hospital's gynaecological clinic. He found himself in a totally unfamiliar world:

> There is nothing like birth. The woman changes and you change. All you care about is whether the pelvis is big enough for the baby's head to pass through easily. Is the

perineum hard or soft? It is the same with the woman: for her the animal functions are all-important. Can she push? Can she contract? And in the actual moments of birth she *is* an animal. She grits and pushes and pushes and pushes. Then, when it is over, the baby is here, she is back to normal. Once more a woman. It is a wonderful moment.

Even though a career in surgery held no further abiding interest, there were still operations to assist at. He developed a dislike of hysterectomy, excision of the uterus, because he believed it was often followed by grave psychological upset.

The unexpected was never far away. One day a respected local gynaecologist referred a patient to the hospital clinic with a clear-cut diagnosis: a huge tumour in the abdomen needed to be removed. Issels was depressed by the case notes. His previous experience told him that the long-term prognosis was poor in such cases. He called the girl into the consulting room.

She was pretty, fair-haired, well-spoken and dressed as befitted the only daughter of one of Düsseldorf's oldest families. She took off her coat, and the tumour site was clearly visible. Even beneath her smock it looked like a full-term baby. But something else immediately struck Issels. Her face, especially her lips were puffed.

He recorded what followed:

> I quickly scanned the case-notes. The diagnosis was quite clear. A tumour. If it was malignant then the girl had no chance. I began to question her gently. Did she know why she had been sent to the hospital? Yes. I waited, not quite knowing how to ask the next question. Could there be any other factor?
>
> She looked momentarily confused. The suspicion at the back of my mind grew. When had she last had a period? Nine months earlier. I looked down at the case-notes. No mention of that there. I asked the girl one more question: was it just possible that she was pregnant? Shock and astonishment came into her face. Impossible, impossible! How could I say such a thing!

If I was wrong, God knows where it would end! I asked her to let me examine her. The breasts were full of milk! The tumour was undoubtedly a baby, and a baby very close to being born at that. Still the girl resisted any suggestion that this could possibly be the case. She was of a good family, had been well brought up . . . I let her run on and on until she ended by reminding me that the original diagnosis had been made by a gynaecologist of high reputation. It was true enough—at least the part about his reputation. I was flummoxed. While I had no doubts as to my own findings there was no escaping the well-documented case history. There was only one way to resolve the case. I had the girl X-rayed. The negative showed a perfectly formed baby.

I went to the clinic's chief and explained the whole story. He telephoned the gynaecologist—who was stunned by the news. So stunned in fact that he could offer no explanation.

I returned to the girl and showed her the X-ray print—and waited. The whole story came out in the end. Yes, she was pregnant by the son of another local ruling family. But her parents did not approve of the relationship—and would never allow a marriage. Early on in the pregnancy she had gone to the gynaecologist and complained of symptoms that *somehow* led him to believe she had a tumour. She had actually hoped that once she was operated on it would be possible to remove the baby without anybody outside the theatre knowing. I gently explained that was certainly not possible, that we could not pretend any more that the baby did not exist.

I thought over the next move carefully—knowing that it probably extended well beyond the normal doctor-patient relationship. But, if all the girl had said was true, then it was worth taking a chance. I sent for her young man and told him what had happened. Then I asked him two questions. Did he still love the girl? Yes. Did he want to marry her? Yes.

So far, so good. But now I faced the biggest problem: the parents. I sent for them. They were all I had expected: wealthy, reserved—and mortified when they heard the full story. I gave them time to get over the hurt to their pride—

for that is what it really was—and then talked some hard sense to them. Their daughter was going to have a baby no matter what they said. The young couple were very much in love. Why not let them marry?

In the end they agreed. But only just in time, for I had to rush away and deliver a bouncing baby boy—their first grandson. The young couple were married soon afterwards, and all was forgiven.

Life was not always so sweet. Periodically Issels recognised an odd feeling that medicine seemed to exist largely for itself; that sometimes the saving of lives was often linked with the advancing of reputations; behind the well-developed bedside manner of some colleagues could be detected the postures of ambition.

Once, when on duty as night doctor he admitted a local factory owner and diagnosed a classic case of appendicitis. During the examination Issels learnt the man was a private patient of a senior consultant at the hospital—who arrived, bleary-eyed, shortly afterwards. Issels explained the symptoms and diagnosis. The consultant exploded: *junior doctors did not make a diagnosis on his private patients*. The consultant examined the man, and said surgery was uncalled for until further tests had been carried out in the hospital's private wing. Two days later, in between the tests, the patient collapsed with peritonitis. Emergency surgery failed to save him. Issels wrote a bitter footnote to the case in his diary:

> If this man had been a simple workman he would have lived. But he had to have all the tests that the consultant thought right for a private patient. I remember the words of Orator: 'If I get sick, please treat me like a simple workman, a *Kassenpatient*.'

His note-books filled more and more with a now familiar cry: when would many of his colleagues recognise that *cause* was as important as effect?

That question remained unanswered until the lunch hour of July 5, 1936, when into the doctors' dining room at the hospital came Dr. Ferdinand Huneke.

The unreality of that meeting came clearly through in Issels' later account:

> He said: 'I am the famous Huneke. Who are you? Issels? Never heard of you. But you must know me—the discoverer of neural therapy.' I had never heard of the man or his discovery. Huneke soon changed that. Nor did it take long for me to realise here was a personality so utterly unlike the conventional image of the medical man.

If Huneke intended to impress, he succeeded totally. Issels was captivated by the tall, slimly built man with a dent on the left side of his greying temples. He spoke a language Issels never had heard a doctor use before, and described a treatment no standard textbook even hinted at. Huneke had a ready explanation for that. Since making his discovery he had become an object of uneasy suspicion and often undisguised dislike among doctors. He was utterly perplexed by their attitude. Nor could he understand why his colleagues and medical societies did not recognise his claims. Initially, it was no more than curiosity which later brought Issels to Huneke's surgery near the hospital. By the end of that meeting Josef Issels was genuinely confused and troubled.

The whole concept of neural therapy was so utterly ridiculous when measured against conventional medical teaching; the claims Huneke made were preposterous for somebody who had graduated with distinction from one of Germany's more respected medical faculties. Indeed, the whole story of how Huneke came to his discovery smacked of the quackery that teaching professors constantly warned their students to avoid.

Until 1929 Huneke was a little-known family doctor in Düsseldorf. One day his sister came to his surgery complaining of acute migraine and local pains in the arm. Thinking to temporarily ease the local pain, Huneke injected her with a small dose of Novocaine, a fast-acting local anaesthetic. By mistake he injected directly into a vein. In that moment, he told Issels, the migraine disappeared—never to return. Huneke tried it on other patients, and claimed the same results. He felt he was a man of destiny in medicine; no amount of ridicule shook him from such a belief.

That attitude also intrigued Issels. He wondered at the sheer energy that kept Huneke going in the face of universal opposition. Issels tried later to rationalise his thoughts on paper, to apply the logic his university training taught him to use for any problem. He failed. There was no precedent in anything he had learnt which allowed him to demolish Huneke's claims. His bewilderment was clear:

> Huneke says what he calls the 'disturbance field' of the body (what the textbooks call the sites of the lesion) was very important. Dead, or suppurating teeth, infected tonsils, and also old body scar tissue could be the cause for asthma, migraine, visual disorders, rheumatism and many other illnesses. He offers no explanation that would be accepted, or understood by orthodox medicine. He just says that it works! I have asked repeatedly how the Novocaine works and he gives an explanation that I simply cannot follow or understand. My head is reeling from what he says. Nobody who believes in the principles of conventional medicine could grasp Huneke's arguments and claims. Yet, I have the feeling that just because I do not yet understand it, does not mean that I should dismiss it, or that he is wrong.

Issels canvassed support for this theory among hospital colleagues. At first they laughed it off as no more than the fad of an enthusiastic doctor with an inquiring mind. But when Issels persisted with his questions, more than one doctor gave him a wide berth.

Increasingly Issels spent his free time around Huneke's surgery, and wrote:

> I have learnt something that I can understand. Huneke is as firm a believer as I am that the *cause* of an illness is what really matters.

Then:

> Huneke injects all parts of the body—and the pain is away. I saw it myself today. An old man came in with a migraine.

> Huneke injected into an old scar behind the ear and the old man was free of pain. Just like that! Huneke explained to me that the scar was the 'disturbance point' of the body and could change the 'electric field' of the body. The Novocaine normalised the electric field in the scar tissue—and the disturbance went away. He does not know exactly how the Novocaine works within the scar tissue. But it does work. That old man was certainly freed of his migraine. My God, I wonder what my professor would say about that.

It was likely they would have said it was mumbo-jumbo; that it all belonged more to the age of sorcery than to an era of scientific medicine.

Issels did not discuss the matter further with anybody. In his summer holiday he worked as a locum in Huneke's surgery. It completed his conversion; the cases he saw being treated by neural therapy were:

> A further blow for me and my beliefs that only orthodox medicine knew the answers. Huneke showed me that in even severe cases of rheumatism and asthma he could get a response. Sometimes he needed five or ten injections in the same scar tissues over two or three days to get a result. And here is something extraordinary. My first patient, a man, with a blinding headache. I prepared an injection and gave it in a scar in the right temple. Nothing happened. The headache was still there. Huneke examined the man and located a small scar, very old, on the neck. He injected there—and the patient was instantly free of pain. Huneke said it all came from experience. Intuition was as important to him as anatomy.

In the month he spent working in such an unorthodox surgery Issels said he learnt to successfully treat a number of cases that totally convinced him of the validity of such a generally unacceptable therapy.

When he returned to the Marien Hospital and tried to describe his experience, his colleagues looked embarrassed; they were uncomfortable that Issels, a man with such a promising future in medicine, appeared to have taken a definite step into a world beyond the discipline of normal science. Thirty years later, in the 1960s, neural therapy was a recognised treatment in many German hospitals and clinics. But in the summer of 1936 Josef Issels was the first doctor to secretly introduce it to the Marien Hospital in Düsseldorf. Without the knowledge of the consultants he treated patients suffering from a variety of chronic illnesses with neural therapy. In many cases he claimed positive results.

These experiences were the first steps along the road to empiricism. Huneke had released something in him. He felt himself to be no longer inhibited by the rules of standard medical practice, nor hindered by the restrictive attitude that if it was unacceptable it must be no good. The experience and ability which he had gathered in nearly four years of surgery and general medicine were no longer enough. He was thirty years old, approaching the time when for most men the road ahead is clearly sign-posted: for the vast majority it is a dull, but safe, road with pensionable obscurity at the end of it. For a brilliant few there is a sign-post leading down a narrower path, one more difficult to negotiate, that ends in success and recognition.

For Josef Issels there was no sign-post. He had not the vaguest idea what would be the eventual outcome of his decision to pursue the unorthodox.

It was almost a natural progression that Issels moved in the autumn of 1936 from Düsseldorf to work as an assistant for Dr. Karl Ruhmkorff, a greying giant of a man who treated the country folk around Hanover with highly unorthodox methods. His reputation had spread until in middle-age he was a minor legend in northern Germany. In some ways he was in advance of his time with his insistence on diet control and the use of high fevers to knock-out an infection. In other things Ruhmkorff belonged to a byegone era with his library of eighteenth- and nineteenth-century books, and an abiding love for the largely forgotten men of medicine.

Night after night, when they completed a daily car trip around a practice scattered over twelve villages, Issels listened, enthralled, to Ruhmkorff expounding the theories of such men as Carl Spengler, the German specialist on tuberculosis, that chronic diseases afflicted the whole body. Spengler had developed a serum with an antigenic function, that he said stimulated and built antibodies against infection. The treatment never caught on.

To his mother Issels wrote in October, 1936, a long letter which revealed how far he had departed from accepted thinking:

> I am learning every day the true *causal* effects of disease. Increasingly I see the importance of the *krankheitsbild,* the full picture of an illness, its history, and also the history of the patient's parents and their constitutions.
>
> I have learnt to trace back an illness through the generations. A grandfather had stomach pains. His son had an ulcer—and now the grandson has cancer in the stomach. That cancer progressed through three generations.
>
> I didn't learn that at university. Nor did the textbooks show me something else that I have learnt here. Everybody from birth has a weak part of general body resistance. It is that which acts as the focal points of the illness. I have found the very same focal points can be traced back through a whole family. You won't find that in the orthodox textbooks. Why don't we hear anything in the universities of such things? Only hard experience has shown me that is true. The work here is very hard; it is nothing to spend twelve or fourteen hours with patients. Ruhmkorff eats very little and then it is a question of snatching something when there is time. But I have never felt better. The air is clean, the people have a much gentler tempo than city people. Only the illnesses do not change.

When a patient with an incurable disease returned from hospital to one of the villages to die, it brought home again to Issels not only the limitations of available treatment, but also the importance of having a dignified relationship with the dying. He gave up precious free time just sitting and talking with a man or woman written off as incurable. From such contact he learnt a great deal about the patient and his family and used that knowledge in better management of the situation. He found that genuine concern was always as valuable as a syringe filled with an analgesic; most people, when they realised the time had come, preferred to die at home surrounded by their loved ones. Often conditions were clearly imperfect, but the rewards for a patient and relatives were tremendous. A dying person benefited from the care of an affectionate family; he retained his individuality and was not in danger of becoming an anonymous hulk in some institution.

Ruhmkorff introduced Issels to homoeopathic medicine. He grasped its principles with an eagerness that never dimmed. He was especially attracted by the way it had survived formidable opposition, including that of his own university professors.

The principles of homoeopathy were first expounded in 1796 by a German doctor, Christian Samuel Hahnemann, who was born in Meissen in 1755 and died in Paris in 1843. He finally enjoyed an international reputation as physician, scholar and chemist. While translating Cullen's *Materia Medici* he found himself disagreeing with the author over the action of quinine. Testing the drug on himself, he found that it produced symptoms of the malaria it was supposed to cure. Hahnemann sensed that here was the law of drug action he had sought for so many years. He tested remedy after remedy. In each case he found that drugs which produced certain symptoms cured sick people presenting similar symptoms. The phrase which he adopted and proved to be true in a life-time of research, *Similia similibus curantur*—'Let like be treated by like'—became the fundamental principles of homoeopathic medicine. He was hounded from one town to another in Germany, chiefly by the apothecaries. They rejected his prescriptions for specially prepared infinitesimal doses which, he argued, removed the underlying causes of disease; the apothecaries feared such medicaments could ruin their lucrative businesses.

Everything that Issels read about homoeopathy convinced him that here was a gentle yet effective system of prescribing; it was based on the principle of stimulating the body's own natural resistance to disease and not merely attacking the disease symptoms, or just destroying germs and viruses within the body. To Issels:

Homoeopathic medicine is based on the sound principle of co-operation with nature. Its emphasis on countering hereditary disease is excellent. The patient is studied as a whole, and as an individual, and not just as somebody to be given routine treatment according to what the text-books say.

He recorded other observations about homoeopathy, writing them by the light of an oil lamp late at night in the winter of 1937–38:

A patient often has symptoms before detectable pathological changes can be seen: the aim of homoeopathy is treating that pre-detectable stage of the disease, so saving the patient from progressing to more serious illness. By division and dilution a drug may be turned into a very powerful agent which, when applied by homoeopathic principles, stimulates the body in its fight against disease.

Or:

Homoeopathic remedies derive from such dissimilar substances as bee stings and snake venoms. Arsenic, gold and even diseased tissues can be used. In using them each remedy presents a different characteristic which needs skilled preparation in making the 'mother' tincture: (θ)

He copied out the baffling process of potentisation—diluting a drug in proportions of one in ten, or one in one hundred, with the essential vigorous shaking at each stage. Later, he saw the effects of such remedies, and wrote enthusiastically of relief in even chronic illness.

From the day he began the practical side of his medical training. Issels had kept a thick ledger book in which he entered useful tips handed down by his professors. The early part of the book was filled with hints on bandaging, splint-setting and diagnosing minor ailments. Later came case details of surgical procedures. Apart from showing something of the diligence of Issels, it was all unremarkable. But from January, 1938, entries appeared that revealed the true width of the gulf between what he had been taught and what he now believed. There were constant reminders of the need to prescribe for the sick individual as a whole, the necessity of knowing what constitutional type a patient was, both emotionally and physically. There were carefully entered details of diluted solutions of belladonna which could be used for burns and scalds *and* scarlet fever; chills and colds could be helped by remedies such as Aconitum D–30 and Arsenicum D–30—neither of which would ever be found in the pharmacies of the great teaching hospitals of Germany. The ledger book showed they were valuable resources in Issels' new armoury of medicaments. By March, 1938, the divergence from the rote and example of conventional medicine widened further:

> Personal characteristics of a patient vital in making the best choice of available remedies. Thus: *Lycopodium :* best results in a patient who has a history of steadiness at work, who is intelligent, but not too strong physically. Probably does not like gay social life, but not eager either for total solitude. Feels the cold in winter, and cannot stand excessive heat.
>
> *Arsenicum Album :* positive, often quick results in cases of nervous tension in a person who is usually elegantly groomed, unduly complains of the cold, and worries about almost everything.
>
> *Pulsatilla :* works best for the placid type of personality. The type of patient given to tearful outbursts and signs of self-pity.

All through the warm summer of 1938 Issels worked and studied the principles of homoeopathy and its associated schools of diet control and fasting under the watchful eyes of Ruhmkorff. Issels was a good pupil—and in time would have undoubtedly taken over the old man's practice.

But he had other plans. He wanted to practise on his own in Mönchen-Gladbach; in part he wanted to show his mother and the family what a good doctor he had become.

Standing, as it were, in the audience of the mounting tragedy around him, Issels became aware that the Nazis were a gang of demolition men ripping out the very foundation of civilisation; a sludge wave of hate was spreading across the land. The train home to Mönchen-Gladbach had a sprinkling of men in Luftwaffe blue or the *feldgrau* of the *Wehrmacht*; the newspapers and radios carried lengthy reports that indicated the Führer's preoccupation with *die deutsche Raumfrage*, Germany's problem of space.

Issels' return home provided a new, and welcome, topic for dinner-table discussion. Everybody chipped in with advice on where he should open a surgery.

Finally he chose 38 Bismarckstrasse, a tall, narrow building, not far from the town centre. There were four rooms on the ground floor and a small apartment above. He borrowed RM 17,000 from a local bank—the first time he had been in debt in his life, but not the last—and converted the ground floor into a waiting room, consulting room, treatment room and small laboratory. All were adequately equipped. On September 15, 1938, Issels was ready to practise on his own for the first time.

In spite of his genuine belief in the healing powers of homoeopathy, neural therapy and other unorthodox treatments, Issels decided to rely largely on a conventional approach in treating his patients. He was uncertain that he could successfully carry out an unconventional regime without the guidance of a Huneke or a Ruhmkorff on hand. He was also concerned with establishing a reputation; it would undoubtedly be easier to do so by prescribing drugs and pills that the local chemists stocked.

Instead, he planned to make his reputation in the consulting room. His greatest asset was boundless confidence in himself; properly applied, he reasoned, it was a most powerful therapeutic weapon. Added to that, he believed he had a more exact knowledge and understanding of medical problems than many of the other doctors in the town.

His first patient arrived soon after he opened the surgery. It was his small nephew, complaining of ear ache. Issels took a history and examined him carefully, and gravely reassured the child that the trouble would soon pass. For the rest of the day he did not see another patient. He sat for hour after hour in the consulting room, listening to the traffic outside, or fending off salesmen peddling medicaments and surgical appliances. The next week was little better; a handful of people, mostly old. Issels wrote in his private diary:

> Each said, in his own way, that they had really come to give me a try—to see if I was any better than all the other doctors in town they had been to! Late in the afternoon a chronic case of asthma presented himself. After a lengthy examination I prescribed a series of standard tablets from my 'recipe book'. The patient looked at me scornfully and said: 'Doctor, I thought you would know more than all the other doctors? I've tried all this stuff before!' I went home and talked it over with Mother. She said: 'You studied long enough so you should know more about it.'

His sense of inadequacy remained a constant factor in the following weeks. The patients came, he prescribed what the textbooks recommended, and the signs of improvement of chronic diseases were few and far between. It did not help to know that other doctors were getting similar results with the same treatments; more than one colleague meant well in telling Issels that he should not expect too much. His depression increased to the point where:

> Patients are now telling me what they would like! One came in this afternoon, presenting a bad case of angina pectoris. The conversation went like this: 'You're the new doctor?' Yes. 'You're young.' Yes. 'My old doctor was an old man.' Yes. 'He was very experienced.' Yes. 'You're young.' Yes. 'You must have learnt a lot of new things.' Yes. A pause, then triumphantly: 'But you can't know as much as my old doctor did about my condition. You see he died from it!'

At the end of his first month Issels had earned RM 90; in the second his income was RM 120. By November, 1938, it had increased to RM 300—still substantially less than his monthly allowance had been as a student. He refused to allow the family to help. There were six other children to educate and he knew his parents could ill-afford to subsidise him. His father was in better health and a good relationship developed between the two men that remained until Herman Josef's death at the age of ninety years in January, 1960.

With time on his hands and a feeling of having failed with orthodox methods to treat chronic diseases, Issels turned back again to the world of the unorthodox. He re-read the theories and methods Huneke and Ruhmkorff had defended with well-argued partiality. Once more his outlook altered. Where the routine use of modern medicaments had largely failed to remove the underlying causes of diseases, he now sought the methods of another school. He became absorbed in dieting as a way of helping the body's natural resistance to illness. Chronic asthma and arthritic sufferers found that consulting Issels meant following a regime of no meat or milk and eating plenty of roughage. Others were sent for hydro-therapy treatments. By January, 1939, Issels reported in his diary:

> The New Year begins on a wonderful note. Many of the chronic patients are now responding well to the new regime. And more are coming every day for treatment. On *Silvester* some of my colleagues said they had heard what I was doing, and they had refused to believe it. I said it was all true, and they looked really shocked. One of them said: 'But Issels, you simply cannot behave like this as a doctor.' My God, if he stopped thinking less about how a doctor should behave and more about his patients it would be better. No matter what they say, I know I am doing good for my patients. That is what matters to me, and I told Mother so, and she totally agreed with me.

By the spring of 1939 Issels was earning RM 2,000 a month, a very high income. He spent a large portion of it in building up a library of books by Spengler, Huneke, Aschner and other medically qualified proponents of the unusual. At weekends he sought out homoeopathic doctors in the area; they were flattered and surprised at this knowledge and passed on their own particular remedies to him.

From his reading and clinical experience, he drew what was to him a genuine irrefutable conclusion: medicine had lost some important fundamentals as it made its spectacular advances. It was an unfortunate fact, Issels argued, that the routine use of modern drugs could itself be the cause of drug-induced sickness. Popular medicine had found no panaceas for many of the diseases which still beset mankind. The germs or parasites attacked by some new compound had a way of becoming immune to the drug, with the result that a newer, and more powerful, method was needed to deal with the problem. Issels saw that as a vicious circle. He also abhorred the 'blunderbuss' techniques of some doctors and their concoctions of drugs which he believed only alleviated the symptoms and not the causal effects.

By the first day of official summer in Germany, June 21, Issels sensed that war was inevitable. Czechoslovakia had fallen. Poland was being threatened. The D.N.B., *Deutsches Nachrichtenbüro*, the Nazi news agency, showed a daily increase of menace. The Munich Pact of September, 1938, with its promised 'peace in our time' became still-born nine months later in the hot summer of 1939.

Issels had toyed with the idea of leaving Germany to go to Zürich, Switzerland, to study further implications of diet control. By July, 1939, it was too late: exit visas from Germany were virtually unobtainable for such a purpose. Only a few shiploads of Jews were allowed to go in return for vast quantities of American dollars.

Some of them were patients of Josef Issels. He had continued to treat them in face of mounting hostility. To Jews and Nazis he gave one answer: he made no distinction with patients.

The authorities had already acted in August 1938. Issels was summoned to S.S. Headquarters in Mönchen-Gladbach. A *Sturmbannarzt*, an S.S. man responsible for all doctors in the area, subjected him to an unpleasant interview. Issels was ordered to remove all Jewish patients from his practice. He refused. He was warned that he placed not only himself, but his entire family at risk. Issels recognised the dangers—but still he could not disobey the dictates of his conscience and Christian beliefs. He discussed the situation with his mother. She bolstered his own resolve that: 'If I am a real doctor, with all the humanity and humility that entails, I must allow nothing to influence me when it comes to my patients.'

A few days later the S.S. *Sturmbannarzt* called on Issels at his surgery. He was more unpleasant than before and ordered Issels to show him around the apartment over the surgery. In the bedroom was a crucifix on the wall. What followed made a lasting impression on Issels:

> The S.S. man shouted at me: 'You believe in Him?' I said, yes, I did believe in Jesus Christ. The answer enraged him further. He called me a 'Jew lover', unworthy of the S.S. and went on and on for some time. Finally he said I must make a choice—the Church or the S.S. I had three days to make a decision—and it had better be the right one, he said. I told him I did not need that much time. I could give him the answer there and then. I would never give up my religion. Then he really erupted: 'You are finished with the S.S. Do you know what that means for your future?'

Issels 'resigned upon his own petition from the S.S. because of confessional and ideological reasons' according to available S.S. documents. He sent back his uniform. Soon afterwards he learned through a friend that his name was on a special S.S. file as a man to be carefully watched.

All his life Issels faced smears and innuendos over his S.S. membership. The B.B.C. felt it necessary to carry out inquiries, using an employee with good connections among British and German intelligence organisations to conduct them. A senior B.B.C. executive justified such unusual behaviour for the Corporation by stating: 'The B.B.C. does not give air time to anybody who might have been a real Nazi.' Happily, it is not necessary to rely on the word of Josef Issels alone. Independent confirmation can be found in a slim folder of affidavits from patients and a doctor who practised in Mönchen-Gladbach in 1939. The patients were all Jewish. The doctor was a member of the S.S. After the war, in 1946, they voluntarily went to the Allied Military Government in the Rhineland and testified that even after Issels had been dismissed from the S.S. he still continued to treat Jews. Those statements of Wilhelm Brandts, Josef Kremer, Kurt Köchlin, Paul and Käthe Königs, and Dr. Eduard Deicke awaken painful memories of that time when Germany seemed gripped by a national madness.

On July 19, 1939, Issels and a friend drove six hundred miles south to Tegernsee in Bavaria for a holiday. Three days later he was introduced to Irmengard Linder. She was rather tall, ash-blonde, lissom, twenty-three years old and a Catholic. Within a week he was deeply in love with her. To his diary he confined:

> I have, never, ever felt like this before about any woman. She is unique. We walk by the lake and talk and talk and talk. Irm has a wonderful mind. She has read so much about so many things. She is the woman I would dearly love to have as my wife.

Irmengard was also attracted to Issels. But she wanted time before finally committing herself. She had the sense to realise that a holiday romance often faded.

Issels returned to Mönchen-Gladbach in early August, clutching a photograph of Irmengard and suffering the pangs of the love-lorn. He showed the picture to his mother. She studied it carefully and said: 'That is the girl for you to marry.'

His happiness was complete.

Next came a postcard from Irmengard. He again showed it to his mother who commented: 'The girl has excellent handwriting.'

Shortly afterwards a more formal letter arrived for Issels. He opened it and learned that his life and history had merged. He had been called-up into the army on the eve of war.

5

War and Peace

ISSELS SPENT THREE MONTHS AT DETMOLD, GERMANY'S national barrack square. At the end of basic military training he was posted as an *unterarzt* to 365 Company of the 10th Panzer Division. His medical rank carried the lowly privileges of a *feldwebel*. His arrival at Division Headquarters near Koblenz, on the Rhine, was followed by an order from Army Medical Corps H.Q. in Berlin for the company commander to file a monthly confidential report on the new doctor's military and political attitudes. Issels told him the story of why he had left the S.S. The officer was sympathetic and promised his reports to Berlin would be fair.

By the spring of 1940 Issels still had not heard a shot fired in anger. On the eastern front Hitler's grey steel juggernaut had flattened Poland, and the D.N.B. carried full accounts of the Kremlin banquet where Ribbentrop and Stalin politically sliced up Poland. At 11 a.m. on October 10, 1939 Hitler had issued his War Directive No 6, ordering preparations 'For an attacking operation through the areas of Luxembourg, Belgium and Holland'. The winter passed with the 10th Panzers on alert to push westwards into the Low Countries or to repel a French thrust from the south.

Issels was barely affected by the strategic planning at Division Headquarters. His company was a mobile casualty clearing unit designed to operate at the front line; he had responsibility for a field ambulance and its three-man crew. There was little for them to do until battle began.

He passed the time writing to Irmengard and his mother, reading their letters, or studying from a large trunk filled with medical books he had taken to war.

The correspondence between mother and son remained warm and affectionate. Their concern about each other was intense. He worried over the strain for her of working almost a full day in the shop and running the house with no staff. He urged her to cut down. She promised to do so, and in turn, asked if he still did morning gymnastic exercises. On another occasion she reminded him about nightly devotions and added she prayed constantly for his safe return home.

The letters between Irmengard and Issels had that special quality of two people in love exploring each other's minds with the certainty they would become husband and wife. The entire courtship was now conducted on paper. Clues were dropped with increasing frequency, and both swiftly ran them to ground. Did she want to start a family at once? She did, believing, like him, that parents retained a youthful outlook on life if children were there from the first year of marriage. She loved reading, walking in the countryside and collecting Meissner porcelain. Had he noticed how much they had in common? The same love for good food and wine, an almost identical taste in the arts and sports. Did he know what she had really thought of him at that first meeting in Tegernsee? That he looked like a blond lobster from the sun!

The first letters set a pattern which remained; both found they communicated their inner thoughts more easily on paper. Expressions of love and unabashed sentiment flowed over the pages. He was clearly enthralled by her intellectual soarings, just as she was utterly fascinated with his long descriptions of neural and homoeopathic treatments. He learnt about those parts of her life which he had not known at Tegernsee. The Linder family trace their lineage back to the fourteenth century. Her father had been a High Court judge until 1938, when the Nazis sacked him because he insisted the laws of the land applied equally to the S.S. and S.A. The family moved to Stuttgart shortly afterwards. Irmengard's letters increasingly revealed facets of her character. She had definite ideas about everything—and would not easily relinquish them. Only in the matter of medicine did she acknowledge his supremacy. Yet, while clearly feeling herself the equal of any man, Irmengard had the genius to make her dependence within their relationship very clear to Issels. In the more mundane parts of his letters, he launched into details of his family life until, in the end, Irmengard felt she knew them almost as well as her own parents and three brothers. Yet, whether he consciously knew it or not, Issels revealed little to her of the close relationship he had with his mother; that was something precious between them. In so many ways this was one of the happiest periods in his life.

Then, on a brief visit home, Issels put it all at risk by rekindling an affair that was a hangover from Düsseldorf. The girl was pretty and sensual. But Adelheid Issels warned her son she was unsuitable as a wife. Inexplicably, he pursued the affair in spite of that advice; it was one of those times when his 'other side' exerted undue influence. By early May, 1940, he found himself in a situation familiar to many bachelors—juggling with the emotions of two girls in love with him.

On May 5, 1940, the war finally intruded into his private life. The 10th Panzers received orders to breach the frontiers of Luxembourg, Belgium and Holland—three small countries whose neutrality Hitler had just publicly promised to recognise. Issels vaccinated his company against typhus as laid down in Wehrmacht regulations: each man was jabbed in the left breast. Then Issels injected himself, and the needle pierced a vein. In minutes he broke into a cold sweat, followed by violent trembling. He collapsed on to a field-bed and rocked it across the room in his fever. There was a sudden, blinding pain in his chest, and he woke up in the military hospital at Koblenz. At midnight the hospital was evacuated for fear of a French attack on the town. The patients were put on a hospital train and shunted eastwards to Berlin. Issels had completely recovered when he reached the city—and boarded another express train heading west for the war.

The 10th Panzers were in the vanguard of a great arc of *feldgrau* uniforms and coal-scuttle helmets stretching some 160 miles from the Frisian Islands in the North Sea to the

Maginot Line. The Panzers crossed the Meuse near Sedan at dawn on 15th May. By dusk their bridgehead was twenty miles deep and thirty miles wide. It sealed the fate of France; within the next three days, seven Panzer divisions raced down that bridgehead westwards to within fifty miles of the English Channel, regrouped, and began to pincer out the British Expeditionary Force and the remnants of the Belgian and three French armies. Trapped in a tightening net of German steel, the Allies fell back to Calais and Dunkirk.

Issels finally caught up with his company in Belgium. He learned that shortly after he had been taken to hospital a French plane had bombed the company, destroying his ambulance and killing his crew. Calais was still partially defended by the British when he drove another ambulance into the town. It came under heavy sniper fire, which outraged Issels until he realised the English soldiers mistook him for an ordinary infantryman in his steel helmet and *feldgrau*. He reached the town hall, and found it crammed with Allied soldiers. It was his first glimpse of the enemy and he was impressed by their dignity in defeat:

> An English nurse [he wrote later] came out of the ruins. She was very tall and regal, and she reminded me of photographs of Queen Mary. She had the same look of calm authority. She spoke good German, and told me that in another part of the building were some wounded German officers. With them was an English major, severely wounded. I put him in the ambulance along with the more badly wounded German officers and drove back to the field hospital wishing to God the snipers would look for another target. The Englishman received the same treatment as anybody else.

The days became a blur of emergency operations and amputations. A legend of that time later received wide publicity. It claimed Issels was constantly in conflict with his superior officers because he 'treated *all* wounded soldiers whether British or German and secondly because he refused to amputate unless it was absolutely necessary'. The facts are more prosaic. It was standard Wehrmacht policy to treat all wounded equally at that stage of the war. Issels expressed an opinion that in some cases amputation might be avoided; but he was a very junior doctor and in no real position to argue with superior officers.

After the British evacuation of Dunkirk the Germans prepared for Operation Sea Lion—the invasion of England. For weeks Issels waited on the Normandy coast to load his ambulance on to a boat. But the embarkation order never came. After rattling southwards in July through the vineyards of central France, the 10th Panzers came to a final halt near Paris. It was time for Issels to relax—and to face the problems of his love life.

He believed he still loved Irmengard. But the Düsseldorf girl exercised a *traumfrau* fascination for him. He found himself in a miserable situation which he resolved by writing Irmengard a long letter explaining the whole situation and begging her to understand why he was ending their relationship.

Irmengard was broken-hearted. It was the second cruel blow in a few days: her brother, Kurt, had just been killed on the eastern front. She finally calmed herself to write to Issels:

> I do understand the anguish you must be going through and I was very impressed by the honest way you saw the problem. I remember, as you say, that we had talked about this other woman before, though then you had assured me that the relationship was over. But I will try and understand why you feel it necessary to resume it. I do see all the problems you face; our separation, that we only have our letters and not the personal contact we both know is so important. I can see, and understand, that she is nearer at hand, and I am indeed sorry that I could not be physically near to you. In my mind I have always been with you, and that is why I understand what made you write such a letter. But even though our future plans can now be no more, I feel that we should at least remain friends. We have, as we both know, so many common bonds, and it would be very sad if we broke them for ever. I hope we can remain friends, so that when the war is over we can meet again, and talk about all those things that are

dear to both of us. You will always be welcome here, and you must always remember that. Dear Jupp: what more can I say? It is not easy to let you go, to suddenly find that all your dreams and hopes have gone forever. To say that I still love you is only to open the wound for both of us. So, I will close with the sincere hope that you will find the true happiness you seek.

The letter deeply moved Issels. Yet he felt unable to respond to it. But soon afterwards he ended the affair with the Düsseldorf girl.

After a spell of home leave he was posted to the 78th Sturm Infantry Division with an officer's rank as *truppenarzt*. The winter of 1940 found Issels muffled on the frozen Polish steppes.

But leave was granted, and when he returned home Issels found all the family reunited for the second Christmas of the war. Maria and Margot were married and both their husbands had also managed to get leave. Helmut was in the Wehrmacht, looking very smart in his new uniform. In spite of rationing, Adelheid provided the traditional dinner of *bleu carp* for December 24. It was all too much for Issels. The emptiness of his love life brought on a wave of self-pity and depression. His mother took him aside before dinner and said: 'Go on, go and telephone her.'

Irmengard was stunned by the telephone call. Later she remembered:

So many times in those first months after his letter I had felt sick when the telephone rang. But it was never Jupp. Now, when I thought I was over him, there was his voice. He sounded tired and depressed, but there was a quality about him, a sort of pleading, that I told him to come and see me. He kept on saying, 'there's nobody else I want to talk to except you', and I said, 'it's all right, Jupp, you just come on the first train possible.'

Before going to Stuttgart, Issels tried to lose his pallor with an ultra-violet lamp. But he exposed himself too long to the rays, and arrived in Stuttgart in much the same condition as Irmengard saw him on that July day in Tegernsee

—red faced and peeling. By the time they reached her home, she wondered how her family would react to the man she was once more hopelessly in love with. That Christmas Day of 1940 the Linders found it easy to include Josef Issels in the general spirit of goodwill—though there was one tricky moment when under Judge Linder's skilful questioning Issels revealed his days as a circus clown. There was a definite silence. Issels said smiling: 'It was a very good circus.' Finally Judge Linder nodded, adding for Irmengard's benefit: 'Please don't keep kicking him. He's right. It was a good circus.'

The next three days Irmengard later compressed into:

> Jupp gets on well with Mother and Grandmother. Mother talks to him of her days in the Opera. Mother likes him and I am sure Father does too. But what is so important is that we have found each other again.

There was a flaw in that blissful reflection. It was one Irmengard never discussed with Issels. It would be 1972 before she expressed what she felt, but could not speak about in 1940:

> There was a quality about his love which made me sometimes feel he wanted me to be a second mother for him. I had the feeling he had put me on a pedestal and did not want to take me down—but preferred to love me from afar.

Even in the first heady excitement of renewed romance, Irmengard was uneasy at the way Issels compared her to his mother. That the comparisons were favourable made them no easier for her to accept. She longed to be a *junge frau* in her own right, and not the carbon copy of a formidable *erdenmutter*.

When Irmengard first visited Alter Markt in January, 1941, she was immediately struck by the closeness of mother and son. Yet from the outset Adelheid Issels accepted her—and did her best to put some meaning into the cliché that she was not losing a son but gaining a daughter. It was enough for the older woman that they both shared, in different ways, a real love for the same man. On that basis Irmengard was immediately welcomed into the family by Adelheid Issels.

But she felt her future sisters-in-law were reserved; for her many of their initial questions had an edge to them. Did she realise how lucky she was to marry their brother? Was she aware he was one of the most popular bachelors in the area? Had she yet fully grasped the special social position that went with a doctor's wife? Irmengard answered the questions coolly, believing they came from that old feeling of superiority many Rhinelanders display towards the southern Germans. She made it clear she was no country girl but came from a cultured background able to meet any challenge. Later she decided the questions sprang from a resentment that Josef Issels, a hero for his sisters, was being cosseted by another woman:

> I don't think any woman [Irmengard said later] would have fared otherwise. All the girls looked on Jupp as somebody special. They didn't mind how many girl friends he had. But a woman who wanted to marry him was something different. It would have been hard on any woman he married.

Josef and Irmengard married on May 15, 1941 in Stuttgart. They exchanged gifts of a bracelet and cuff-links. After a five-day honeymoon, Issels returned to the eastern front. A taste of what lay ahead came in the Führer's Order-of-the-Day to Feldmarschall Walther von Brauchitsch:

> The war against Russia will be such that it cannot be contained in a knightly fashion. The struggle is one of ideological and racial differences, and will have to be conducted with unprecedented and unremitting harshness. Russia is not a party to the Hague Convention and therefore has no rights under it.

Next day, June 22, 1941—the anniversary of Napoleon's crossing of the Niemen in his drive on Moscow—the German legions swept across a two-thousand-mile front; *Fall Barbarossa,* the crusade against evil in Nazi minds, was under way. Shocked and ill-equipped, two million Russian troops fell back. They tried to rally at the Korosten fortified line in the Ukraine. But the Germans smashed through the concrete blockade in five weeks. In the north, Ritter von Leeb's Army Group sledge-hammered its way into the suburbs of Leningrad—and became bogged down in a siege that lasted two years. It was an omen. Another came in the centre of the buckling front line. Panzer thrust after panzer thrust was thrown back under the brilliant guidance of red army Marshal Semyon Timoshenko. Moscow was saved, and the winter of 1941 found the 78th Division holding a defensive position west of the capital.

Issels wrote long, daily letters to his bride and received similar ones from Irmengard with gossip about her search for their first home, the problems the war brought on the Home Front—'you can't buy a good candle anywhere'—and of her sheer happiness at being addressed in the local shops as *Frau* Issels. In March, 1942, she found a flat in Mönchen-Gladbach. She filled each of the five rooms with antique furniture, expensive porcelain and oil paintings. The floors were covered with real Persian carpets. It all came from her family.

Issels was overwhelmed nearly to tears when he came home on leave and saw the loving care put into everything.

Irmengard had never been happier. Yet Issels felt an uncertainty within himself. He could not isolate the feeling—or indeed even find a general cause for it. Irmengard noticed his moodiness, tried to laugh him out of it, and found his mood grew blacker. As he left to return to the front she told him: 'We have to get used to each other. We love each other—and that is the most important thing. It overcomes all things.'

The next leave several months later had been eagerly looked forward to in their letters to each other. Yet, within a few days of being together, they found there were awkward pauses in their conversation. Both were troubled by the situation, yet both were incapable of exploring together the cause of their problem. Irmengard tried hard to maintain the pleasant fantasies she had so eagerly written about, and he made an equal effort to turn the promises of his letters into reality. Both failed because they never developed real verbal communication with each other. Yet neither was to blame; the fault lay in a reticence felt increasingly in each other's presence. It was with a feeling of silent thankfulness that the leave ended, and they returned to the relationship they knew and understood—one conducted at a distance by letter.

Irmengard's letters through the summer took on a definite theme: they charted the various stages of her pregnancy. Issels wrote encouragingly of the joy ahead for both of them. On December 21, 1942, their first child, Ruthilde Maria Issels was born. They shortened her name within the family to Uti.

Issels returned from leave to Russia after the fourth Christmas of war convinced Germany would not win; at best there could be a negotiated peace.

On January 10, 1943, Russia launched its great counter-offensive. Ten thousand cannon erupted in one shattering roar. The effect was devastating. At Stalingrad alone, twenty-two German divisions were decimated; of 330,000 men only 80,000 survived the twenty-four days of continued Soviet salvos which turned the city into a scorched lunar landscape. The Germans fell back on all fronts. Hitler proclaimed three days of national mourning. In Mönchen-Gladbach Irmengard nursed baby Uti and shivered as the radio played the *Siegfried* funeral march and the haunting *Ich hatt' einen Kameraden:*

> His hand he tries to reach me,
> As I my charge renew;
> My hand was never given,
> But he will be in heaven,
> My comrade tried and true!

Only the confidence of her mother-in-law sustained Irmengard. Adelheid Issels visited her daughter-in-law daily with the comforting news that the previous night she had dreamt again that Josef was still alive. Then, together the two women prayed for his continued safety. Their devotions were regularly interrupted by the sirens, followed shortly afterwards by the barking of the *Flieger-Abwehr-Kanone,* the flak guns ringing the Ruhr against Allied air attacks. Irmengard clutching baby Uti, and Adelheid prided themselves on reaching a nearby air-raid shelter before the first bomb fell.

Far to the east of that bunker Issels spent his days and nights working under almost continuous Russian attack. He also suffered considerable pain from stones in the kidneys: twice previously in the campaign the pain became so excruciating that he had been hospitalised and medically recommended as being unfit for further active service. On each occasion, Issels believed, the long arm of the S.S. reached out and arranged for him to be sent back to the battle zone. He found himself working almost at the elbow of the infantrymen in the thickest of the fighting. His world became an endless succession of splintered bones, severed blood vessels and torn muscles. There was a savagery about the war in the east which numbed Issels. The wounded were moved in open carts. Those who could not be moved begged to be shot rather than fall into Russian hands. The request was invariably granted—though Issels could not bring himself to end a life. Instead he led a convoy of horse-drawn carts filled with wounded from one battle-field after another. It was a desperate time for all involved. Because of valour under fire Issels was decorated with the Iron Cross First and Second Class and the War Cross Second Class.

In a brief respite Issels found himself in the spring of 1943 attached to a field hospital well behind the battle zone. It was filled with a stench from the appalling effect of powerful explosives on the human body. Many of the wounded were half-frozen by the sub-zero temperature. In the comparative warmth of the hospital the surgical teams waged a fight against massive destruction of human tissue and infection; there were cases of septicaemia, tetanus and gangrene. Issels saw the problems clearly enough:

> It was not just the terrible effects of gun fire [he said later]. There were also serious side effects from open wounds being infected by soil and scraps of clothing. The sheer impact of a high velocity projectile drove earth and cloth deep into a wound. Often, too, a man lay some time where he had fallen before stretcher bearers reached him. By then the extensive damage already done by a shell or

bullet would be further compounded by microbes that found the necrotic tissue an ideal breeding ground.

The German surgeons operated until they almost slept on their feet. But even their speed and skill often came too late. Truck loads of wounded died before they reached the field hospitals. Issels noted his own attitude towards the situation in May, 1943:

> The frequent and increasing losses have blunted any outward expression or display of grief. If you still feel it—you don't show it. There is no place for such emotion here. The dead have become numbers. Thirty on Sunday; 52 on Monday; 45 on Tuesday; 70 on Wednesday. God knows how many by the end of the week. They are not people, or comrades—at least nobody outwardly acknowledges they are. They are bodies, numbers. And it helps to think like that. When the first deaths came it was painful. We knew the men. They were often friends. We shared things with them—a joke, a cigarette, a bit of news from home. But after a hundred deaths, the losses become accepted as inevitable. It is always somebody else's turn. Never yours. That's what keeps you from going mad. They are killed and replaced, and then the whole process is repeated, killed and replaced, killed and replaced. A fearful cycle. But it causes the blunting that is so essential. I know some colleagues who feel positively grateful that this blunting has occurred. It gives them a real sense of relief. War makes no sense to us doctors. We spend all our lives trying to prolong life for worthwhile reasons. In war we just save a man so that he can go back and be killed. It is all so futile.

Through the summer of 1943 Issels retreated in a series of moves reflecting a wider strategic picture of German losses. In North Africa, Rommel's Afrika Korps fell back. Italy was threatened with invasion. On the French side of the Channel, German forces waited anxiously for an Allied armada. But the grimmest fighting was on the eastern front. In Russia nearly 700,000 Germans had died in eight months. The Red Army crossed the Donets and in a savage thrust recaptured Kharkov, and advanced on all fronts. Then, suddenly, came a respite. The Russians lost their impetus as supply lines were over-stretched. On the Dnieper, General Fritz Erich Manstein, the new commander of the Germany Army Group South—a phalanx of thirty-seven panzer divisions, eighteen infantry and two motorised regiments—counter-attacked. Once more Issels found himself advancing into the carnage from 6,000 tanks locked in a battle punctuated with mighty artillery barrages. By July 22, 1943 the Germans had lost 70,000 soldiers killed and 200,000 taken prisoner. It was the death knell of German success in the east. By the end of the year Issels found himself in the middle of a mass retreat from Soviet soil.

He snatched a brief leave home and found Mönchen-Gladbach gripped in the Wagnerian murk hanging like a pall over the entire Fatherland. The Allied air attacks were heavier, cutting a swathe of rubble through a dozen cities on either sides of the Rhine. Issels found all semblence of ordinary life no longer existed: life was something out of a Brecht play, with the Lancaster bombers controlling the length of each act.

One night he and his brother Helmut visited one of the few bars still open in Mönchen-Gladbach. Both wore their officers' uniforms. They found the bar filled with soldiers—who jeered and catcalled at them. The rankers typified the resentment many soldiers felt towards their superiors at the way the war was being conducted. Issels persuaded his brother to avoid further trouble by leaving. Outside they were confronted by another gang of soldiers, bent on violence. Standing back-to-back the brothers fought them off. An air-raid warning sent the assailants scurrying for shelter.

He didn't mention the episode to Irmengard for fear of alarming her further. Life for his wife and daughter was grimmer by the day. Irmengard and Uti eked out their rations with an occasional cupful of bacon fat or a pinch of sugar Adelheid Issels bartered on the black market. Issels was distressed by the obvious signs of strain in his wife that resulted from the nightly bombing raids. He was even more shocked at the physical changes in his mother. Adelheid Issels was wasting away from not having slept a full night for months. She had not eaten properly in that time: she gave most of her rations to the children remaining at home, Charlotte and Reinold. There was the further strain in having Helmut fighting on the Russian front. Already the family had been touched by one death from that battle-field: Irmengard's second brother, Rolf, had died during a recent Soviet attack. It brought the two women closer together: Adelheid looked on Irmengard as a favourite daughter.

The relationship between Josef and Irmengard followed a now familiar pattern of periodic silences broken with small talk. Irmengard put it all down to the war, and there was considerable truth in that deduction. Issels' elation at coming home on leave had steadily been evaporated by what he saw. This was not a war his intellect could easily rationalise, with its nightly air raids and the dawn count of bodies among the ruins that stretched for kilometre after kilometre. The war at the front had been numbing in its savagery. But nothing matched the sheer massiveness of the destruction in Mönchen-Gladbach. This was the war of Goya and not Constable, and the enormity of it all weighed heavily on Issels. Perhaps if Irmengard had left him to his thoughts it would have been better. Instead she chose to offer him numerous examples of how her family down the centuries had coped with other crises—and how she would do the same. She meant it well. The effect was disastrous. She failed to recognise that her husband grew increasingly irritated at what he fancied were pointed references to the aristocratic and long lineage of her family at the expense of his own. For him the parade of five centuries of Linders became too much to take when he could only muster comparatively few generations of honest shopkeepers. Unwilling to bring the matter to the boil, he fell back on morose silences. Other factors also strained the marriage. Issels had never severed his close ties with his family. He saw nothing unusual in spending several hours a day of his leave with his mother and sisters. Irmengard was deeply bothered by such behaviour; she felt it reflected on her ability to provide all the comfort he needed. But she could not bring herself to discuss it openly with her husband. So another barrier remained erect between them that might have been dismantled by open discussion.

Josef Issels returned to the war anxious over their marital situation. He still loved Irmengard and wanted to be a good husband; it was a theme he dwelt on at length to her in his letters. But he did not write about his growing feeling that it was simply not enough to be in love, that a relationship must have a basic compatibility. It depressed him that the chemistry of their marriage lacked such a quality.

In the late spring of 1944 Irmengard salvaged what she could of her antique furniture and porcelain following a particularly heavy raid, locked the apartment door, and took a train south to a small village near Stuttgart where she hoped she and Uti would be safer from the bombing. Her relief at leaving Mönchen-Gladbach was not entirely due to escaping from the flight paths of the R.A.F. bombers. She saw that living in the countryside of south Germany meant that when her husband returned home on future leaves she would not have to share him with his family.

In May, 1944 Issels received a telegram from Charlotte with the news that a direct hit had destroyed 1–4 Alter Markt. The family had all survived and were camped out in the rubble. Another bomb had gutted his surgery in Bismarckstrasse. On the day Charlotte sent that telegram came the news that Helmut had been killed in a Soviet attack. The family bore the tragedy stoically.

But in early June, 1944 Issels received the news he had long dreaded. His mother had suffered a serious heart attack and was in the Maria Hilfe Hospital. He got compassionate leave and rushed home. He found his mother in a bed in the hospital air-raid shelter. It was a dark and depressing place and her cot was regularly rocked by bombs falling nearby. She had developed a chronic infection of the gall-bladder; coupled with the heart attack was a general debility and her doctors did not expect her to recover. The news stunned Issels with the same force as if he himself had been told he must soon die. Professionally he had come to terms with the situation of the fatally ill patient. He had established his own rules, for war and peace, in coping with a person suffering from such an illness. He had developed a necessary armour against tragedy. Now he found it all of little use. Faced with his mother's condition he found himself gripped by other emotions that approaching death often brings—a feeling of anger, of despair, of helplessness and of deep resentment that she, of all persons, should be in such a situation. He refused to accept that a precious life must be lost. His mother begged him to have her moved from the stifling gloom of the bunker. In a matter of hours he accomplished the considerable feat in a crumbling society of having her transferred from Mönchen-Gladbach to a small but well-equipped hospital near Irmengard. Then on June 6, 1944 he travelled east as the first Allied soldiers came ashore on D–Day on the Normandy beaches.

Irmengard spent her days, and most of her nights, seated beside her mother-in-law's bed while a family friend minded Uti. For a while Adelheid Issels rallied. Then in the first week of July she relapsed. Irmengard sent for Hermann Josef Issels and his daughter, Charlotte. A priest was summoned to give the Last Sacraments of the Roman Catholic Church with Penance, Viaticum and Extreme Unction. It was too late. Adelheid Issels died in her sleep shortly after collapsing.

Issels arrived home after the funeral. Nothing before, or since, affected him so greatly as the death of his mother. He questioned the doctor carefully about the cause, and noted that:

> Mother had a latent chronic infection of the teeth that affected the last stages of illness. This infection had spread and so further lowered her resistance. In turn a new, and for her, intolerable, strain was placed on her heart. The cause of her final heart attack could be directly traced back to the focal point of infection, her teeth.

Firmly planted in his mind was an unswerving reaffirmation that when peace came he must intensify his search for the focal points of illness in every patient he treated.

In December, 1944 a doctor confirmed Irmengard's suspicions: she was pregnant again. She had no way of communicating with her husband: the postal system, like much else in Germany, was severely dislocated by saturation bombing.

Issels' regiment, the 278th, retreated through the icy winter of 1944 into Czechoslovakia, pursued by the Red Army. He found himself in the customary position of *Bataillonsarzt*, dodging the bullets as he tended the wounded. Several times he narrowly escaped death. On May 8, 1945 the war in Europe officially ended. But for Josef Issels and his comrades it was a day like any other—spent trudging towards where they hoped the American Army was; they wanted to reach the Americans before the Russians overtook them. The Germans had no wish to endure the rigours of Soviet captivity. But, on May 11, a Red Army unit surrounded them. Issels found himself in a forced march to Prague. Near the city they were interned in a prison camp and subjected to a hard time by partisans with bitter memories of S.S. behaviour. After a couple of weeks Issels was shoved aboard a cattle truck, one of a long train filled with prisoners, and moved to within sight of the ruins of Dresden. The engine was uncoupled. The trucks were surrounded by heavily armed Russian soldiers. For fourteen days and cold nights hundreds of prisoners remained caged with no food and little water. They were allowed out once a day to perform their toilet. At the end of two weeks many showed symptoms of severe malnutrition. There was little Issels could do, apart from making the more seriously ill as comfortable as possible. In June the prison train moved to a huge camp north of Dresden. It held 55,000 German prisoners; Issels found himself one of 150 captured doctors. Many were specialists, and they were all shipped off to Russia. Issels escaped the Soviet net by posing as a physical fitness instructor. But with only a handful of doctors left he found his time fully occupied dealing with his fellow prisoners.

The harsh circumstances of exhaustion, little food and widespread dysentery in the camp were breeding grounds for apathy and depression. Many prisoners gave up the continuous struggle to care for themselves and they died. Over the next months Issels did his best to relieve mass depression with psychotherapy and the effect was demonstrably beneficial. He found that emotional balance directly affected the chances of survival. Depressive symptoms could hasten death. Men died around him because they no longer had the will to live. Issels stimulated a determination to live in others by encouraging them to make light of their hardships and to retain their sense of individuality. He led them in walks around the prison compound, forcing them to always reject not only a feeling of defeat, but also of illness and death.

So steadfast was his belief in his own survival that he made a sketch of what his future surgery would look like: the blueprint showed a complex of eight consulting, treatment and administration rooms. He also had other assets in his make-up that enabled him to look to a future beyond the barbed wire. He believed he had survived so far through a mixture of luck and determination; he saw no reason why those qualities should desert him. He had a sense of humour that was spirited enough to offer another form of salvation. He laughed at situations that others found oppressive. Finally he had his faith which sustained him more than anything else in the incessant struggle against the apathy and disease of camp life. Many years later that period as a prisoner was crystallised by a passage he read which Einstein wrote:

> Strange is our situation here upon earth. Each of us comes for a short visit, not knowing why, yet sometimes seeming to divine a purpose. From the standpoint of daily life, however, there is one thing we do know: that man is here for the sake of other men, for the countless unknown souls with whose fate we are connected by a bond of sympathy. Many times a day I realise how much my own outer and inner life is built upon the labours of my fellow men, both living and dead, and how earnestly I must exert myself in order to give in return as much as I have received and am still receiving.

On August 5, 1945 Josef Issels and fifty other fellow prisoners were freed by the Russians on medical grounds. Issels weighed 120 pounds and still suffered from stones in the kidney. When his sister, Margot, met him at Chemnitz, she was reminded of a walking scarecrow coming towards her.

When he finally arrived home he found Irmengard had given birth to a son, Peter Hans on July 18, 1945. Within weeks the baby developed encephalitis, inflammation of the brain. Shortly afterwards Uti contracted glandular fever. Irmengard camped out between two hospital wards.

Issels was not allowed to stay with his family. He was ordered to Mönchen-Gladbach by the Allied occupiers to help clear the streets of bomb-damage. He worked at that task for weeks; later he cleaned out lavatories, and finally was transferred to the local NAAFI as a tea-boy. Shortly afterwards Irmengard wrote with the news that Peter was dying. Issels obtained special permission to travel south to Stuttgart. He went to the hospital—and found Peter desperately ill. There was nothing the German doctors could do. Issels argued and pleaded that *something* must be available to save the baby's life. In the end a doctor suggested he tried an American medical unit which occupied half of the hospital. He talked his way past armed G.I.s to the desk of an American major. Issels explained he was a doctor and begged for penicillin for his son, believing it would help him. The major looked at him and said: 'Get out of here. We don't give drugs to Germans.' A few days later, on October 28, 1945, Peter Hans died. He was three months old.

Uti recovered from glandular fever. By Christmas, 1945, Issels was allowed by the occupying powers to open up his practice again. On January 2, 1946, he fetched his wife and daughter to begin a new life in Mönchen-Gladbach. He loved his daughter deeply. But the common tragedy he had experienced with Irmengard had brought him no closer to his wife. That much they both recognised.

6

Into the Unknown

THE FIRST MONTHS OF PEACE BROUGHT THE COMFORT OF overwork. There was the thrill of opening a new surgery in Humboldstrasse and equipping it with borrowed instruments. There was the excitement of greeting patients and discovering he had lost nothing of his skill at making positive relationships. Finally, there was the joy of supplementing his considerable knowledge of textbook treatments with other remedies. The influence of Huneke and Ruhmkorff was as strong as ever. But circumstances governed how far he could follow their methods. Dieting was impossible: most of his patients were starving. Medicaments were strictly rationed by the Allied Control Commission, who gave priority to hospitals. Issels scoured the countryside for homoeopathic remedies. He found a cache of leeches, and used them for blood letting: when they had gorged themselves on a patient the worms were stored for further use. He used old-fashioned hot-and-cold water treatments for the aches and pains of the old and infirm. He charged them all modest fees, often asking no more than he had before the war. Money held no real interest for him: anything to spare was spent on replacing his library of books destroyed in the war. Within months every major bookseller in northern Germany knew of his need for nineteenth-century medical volumes. On Sundays he read, applying the same technique he used as a student to memorise whole chapters. He was oblivious to almost everything which did not impinge directly on his work.

Yet it was a period of hardship for his wife and daughter, not made easier for Irmengard by the affluence of her in-laws. For her:

> The situation is impossible. Coffee is the equivalent of RM 500. A packet of cigarettes for Jupp costs 200 marks. A pair of shoes for Uti costs almost as much as a car did before the war. Jupp's family have a new shop selling textiles and linen. Charlotte runs it. She barters her goods on the Black Market for food. By our standards they are well off. They have meat while we often only have dried potatoes and gravy. Jupp does not understand that I have nothing to barter so I can't afford much else. I know he feels if Charlotte and our other friends can do it, why can't I?
>
> I don't blame him. He works at a tremendous pace. He will not, and cannot, barter his medical skills under any circumstances. His sense of ethics is too well developed for that. He has been offered money for abortions, big money. He refused. I agreed with him entirely on this matter. There has been enough killing already in the war.
>
> The war, I am sure now, is really to blame for much of the trouble between us. I see that we don't know each other in so many ways. For instance, he is a person who feels a real need to go off on his own. I find that hard to accept. But he goes. When he comes back, things are better for a while. Then he feels the need to do it again. He has tried to explain about his 'other side', but it is like being on an emotional see-saw. I don't want to be possessive, but I do find it difficult to understand.

Issels saw no harm in his behaviour. The regular escaping to the company of casual friends was a very necessary relaxation from the strain which eternal preoccupation with his work brought. He could not find such relief in his marriage. Returning home in the small hours he plunged afresh into the theories of Spengler, Hollos, Raven and all the other medically qualified practitioners of the unusual whose treatment ideas had failed to attract general attention. Much of what they advocated would have seemed archaic to post-war German doctors excited by the major advances in treatment coming out of America and Britain. Issels never rejected those developments, and whenever possible made use of them. But he felt there was a danger in the indiscriminate use of drugs. For him the constant clamouring for what was 'new' provided no substitute for his tried and trusted homoeopathic remedies. The theories of Carl Spengler particularly attracted him. Before the war he had read and observed something of the effects of *Spenglersan* in his time with Ruhmkorff; he saw the serum brought relief in a variety of chronic illnesses—asthma, rheumatism and bronchitis had all responded to drops of *Spenglersan* either taken orally, or rubbed in the skin. Faced with post-war patients suffering acute symptoms of those illnesses, Issels studied Spengler's work again.

Carl Spengler had been no back-street quack. He had worked under the distinguished German bacteriologist, Robert Koch, before continuing his own research into the cause of tuberculosis. In 1888 he published his theory on 'masked tuberculosis'. From his considerable clinical experience he concluded that residuals of active or latent tuberculosis in man led to a sensitisation of the body cells which he defined as 'masked tuberculosis', that in later life often produced one of the chronic type illnesses. Spengler argued it was not enough to treat the symptoms of those illnesses, but an attack must be made on the 'masked tuberculosis' itself. He claimed *Spenglersan* did that, and offered a respectable number of case histories to support his contention. He was ridiculed by the powerful Swiss sanatoriums offering expensive mountain air as the cure for tuberculosis.

For Issels, Spengler's arguments made sense. He tracked down a supply of the serum in Bonn and began to dispense the ampoules for a wide variety of chronic illnesses. He found the same result whether he rubbed the serum on their skins or trickled it down their throats; by early 1947 he observed: '*Spenglersan* is slow acting. Three to four months needed for an effect to be noticed. Combined with homoeopathic remedies it is very successful in cases of anaemia, rheumatism and other similar complaints.'

His success in some cases is impossible to explain in

terms of accepted medical beliefs: a young girl was cured of unsightly body hair after a three-month course of *Spenglersan*. An older woman suffering from alopecia had her hair restored after four months of treatment with the serum. A child with a history of sleep-walking was treated with *Spenglersan* and after four months slept soundly every night. He documented each successive case in minute detail, and found a common factor in all of them—Spengler's 'masked tuberculosis' had been present in each patient.

By 1947 it was routine for all his patients to have dental X-rays and dead or infected teeth extracted. Those who refused were asked to seek treatment elsewhere: if a dentist baulked at the instructions to extract, Issels demanded he signed a paper 'guaranteeing' the patient's future health. No dentist was willing to sign such an undertaking—so they extracted the teeth. Issel's insistence on such treatment came not only from his reading: he also had become a passionate believer that devitalised teeth were a key focal point of infection in the body since that day his mother's doctor told him her death was linked with a set of infected teeth. Later, chronically infected tonsils were also removed for the same reason. Any focal point of infection was attacked because:

> My experience shows it is essential to approach an illness, especially a chronic one, from the basis that the damaged organ is only a symptom of a number of deeper factors. There is, for instance, clear evidence from my own clinical experience, that the effect of poisons on the body over many years, often over a life-time, causes severe damage. This secondary damage had been clearly defined by Grothe and Rossle (two nineteenth-century exponents of causal treatment). These toxics must be removed by regenerative measures of a general and specific nature until such time as the patient's body has been built up to provide its own resistance. Proper diet is important. The usual foodstuffs of our civilisation must be replaced by biologically adequate foodstuffs adjusted to suit the organ conditions of individual patients. Points of focal infection must be noted and acted upon. Dead teeth must always be removed. So must diseased tonsils. The whole body

must be treated according to the needs of individual cases. Most chronic patients need a ferment substitute to compensate for a loss of efficiency in their digestive system. Tobacco, alcohol, coffee, tea etc.—all such exterior factors must be removed. So, too, whenever, and if at all possible, must long-standing mental stress be helped. While all this is being done the diseased organ itself can be treated with the confidence that the *cause* of the illness is also being properly treated.

Those words were written in January, 1948. They marked the laying of the final foundation stone in the *ganzheit*, or whole body, approach to medicine that Josef Issels henceforth followed.

He had not discovered it over-night. Rather it had been a slow evolvement over a lengthy period of time and many cases. The old man with migraine he treated as a locum in Huneke's surgery before the war; the case of arthritis he prescribed homoeopathic medicine for in Ruhmkorff's practice; the chronically ill men and women he treated with *Spenglersan* before and after the war: all played their part in the development of an unshakable belief he finally reached about how *any* acute and progressive disease should be treated. There was one exception: cancer. As the cause of cancer was unknown, he felt it impossible to apply an effective causal treatment for that specific disease. But for every other chronic disease he passionately believed *ganzheitstherapie* was the answer. He freely acknowledged the help of many others. Men like Spengler and Aschner had rung a bell in his mind for a decade before he fully heard it.

Issels wanted to share the full significance of his discovery with his colleagues. Issels preached the *ganzheit* gospel to the family doctors of Mönchen-Gladbach. They rejected him flatly. For some of his thinking fell little short of medical heresy; even his milder opponents seriously wondered whether Issels suffered from some kind of delayed shock from his war experiences. He was deeply wounded by their reactions. His mother was no longer there to soothe his hurt and confusion. He turned to Irmengard and made a pleasant discovery. She offered him fervent support, and was able increasingly to converse intelligently on the subject of *ganzheit* therapy. She wrote in a Christmas letter to her parents in 1948 that:

> Jupp's colleagues just do not see the positive side of his theories. They cannot grasp why a man with a bad heart needs to have his infected tonsils taken out. Yet it is obvious that the tonsils lower the body's resistance by draining poison into it. Proof of his success is in the fact that Jupp now has one of the largest practices in town. Most of his patients are chronic cases. But under his care many of them show remarkable improvement. Jupp, being the man he is, goes on talking about the success of his methods to his colleagues. I have said to him that it is best if he did not do this; it only makes some of them positively jealous of him. But his patients adore him, and that is all that matters, because Jupp lives for his patients. He never treats them as discards. Instead he takes a very positive attitude to every one who consults him.

That was true enough except in cases of cancer. For those patients he offered little else except sympathy and pain-killers simply because he knew of no other prescription.

All he had observed indicated the disease only responded to surgery and radiotherapy, and then often not very successfully. He dipped anew into the literature and what he read made it clear that no cause had ever been established why cancer afflicted all living things: plants, insects, birds, mammals, humans were all attacked and destroyed by one or another kind of cancer. His books told him that it was an ancient disease: two thousand years before the birth of Christ Indian physicians treated it with an arsenic compound. Hippocrates, borne in 460 B.C., treated the disease by cauterisation; John of Ardeone, born in 1307, and said to have been the first English surgeon, urged his colleagues to avoid treating the disease as it was incurable—and would only damage the reputations of those who tried to treat it. Issels was appalled by the widespread destructive nature of cancer. Percival Pott (1714–1788), a surgeon at St. Bartholomew's Hospital in London had observed and described cancer as an occupational malignancy—he had found it in the scrotums of young chimney sweepers. Thomas Hodgkin (1798–1886), a pathologist at Guy's Hospital, London, characterised the disease as causing 'certain morbid alterations of structure', which later became known as Hodgkin's disease. His suggested treatment sounded highly unorthodox by the standards of the mid-twentieth century: 'It is essential for the utmost protection from the inclemencies and vicissitudes of the weather, to employ iodine externally, and to push the internal use of caustic potash as far as circumstances might render allowable.' The German pathologist, Rudolf Virchow (1821–1902) discovered 'white blood . . . and the body may be regarded as a state in which every cell is a citizen; disease is a civil war, a conflict of citizens brought about by the actions of external forces'. A few years after Virchow died, two Japanese professors at Tokyo University, K. Yamagiwa and K. Ischikawa, induced cancer in rabbits by the persistent application of coal tar. Fifteen years later, Ernest Kennaway and his colleagues at the Royal Cancer Hospital in London produced the first chemical carcinogens—substances capable of inducing cancer—and, for the first time, identified a chemical capable of causing cancer: 3,4–benzyrene; later it was found that this carcinogen was usually present in smoked foods and fish, tobacco smoke and polluted air. Yamagiwa, Ichikawa and Kennaway all made important advances in cancer research with their carefully controlled experiments. But little new followed their pioneering work, and in 1948 the cause of the disease remained as mysterious as it had half a century earlier.

Issels turned away from his reading again convinced that nothing could be done to find an effective treatment until the cause of cancer was known. He had experienced the limitation of surgery, and had seen the all-too-poor effects of irradiation on many cancers. He felt a deep sense of sorrow that there appeared to be nothing available either in the heterodixic world to alleviate cancer suffering. It was one thing to treat a chronic case of asthma when he believed he knew the cause—it was quite another to attack a malignancy of the cellular system that nobody seemed to really understand. Unable to help such cases, he worked all the harder for those patients he felt he could make better.

By 1948 his work load was phenomenal. Patients came from all over West Germany. He regularly worked a twelve hour day, six days a week. On Sundays he studied until the small print swam before his eyes. He failed to see the effect it had on his marriage. By February, 1948 Irmengard was desperately aware that: 'We both need good will to make our marriage work. But Jupp is selfish. Outside his work he is influenced by his family.'

It had been a difficult winter for her. She was pregnant again, and suffered more than the usual bouts of morning sickness and cramps. She tried, and did not succeed, to convince herself that a doctor's wife was the last person who should expect attention from her husband. On April 25, 1948 she gave birth to a healthy boy while her husband was at work. They named him Rolf Dieter Maria Josef.

By the end of the year Issels had a huge, flourishing private practice. Yet it was not a money spinner. His fees remained almost absurdly modest: he charged for a house-call less than other doctors asked for surgery consultations. But he had saved enough to find the deposit for a second-hand car. Irmengard sold a gold bracelet to complete the purchase and the jalopy became a familiar sight bouncing through the streets of Mönchen-Gladbach. Issels once snatched a few days away from his patients to drive the family south to Stuttgart. The car was so noisy they had to shout to make each other heard. After a hundred and fifty miles the motor finally seized-up and they completed the journey by train, laughing their way through the night.

But Issels found less and less time for such personal happiness. He was on a treadmill, driven harder and harder by the demands of his patients. Suddenly, in May, he collapsed at home: by the time the ambulance Irmengard called reached hospital he was unconscious. He awoke three days later to find he was being treated for an acute virus infection probably caused by physical and mental exhaustion. But the role of quiescent invalid was one he refused to play. Within a week he dragged himself back to work, ignoring the emphatic warnings of the hospital doctors.

Irmengard was concerned not only at her husband's apparent disregard for his own health, but also by the criticism increasingly levelled at his treatment methods. She finally wrote to her parents: 'His illness gave some of his colleagues the chance to say "physician heal thyself". Their jealousy is something awful. Jupp is so proud of what he does and tells everybody . . .'

Judge Linder replied to his daughter in a letter which was remarkably perceptive:

> We all believe in him. But it will take a long time to convince people that *ganzheit* therapy is the solution for all illnesses. Helping his own patients will not be taken as proof in scientific terms. I know that Jupp is not especially concerned with that sort of proof because that's the nature of his temperament, and I, for one, would not dampen his enthusiasm, but he must be prepared for criticism from those who like to see everything properly tabulated.

It was sensible advice. Irmengard did not pass it on because she feared her husband would take it as an attack on his methods. It was also doubtful if Issels would have heeded such guidance. His mind once more was filled with the problem of cancer patients. In July, 1948 he found:

> I have no real way of treating the disease. And that is what is so terrible. A husband came to me and pleaded for help for his wife, who had a huge tumour on the uterus. I said I could do nothing. But he pleaded and pleaded. I saw the wife. All I could think of doing was to change her diet and prescribe pain killers. She said: 'If you treat me. I know there is still hope. You see, all the other doctors gave me up.'

He had never before considered the role psychotherapy played in a fatal illness. He now viewed the problem in the wider context of making a relationship with the dying. He saw the beneficial effect of allowing the woman to feel she was still capable of receiving some treatment—however unorthodox. He knew that the diet changes he prescribed could not possibly alter the course of the disease. But the psychological benefit was marked. After fourteen days the woman insisted her pain had totally gone. Issels could not believe it. But he continued to see her, and his very presence seemingly helped sustain her. But two months later she relapsed and died.

By then Issels was managing other cancer patients, trying to ease their pain and improve their general resistance. He saw some effect. But in each case the patient died. Depressing though this was, he felt a glimmer of hope. Once more he returned to his books, and travelled a path others had done, to come to the science of immunology. He began to grow excited at the possibilities of immunotherapy, the treatment of disease by immunological methods, developed by an Englishman, Edward Jenner (1749–1823). He pioneered successful vaccination for a number of diseases previously fatal. Jenner had, of course, found no answer to cancer, but down the years a hypothesis gained favour that the natural immunological defences of the body did respond against cancerous cells; only when the body defences were overran did the disease rampage to its deadly conclusions. The answer clearly was to find an effective immunotherapy agent to reinforce the ailing natural defences. Over the years several vaccines had been tried. Nobody knew exactly how they worked—just as no one knew precisely how smallpox vaccine worked. The more Issels read the more he became convinced that immunotherapy might stimulate anti-bodies to deal with the cancer cells. He found a vaccine, Neo-blastine, made from the tissues of untreated primary and secondary cancer tumours which contained large amounts of a virus-like particle.

With a certain amount of hesitation—for the world of immunology still baffled him—Issels gave a patient with lung cancer a subcutaneous injection of the vaccine. At the same time he treated the man with the full *ganzheit* regime; he removed infected teeth and tonsils; prescribed a diet and generally built up the body's resistance. The patient lived three months longer than Issels had expected.

He now read all he could find on immunology. It was a characteristic approach to a problem as he digested books, scientific magazines and papers at a steady pace.

At the same time he ran an ever expanding practice. His working day lengthened to fifteen and sixteen hours, six days a week. He also found the time to open the town's first sauna bath. He had virtually emptied his modest bank account to do so, and, against Irmengard's advice, borrowed money for the venture. It failed, and Issels found himself with DM 15,000 of debts. He worked even harder. At home, when he was there, Irmengard found him tetchy and restless. He was showing all the signs of strain he so quickly observed in others.

On Christmas Eve, 1949 he collapsed. For two days Irmengard let him sleep, believing that was the best possible treatment for exhaustion. On the third day, unable to wake him, she sent for a doctor. He diagnosed meningitis. For eight days Issels was close to death in Mönchen-Gladbach's Protestant Hospital. He was delirious for long spells. When his mind cleared he found a hospital doctor by his bedside. What followed became a traumatic experience for Josef Issels:

> The doctor's questions puzzled me: 'What day is it?' 'How many days in a week?' 'What is the name of your mother?' 'The names of your children?' I looked at him with growing horror. I realised he thought I was going mad. On my answers depended, I felt sure, whether I would be committed to a mental hospital. I felt desperately low. My own mind asked one question: how had I come to this stage? How, how, how? Then something came over me. Some inner force said that the only way to break this terrifying situation was to deliberately stage a diversion. Anything was better than those quiet, calm, idiotic questions that might just drive me mad in the end. I screamed and shook and screamed. The doctor went away. When he came back I was calm. But I knew I could not stay another moment longer than necessary in that hospital. When I was alone again I walked out in my pyjamas and took a taxi home, and went to bed. I thought they would come and fetch me. But nobody came—and if I had been mad I have no doubt they would have fetched me. I lay in my bed for days, reading my books. I memorised whole passages. Then one day an image

appeared over my bed. I couldn't move, but just lay there, almost transfixed by it. What was incredible was that the image was of me in a previous life.

I was dressed in the period of the Middle Ages. I watched myself walking down a street in the Holland of 400 years ago. My name was Jan. People called out to me. Every detail was startlingly clear. It was like watching a film—only the focus was sharper. I came to a wine cellar. A girl, pretty enough, asked me where her red leather boots were. I went out in a small boat to a bigger vessel anchored in the town's harbour, climbed on board and returned to the wine shop with the boots. The moment I handed them over the whole scene dissolved . . . and I was back in my bedroom. I felt sure I was going mad. Later the whole thing was exactly repeated. I became aware of other phenomena. I could hear people clearly talking four floors below; it seemed to be like the acute hearing animals have. I could smell like I had never smelled before. Some people had a bad aroma that I detected in the way a dog detects a smell humans cannot.

The whole experience was quite terrifying. I knew now that I was not mad—yet if I told anybody they would think that I was. I could not go on like this. I searched my mind for a possible solution. I knew nothing in orthodox medicine that could assist. Then I recalled Huneke once talked about successfully treating with neural therapy a disturbance of what he called the 'neurological field'. I persuaded a doctor to give me an injection in a spot I selected in the back of my neck. The moment I received the injection, my acute sense of smell and hearing left me. Soon afterwards I recovered fully—but I found my powers of listening and observation had been sharpened. I found I could make even better contact with my patients. I had been a patient and could see things as they did. I could look them in the eye and knew I would always tell them the truth—just as I had wanted no lies during my illness.

A psychiatrist could possibly interpret that experience in several ways. Issels in fact did consult one psychiatrist when he had recovered. The specialist took a careful history and pronounced it such a rare case that he proposed to write it up for a medical journal. Perhaps that was the most fitting ending to a strange episode.

Issels returned to work eager to broaden his knowledge about immunotherapy as a treatment for cancer. He found a vaccine called Toxinal, tried it on a patient, and saw it gave modest success. One Sunday he drove to Kreuznach, a small Rhineland town, to attend a conference of doctors who had gathered to exchange experiences with Toxinal.

> A whole new world opened up for me [he said later]. Those doctors had used the vaccine widely; more important, they had a considerable knowledge of the problems of not only treating cancer with the vaccine, but also of the nature of cancer itself. I realised how little I knew. There were forty years of papers alone on the degeneration of the coli to read up. . .

In spite of all his reading and his enthusiasm the result was always the same: the patients died. And after he treated some sixty such cases he became uncomfortably aware of the accusations levelled at him by other doctors in Mönchen-Gladbach. They said he could not possibly succeed with such treatment because the only palliative after surgery and radiotherapy were measured doses of morphine to deaden the pain. More than one doctor added that Issels was in it for the money.

Issels shrugged aside the accusations. Cancer patients were often treated free. He had more pressing things to think about than slanderous accusations of charlatanism. A pattern was clear in nearly all the cancer cases he had tried to help. Patients showed symptoms of a general chronic illness; they responded positively to *ganzheit* treatment. Therefore, cancer was in principle no different from any other chronic disease. The conclusion was stunning in its simplicity; its potential staggering. Every textbook taught that cancer was a local disease, that while a patient may have, for example, cancer of the stomach, his whole body remained healthy until the terminal stage, when the disease had spread beyond the control of surgery and irradiation.

With mounting excitement Issels examined cancer from the stand-point of any other chronic disease. Certain factors, he wrote, became immediately clear:

> The tumour is merely a late stage symptom, accidentally triggered off, but able to exist and grow only in a bed already prepared for it. The 'tumour milieu' is the result of secondary damage to organs and organ-systems. This affects functional, regulative and humoral balance between organs and organ systems with severe impairment of the system for the disposing of the lysed cells. Secondary damage is sustained by causal factors of endogenous and exogenous origin. Causal factors, as in all chronic diseases, may be found pre- and post-natally.

It was an original piece of thinking that encapsulated an entirely new attitude for the management of cancer. Implicit in that theory was a belief that a healthy body could not develop the disease: therefore, it was essential that the entire metabolism of the body must be treated; like other chronic illnesses, cancer might be dormant in anybody, activated only when the metabolism was lowered to a point where the defence mechanism was no longer capable by itself of destroying cancerous cells. Accepting that cancer was a *whole body* disease, Issels saw clearly why conventional treatment was limited. In the majority of cases it offered only a temporary stop; the cancer often returned later in the form of secondary tumours. He now believed that removing the local symptom, the tumour, did not eliminate the threat to the patient: it was still impossible for the body to develop sufficient resistance that ensured freedom from further cancer. He did not reject conventional treatment: he knew that sometimes surgery produced a bio-chemical change in the body which allowed the defence mechanism to produce enough antibodies to combat the danger from further cancer. But he now firmly believed conventional treatment did no more than keep a patient on a razor's edge of survival. He was convinced there was room for another approach—*ganzheitstherapie*, his method.

Issels became increasingly aware of the limitations imposed by a busy family practice in treating cancer patients. Cases were scattered far and wide. He felt there would be definite psychological advantages in bringing them together: they would not be alone with the burden of their illness; he could concentrate on what he believed was essential group psychotherapy; and carry out intensive *ganzheit* treatment while at the same time attacking the specific cancer itself.

To achieve all that meant opening his own clinic. He began to search for suitable premises. In the spring of 1950 he finally found what he wanted. In the Mönchen-Gladbach suburb of Hehn was the *Krankenhaus St. Maria*, a small, run-down cottage-style hospital with almost empty wards. The hospital administration eagerly accepted his offer to take over a ward of thirty beds for chronic cases, including cancer. Nursing assistance and a small examination room went with the ward.

He moved his patients into the hospital, and drove himself several times to the edge of a new collapse. He awoke at 6 a.m. and went to the hospital. By 8.30 a.m. he was in his surgery. For the next four hours he handled a stream of cases. From 12.30 p.m. to 4.30 p.m. he carried out housecalls over twenty square miles. At 5 p.m. he began evening surgery. Around 8 p.m. he showed out the last patient and returned to the hospital to continue treating his chronic patients. By about 11 p.m. he was ready for bed. A succession of such seventeen hour days found him passing the nights on the couch in the examination room.

At home Irmengard fretted. Money was still scarce for all but the essentials of life. She found it difficult to match her husband's enthusiasm for his work.

In the following months Issels treated a growing number of cancer cases. Many came to the hospital with the prognosis that no further treatment was possible. Issels treated them with a combination of ethical and unorthodox remedies. Standard drugs were used to purify the blood, revitalise the liver, kidneys, indeed every organ in the body. Other preparations were given to remove unhealthy bacili in the intestines. Complementing that treatment were special diets of yoghurt, organically grown vegetables and milk-sugar to provide a base for healthy bacili to develop.

The mucous-membranes were treated, and fermentation substitutes given to improve the digestive process. Reinforcing the battery of physical treatment was psychotherapy. Patients were encouraged to come to terms with their illness; they were told the nature of their cancer because Issels had come to believe it was fundamental for their survival that they knew the truth. He saw his role there as:

> To instil a will to live. This can only be done if the patient knows the clinical picture and is prepared to fight with me. It is a two-handed partnership, building this bridge between doctor and patient over which the treatment regime crosses.

He relied on well-tried homoeopathic solutions, such as Homoeopathic Ref. D8, to encourage cellular regeneration, indirectly producing anti-bodies to strengthen the general resistance of the body to fight cancer. The entire discharge system—kidneys, intestines and the skin—were treated to meet the toxic effects of the tumour. Patients drank pints of water and herb tea to irrigate their kidneys. They received mild purgatives to irrigate their colons. At the same time he attacked their cancers with immunological preparations. He saw that it worked, that many patients were given a valuable extension of life. It encouraged him to plunge deeper into the field of cancer treatment.

In October, 1950 he was asked to visit a cancer patient who had been sent home to die from St. Josef's Hospital, Krefeld, a town near Mönchen-Gladbach. Her doctor, and husband's pleading, persuaded Issels to travel fifteen miles to see Käthe Gerlach, a journey he could ill afford because of the pressure of time. He found a forty-one-year-old woman in a terminal state. She was expected to die any day. She looked at Issels and said: 'Doctor, if anybody can help me you will.' Issels made no reply; he had never seen such a bad case. She had a massive tumour in the uterus that had forced its way out through the vagina. Oedems in both legs immobilised her. Her medical history was one of progressive chronic illness; she had suffered excessive menstrual disturbance and constipation. In 1949 she contracted typhus. After three months in hospital a surgeon found a cancer in the uterus. His biopsy showed it was malignant and inoperable. Over the next few months she received radiotherapy. In March, 1950 that treatment was stopped because of her worsening heart condition. Throughout the summer she lingered on in St. Josef's Hospital. In September, 1950 she developed secondary tumours. Her physician, Dr. Lothar Ley, a gynaecologist with considerable experience in cancer cases, wrote on her case file that she was 'incurable'.

There was a quality of quiet courage and faith about Käthe Gerlach which touched Issels. He agreed to treat her—even though it meant a two-hour journey each day.

On October 9, 1950 he wrote in her case file: 'Treatment begins to try and improve what seems an impossible situation.' By October 20, he observed: 'definite signs of improvement in the whole body. She goes to the toilet. Her pain is considerably less.' November 1, showed a further 'good reaction. The oedema is reducing. But the tumour is still very large.' After that visit Issels learnt that the family could not afford to pay him. He said he would treat her for nothing. On November 7, she had progressed enough to be moved into hospital. Unable to afford an ambulance Issels drove Käthe Gerlach to Hehn in his car. In hospital she was subjected to the full force of his combined treatments. The improvement was startling: her blood circulation improved; she perspired for the first time in years; the swelling in her legs reduced; pieces of tumour were passed out through the vagina. Within a week she could walk. On November 25, Issels wrote in her case notes: 'Tumour in the abdomen definitely regressed. On the left-hand side it is quite small.' A month later he observed: 'impossible to feel tumour on the left-hand side. Her whole body has increased its resistance.' Two months later Käthe Gerlach was discharged as having no further detectable cancer in her body. On March 28, 1951, Dr. Ley examined her carefully at St. Josef's Hospital. Afterwards he wrote to Issels:

> From my examination there is no detectable cancer in the patient. I hope I can help you with this finding. You

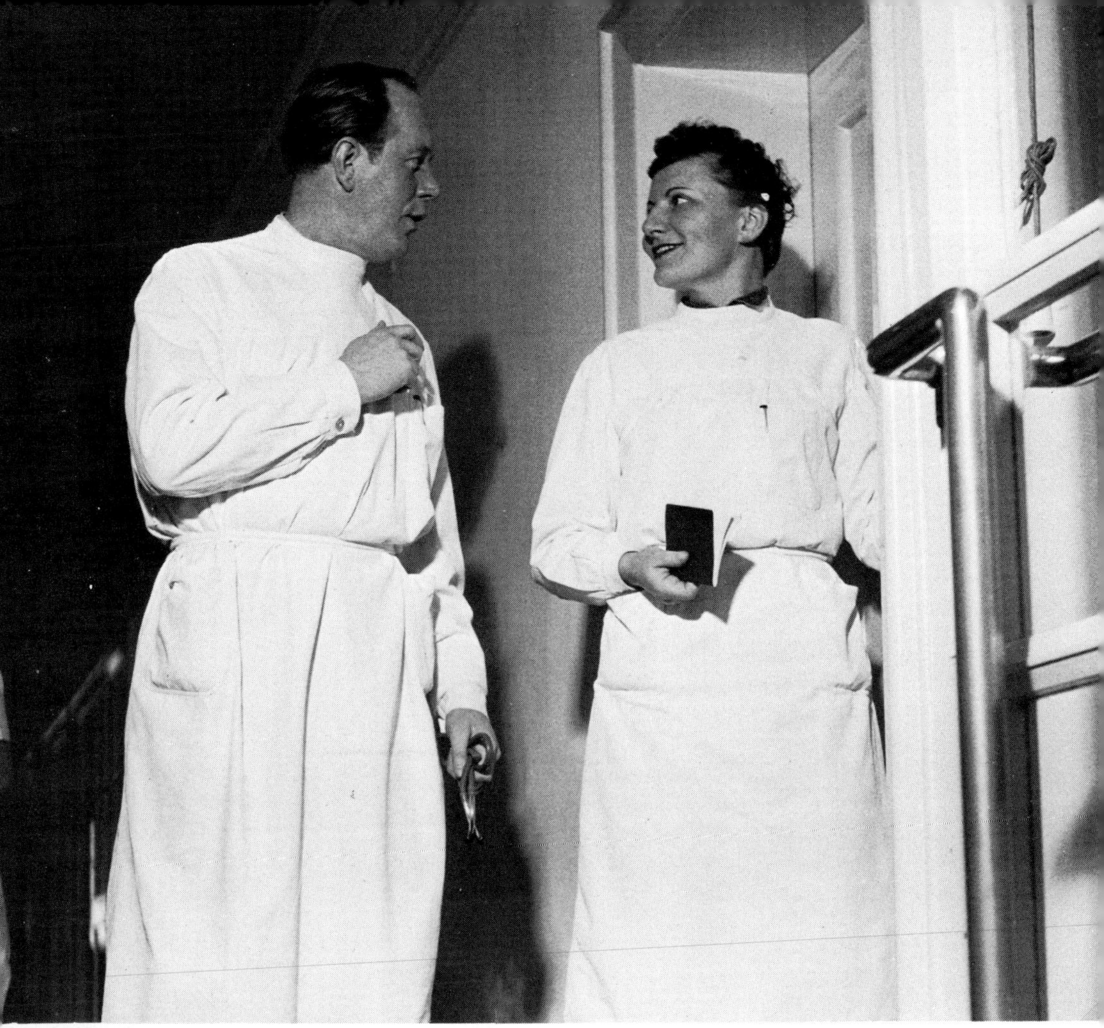

Issels and Irmengard, 1953

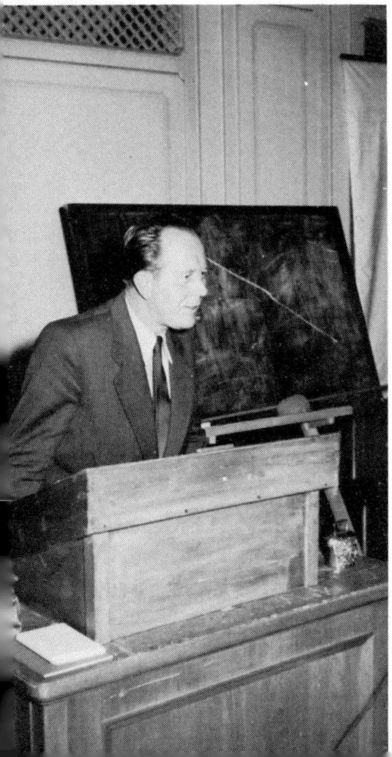

Issels addresses a cancer congress at Berchtesgaden

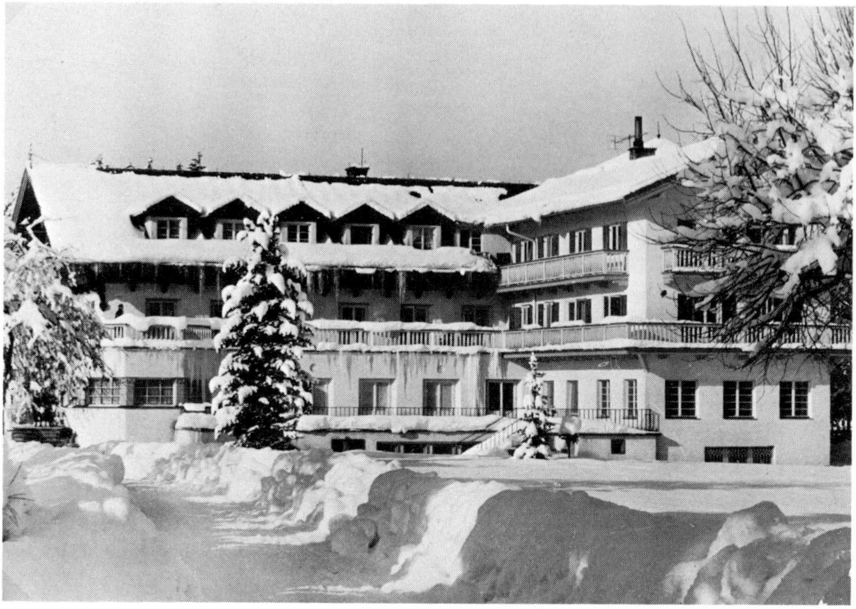

Main house in winter, 1972

Patient's bedroom

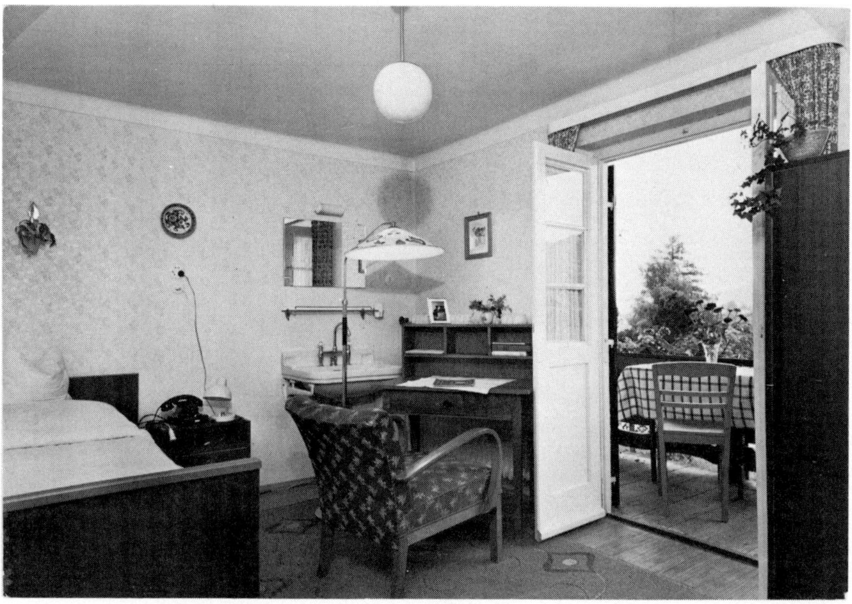

> cannot take this case to judge a treatment because she had previously had many other treatments. But I would be happy to send you untreated cancer patients, and I would be even happier if you would cure them. I am not opposed to your methods, because my opinion is that our orthodox cancer treatment is limited.

Issels was elated enough to write a footnote to Ley's letter:

> I am now totally and fully convinced that I was right to treat cancer as I do. It is a logical progression of everything I have learnt in the last fifteen years about chronic disease. Cancer is just one more chronic disease.

Issels' reputation for offering positive treatment, however unorthodox, resulted in growing hostility among many of his colleagues. For every physician like Dr. Lothar Key there were many more who condemned him as little more than a fraud. When he moved his family into a new apartment, a modest enough place, there was gossip that he had exploited the dying to better his own style of living. Issels ignored the rumours. But Irmengard found them hurtful. She wrote to her parents in March, 1951:

> Our social life in so-called accepted medical circles is almost non-existent. Colleagues ignore us because of Jupp's beliefs. But Jupp in any case has no time for such a thing as a normal social life. His whole life is his work . . .

Though she did not write it, Irmengard felt a premonition that the situation would worsen; she accepted that premise in the same spirit she conceded their marriage was now little more than a shell.

On May 6, 1951 Issels journeyed to Holland to see yet another cancer patient, though Karl Gischler was by far the most important man who had consulted him. He was a director of the Phillip Van Ommeren Shipping Line.

Issels found that Gischler was a classic case of the effect of hormones in conventional management of cancer: he had developed breasts as a result of hormone treatment for cancer of the prostate gland. The course had lasted six years; at the end of that time the cancer had metastasised into the pelvic bones and the whole spine; a side effect had paralysed his right leg, leaving Gischler permanently bed-ridden. In early 1951 he saw specialists from America and England. They told him the cancer was progressive and there was nothing more to be done. But Gischler's wife refused to admit defeat. On the day Issels arrived, an English consultant and an American professor had been flown in to examine her husband; the consultant suggested a course of radiotherapy, the professor urged further hormone treatment.

'And what do you suggest?' Gischler asked Issels.

Issels outlined his combined treatment, explained that it was still new, but that it was at least a positive alternative to what had been hitherto offered. Gischler asked for time to consider what he had heard. Three hours later he told Issels that he was ready to travel to Germany.

He was admitted to a private room in the *Krankenhaus St. Maria* on May 18, 1951. Issels was impressed by Gischler's dignity in the face of grave illness. The fifty-six-year-old shipping magnate was in constant pain yet bore it stoically. After a month there was only slight improvement in his condition. Gischler began to question Issels carefully about his expectations for such a regime in the general treatment of cancer. Issels talked frankly about his theories and beliefs, going into more detail than he had ever done previously with a patient. The two men became involved in a dialogue which ranged far beyond immediate treatment. Issels encouraged such talks in the belief they removed still further the taboos that made cancer an unmentionable word in the usual relationship between a doctor and a fatally ill patient.

For some time Issels had realised there were sound reasons for open discussion in the area of chronic illness that could end in death. He saw that patients felt a sense of relief when they could question or discuss their situation; many said that they had felt cruelly isolated from the reality of their cases by almost a conspiracy of silence among their previous doctors. Issels never concealed from patients that they were mortally ill: he believed there was a spiritual need for the truth, above all else, at such a stage. But he did not speak to them of death, or indicate there was no hope of recovery. Rather he maintained a genuine level of communication, recognising that even if he had no doubt about the eventual outcome, it was also impossible for him to foretell accurately the time of death unless it was very close.

Gischler's questions took on a new and definite slant by June, 1951. Was Issels aware of the opposition he faced within the hospital? Did he know that even his own nurses had little faith in his methods? Was he aware of a growing lobby among the other doctors to remove him from the hospital? Issels was discomfited by such questions, for he knew too well the resentment he generated. One day Gischler said: 'Doctor, the only solution is for you to find your own clinic.' Issels took it at its face value of no more than an encouraging gesture by an appreciative patient. Any question of opening a full-scale clinic was well beyond his financial means.

Early in June the opposition within the hospital hardened to the point where Issels received a formal letter from the administration. It forbade him to admit, or treat in the hospital, any more cancer patients. Issels was shocked.

Then, on July 1, 1951, another incident occurred which settled the future of Josef Issels. Twenty years later it was still fresh in his mind:

> I found Gischler crying in his bed. He was in considerable pain. But it was not just from his tumour. A nurse had slapped him in the face because she felt he was too troublesome. I was shattered that such a thing could have happened. All Gischler said was: 'Now doctor you *must* find a place where you can hand-pick your own staff. What will a new clinic cost?' I was still seething at what had happened to him that I answered almost automatically, not giving any real thought: 'I don't know—maybe DM 150,000.' 'Then you will have the money!' The magnitude of what he had said did not penetrate at first. He repeated his offer: he would provide the money.

When Issels finally accepted that Gischler was in earnest he began to search at once for suitable premises. There was nothing in Mönchen-Gladbach. Besides, he had no further desire to practise a day longer than was necessary among colleagues he felt were bent on professionally destroying him. After a month he had found nothing in northern Germany that could be converted into the clinic of his dreams.

He travelled with Irmengard through the night to inspect one property after another, and then drove back to perform a full day's work. By the end of July, Issels was very tired. On the last Sunday of the month he and Irmengard drove six hundred miles to the Tegernsee valley where they had first met. Friends had told them of a small hotel overlooking the lake that was for rent. But it had been designed by an architect who, for some reason, had not included a kitchen in his original plans. Issels left Irmengard behind to rest and drove back to Mönchen-Gladbach convinced he would never find a place.

Next morning his wife telephoned with the news she had discovered a run-down hotel for rent on the Tegernsee at Rottach-Egern. It was called the Ringberg Hotel. Then, all they had to do, said Issels, was to change one word—and rename it the Ringberg-Klinik.

7

Chefarzt

Issels immediately saw the hotel's potential: it could fairly easily be converted into a clinic with two wards and various treatment rooms. The hotel was built in the pleasing style of Bavarian architecture and stood in spacious grounds bordering the Tegernsee and a protecting circle of mountains, including the Wallberg alp. The therapeutic value of such surroundings for seriously ill patients would be considerable. He agreed to rent the property for DM 1700 a month, with DM 15,000 deposited in advance. The vendor's lawyer insisted the money was to be paid over on the stroke of midnight on September 14, 1951, the moment Issels' lease began.

He drove Irmengard home, and the journey quickly passed in discussing plans for the clinic. But by the time they reached Mönchen-Gladbach, Irmengard's enthusiasm cooled when she realised she had to give up a comfortable home, and leave the children behind, for a small bedroom in the clinic. It was typical of Issels that his schemes included only the minimum personal comfort: all his designs concentrated on the welfare of his patients. Nine, including Karl Gischler, agreed to follow their doctor into the medical wilderness.

The exodus south was planned stealthily. Issels could not bring himself to say good-bye to his practice patients; he keenly felt the wrench of parting from many who had become friends. He told them he was taking a holiday. He searched for a suitable successor and found a young physician interested in homoeopathic medicine, and gave him the entire practice for nothing; it simply never occurred to Issels to negotiate a proper price for the good-will. It was enough for him that the doctor promised to carry on the same regime of treatment.

Handing over the practice finally convinced his family he was determined to pursue an idea they still thought dangerously foolish. It was one of the few times that Irmengard found herself in agreement with Issels' sisters, Margot and Charlotte.

By September 13, Issels had effectively ended his professional connection with Mönchen-Gladbach. His car was loaded with everything he needed to begin immediate treatment at Rottach-Egern. A hospital train coach had been hired to take the patients and two nurses southwards. Irmengard and Margot, who had accepted her brother's last-minute offer to handle the administrative side of the clinic, would also travel in the coach. Issels made a last call—to say good-bye to one of the few members of the local medical fraternity who still spoke to him. The doctor begged Issels to turn back even at that late stage. His words stayed with Issels for a long time: 'You are heading for professional death unless you stop your cancer treatment.' Issels was moved by the man's genuine concern. But he felt a greater force guiding him. In his private diary he wrote on his last night in Mönchen-Gladbach:

> For the first time I feel free from the inhibitions and hinderances of orthodox thinking. At Rottach, with the help of God, I plan to devote myself to my belief that another way is necessary in addition to knife and radiation. I am not the first to say it; I doubt whether I will be the last.

He arrived in Rottach-Egern late in the afternoon to find the hotel carrying on business as usual. The bar was filled with guests. Waiters hurried between the kitchen and dining room. Nobody seemed to know of the impending changeover. Nonplussed, Issels retired to his room on the second floor. Shortly before midnight the vendor's lawyer arrived. Issels handed over the money. The contract he signed made over to him everything in the building: at the stroke of midnight he acquired a respectable wine cellar, a pantry filled with delicacies, a French chef, a staff of waiters, barmen, scullery and chambermaids, a housekeeper and a porter. Issels asked what he could do about the guests. The lawyer shrugged as he disappeared into the night clutching a briefcase stuffed with money. The guests, like the staff, were now Issels' responsibility.

Issels decided to ponder the problem over dinner. He ordered well; as the new owner he felt he could afford a bottle of champagne. After dinner he retired to his room, no closer to a situation, and fell asleep. He was awakened in the early hours by the headwaiter asking him to pay for dinner. Dumbfounded, Issels explained he was the new owner. The waiter was adamant: he knew nothing of a change of ownership—all he was concerned about was balancing his books. Issels paid, wondering what next to expect.

Next morning the unreality of the situation persisted. Guests and staff paid no more than passing interest as hospital cots were moved into the building. They looked surprised when 'No Smoking' notices were posted everywhere by Issels. Only when the convoy of ambulances drew up did realisation come. They gaped at the procession of stretcher patients being carried upstairs.

'Who are these people?' one guest demanded irritably.

'Cancer patients,' replied Issels.

The man paled and promptly checked out. It took several more days for the other guests to finally leave. By then the bar was closed and the French chef had been introduced to the mysteries of diet menus. He found it too great a strain preparing grated carrots, plain salads and yoghurt desserts. He resigned. Before leaving he asked one favour: could he be allowed to cook a farewell dinner for Issels and the staff? It was a magnificent banquet that helped deplete wine-cellar and pantry.

Everybody had a favourite story of that period. Irmengard remembered a waiter answering a call for room service to find a patient wanted a bed-pan. Margot found herself making beds. Issels supervised the conversion of the wine cellar into a pharmacy. New problems arose constantly.

Local shopkeepers called and asked for prompt payment of old bills. Issels explained in vain that they were not his responsibility. With essential supplies threatened he paid up. One afternoon two men arrived to repossess the furniture; the previous owner had not maintained the hire-purchase payments. Issels paid. It was the same with the bills for lighting and heating. They had accumulated, and Issels, the *ausländer* in a clannish Bavarian community, found himself doling out hefty sums of money. But there were compensations: there was something of the artist's enthusiasm about the way he planned colour schemes for the clinic; he had a newly discovered enthusiasm for pastel shades and soft fabrics. An old note-book has survived to give a glimpse of how he involved himself in everything.

> Gischler consulted about laboratory. Says to go ahead. The money will be found . . . treatment cards very important. Must have plenty. Staff and patients must see them as mirrors showing prognosis of cases. Must instil that now . . . Architect says thirty-two beds possible. Plus X-ray and small operating room. Rooms must be bright . . . Long talk with Gischler. He said to me: 'Doctor, this is only the beginning.' Very heartened by his positive support. But he does not know all the problems. Margot wonders if we will fill all the beds. Even at DM 800 a patient a month inclusive she says there will be nothing to spare. I said to her we will manage . . . must have a lift . . . spoke to the Lipps. Very happy they will stay on.

Georg and Anneliese Lipp had been the hotel's porter and housekeeper. Their considerable knowledge proved a God-send in the transition period and afterwards; they would finally become the longest serving members of the clinic staff.

Within a week the clinic was firmly established. It had been granted a licence by the local Bavarian government. Issels followed a German custom and placed a small advertisement in a local newspaper announcing that the Ringberg Klinik was 'a special clinic for treating incurable cancer patients'. He attended a local medical association meeting, and found the advertisement scorned. One doctor after another said it was impossible to offer treatment for such cases. Issels defended himself; his words fell on deaf ears.

Late in the afternoon of September 21, an ambulance arrived at the clinic bringing the first new patient. Margot and Irmengard watched the ambulancemen carry in a wasted body which made them both realise, for the first time, the full horror of cancer in the terminal stage. The patients who had come from Mönchen-Gladbach were in a relatively good physical state. The newcomer, Lydia Bacher, had been ravaged to the point of death by a massive, inoperable brain tumour. The sense of shock at her condition was also shared by the clinic's nurse. She went to Issels and said: 'I cannot touch her. This is a death house.'

'I know how you feel,' he said. 'But it's our job to help such people. Besides, cancer is not a contagious disease.'

Together they went to Mrs. Bacher's room. Her husband explained he had brought her from northern Germany after hearing about the clinic. Issels examined the woman. He noted she was bald from repeated courses of radiotherapy. She was blind, deaf and dumb as a direct result of the rapidly growing tumour. She was also totally paralysed in both legs and the right arm. Her bladder and rectum no longer functioned. Mrs. Bacher lay in the posture of a spastic.

The case notes which her husband had brought from her last hospital confirmed a classic clinical picture of cancer of the brain. The original diagnosis had been made by Professor David Bodechtel, professor of physical medicine at the Academy of Medicine in Düsseldorf, where Issels had studied. Bodechtel had a deserved reputation as a physician; he saw the tumour was inoperable. He referred her for radiotherapy at the Ferdinand-Sauerbruch Hospital at Wuppertal. She received several courses of irradiation; each time the tumour was temporarily arrested, only to grow again. Finally, in August, 1951 Mrs. Bacher was assessed by the hospital's radiotherapist as 'not responsive to further therapy'. Consultant physician, Professor Adolf Reimers, confirmed no further treatment would help. He recommended pain-killing drugs—to be given at home. On

September 3, 1951 Mrs. Bacher was discharged in the condition she arrived at the Ringberg Klinik.

Issels began immediate treatment to improve her natural functions and at the same time treated her tumour with daily injections of the immunotherapy drug, Toxinal. Her case-notes recorded what happened:

> September 21: 'Treatment begins in typical form.' October 1: 'Patient is able to urinate. Rectum is clear.' October 10: 'Patient is a little fresher.' October 20: 'Her speech has returned. She can now also read the headlines in a newspaper. Hearing too is better. She hears noises quite clearly at one meter. Distinguishes words at closer range.' November 30: 'The spastic nature of her movement decreases. Right arm moves a little by itself. Incontinence is better. She now has control over bowel movements.' December 12: 'A general improvement of her situation.' December 15: 'She walks for the first time since admission three months ago.' January 20 (1952): 'A relapse. She cannot walk. Patient is very depressed. But continue with immunotherapy.' February 13: 'She is over the crisis. Daily signs of lasting improvement.' March 1: 'She walks and speaks very clearly. She reads well. Hearing is good. All limb movements are normal.' March 17: 'Patient discharged'.

Lydia Bacher was examined by the doctors who previously treated her. They were astonished and baffled that she had survived. In the end they put it down to spontaneous regression, that somewhat rare situation where an incurable patient recovers totally by seemingly miraculous means. The doctors felt it unnecessary to inquire about her treatment at the Ringberg Klinik. It was a situation Issels became familiar with: if a patient recovered, their doctors sought numerous other reasons for that improvement outside that claimed by the clinic. Lydia Bacher was a prototype of the cases the clinic henceforth treated. She had independently proved reports from specialists showing a conclusive diagnosis of an incurable brain tumour which was no longer treatable by conventional means. She also became the clinic's first patient to express the effectiveness of treatment by surviving the somewhat arbitrary limit of five years without detectable symptoms which the International Union Against Cancer accepted as proof of genuine remission.

Issels believed that his success with her case, as with other patients, came from combining immunotherapy with a battering ram of specific and non-specific treatments that were both orthodox and unorthodox. Unhampered by what he considered to be the constrictions of conventional medicine, he had a free hand to practise his novel ideas. In the overall treatment of the body any of sixty-three German standard preparations were used. All could be found in the pharmacies of any continental hospital, although they would seldom be prescribed for cancer patients. But every day at the Ringberg Klinik patients received them in an attempt to improve their general health. In the clinic's laboratory the effects of these, and other, drugs were monitored. Standard tests, identical to those in any State hospital, were regularly carried out, and the results of such screening carefully entered on each patient's treatment card. Patients were encouraged to read and understand that information. It was another fundamental that all patients became involved in their treatment, playing their part in the constant fight Issels waged against their cancers. They took their own temperature and weight, and talked openly about their symptoms.

Some visiting doctors felt putting incurable patients through such a routine gave them hope, false hope. But many of the patients, whether they realised the psychological implications or not; regarded the detailed recording of their progress meant one thing—treatment was still possible, however unorthodox.

Every week Issels summoned his patients to a two-hour lecture in the dining room; it was a mixture of science, homespun philosophy and shrewd psychology. After attending several such lectures many patients felt their fear of cancer diminished, and that their will to survive returned. At the lectures there were no secrets. Patients' case histories were openly discussed; for those too ill to leave their beds, the lectures were relayed on loudspeakers to their rooms. Much of what they heard was not medically proven. But implicit in everything was Issels' belief that his concept was the correct one. Twenty years passed before the great cancer hospitals of the world began to recognise the potential value of intensive psycho-therapy for cancer victims; there was growing awareness that stress played a critical part in whether such patients improved. At Sloan-Kettering in New York and the Royal Marsden in London specialists saw that peace of mind helped a diseased body. Observers from both hospitals visited the Ringberg Klinik and privately told Issels they agreed with his psychological approach.

From the outset Issels made observations which in later years doctors all over the world recognised, and commended, had real value in understanding better the problems of managing terminal illness. Every one of his patients showed various degrees of emotional distress which needed positive treatment: it came from a belief that death was close. He found it important to listen to such fears, and to alleviate them with honest answers. Pain and physical discomfort had to be also handled from the psychological standpoint. Fear, in whatever form, was almost as real a problem as the cancer tumour itself. It was not always easy to isolate the cause of disturbance.

Often patients concentrated their conscious distress on a relatively minor source of anxiety because their real fears were too frightening to think about. One patient complained from stiffness in the finger joints when he was dying from lung cancer. A woman with a rapidly progressing tumour of the uterus said she could cope with her condition: what brought tears to her eyes was the situation of another patient she had become friendly with. That relationship manifested one of the many problems of managing the fatally ill in hospital: that woman escaped from her own circumstances by believing her very real distress came from being in the presence of another mortally-ill person. Handling such situations was never easy, though Issels grew increasingly adept at it. He saw that a proper degree of love and companionship was an important part of treatment. He encouraged his staff to follow his own rule and never reveal any signs of emotional withdrawal from the dying. Ten full years before that very human reaction was given a label—

'bereavement of the dying'—Josef Issels realised that its symptoms of hollowed cheerfulness and stilted conversation had no part to play in his attitude towards incurable patients. He believed the fatally ill were entitled to genuine emotional support and understanding, even if sometimes their attitudes produced real strain in all those involved in their care. He reduced the risk of tension for his nursing staff by encouraging relatives to be constantly on hand, he abolished visiting hours, and was himself freely available on any topic.

Away from his patients Issels embraced new treatments for their care. Infusions of molecular oxygen and inhalations of hot ether gas became regular components of the medical regime.

The use of ether as a treatment had been recently discovered by a German surgeon, Dr. M. Tiegal, suffering from secondary prostate carcinoma. The rapidly growing swelling was accompanied by severe neuralgia and cachexia. By May, 1948 he suffered from bowel paralysis. He decided to inhale fifty grams of hot ether, heated to the point it evaporated into gas. He believed it might prolong his life for a little while. A few hours later, his bowels opened. Next day his appetite returned. Over the next ten days he repeated the ether inhalations and finally he noticed fragments of his tumour being passed with the urine. Later completely recovered, he treated a number of similar cases to his own and claimed success. He believed hot ether—inhaled at 95°C—dissolved fat substances, lipoeds, in the body. In healthy cells structure lipoeds catalysed cell breathing. He argued that cancer cells probably contained membrane structures easily dissolved by ether gas, and claimed his discovery was an effective and relatively harmless chemotherapy. His work was totally rejected by conventional researchers. A similar story happened with molecular oxygen: claims advanced by a number of *ganzheit* practitioners that it had a part to play in revitalising the body, were dismissed as quackery. Issels accepted that neither treatment had any direct effect on the tumour, but he found that ether gas inhalations removed symptoms of depression in patients and infusions of molecular oxygen did stimulate cellular activity.

In his continued search for an immunological cancer agent

Issels found himself in step with conventional beliefs. Cancer specialists had long recognised that the solution of the cancer problem would have to await the discovery of a means of preventing cancer, such as an anti-cancer vaccine. The idea of an immunological solution had been pioneered by Paul Ehrlich in 1903. But his work was dismissed by later researchers as being valueless because of inadequate experimental methods. He had simply failed to produce evidence that freedom from cancer might involve immunity defences similar to those mustered against invading germs. Later, Dr. Peyton Rous, of the Rockefeller Institute, New York, showed that a virus was responsible for a type of cancer in chickens. Other virus-induced animal cancers were subsequently discovered, including mammary cancer in mice. But viruses were not taken seriously as a probable cause of cancer until Dr. Ludwig Gross, a New York cancerologist, discovered that mouse leukaemia was a virus disease. That revelation was swiftly followed by another one, more significant. At the University of Texas, Dr. Leon Dmochowski proved virus-like agents were definitely present in some cases of human leukaemia. Issels himself had little doubt that viruses were implicated in at least some human cancers. At the end of months of intensive study he postulated a theory that essentially stated:

> The more the antigen effect of the vaccine corresponds to the antigen effect of the cancerous cells, the more effective will the anti-bodies created by the stimulation be against cancer cells, and thus help in their destruction.

It was an acceptable enough scientific premise: it could be heard in any of the great cancer research centres of the world. But Issels went beyond what was medically acceptable theorising in his belief that effective immunotherapy agents already existed. Toxinal was one. A vaccine called Blasto-lysin was another. Both had been recently rejected as having no proven value. Issels weighed that against a factor more important to him: he believed he saw clinical success with the vaccines. That was enough for him.

By the end of 1951, forty-three patients had been treated

at the clinic. Twenty of them had paid the full amount of DM 800 a month for board and treatment. The others paid what they could afford. Of those treated eleven had died, including Karl Gischler, whose faith and money founded the clinic. Shortly before his death, the shipping magnate told Issels:

> You cannot help me. It is too late. It will be too late for many others as well, simply because they will not have come to you in time. But you must not let that stop you. You must promise me that you will never give up. I know something of the opposition you have faced now, and will face. But you must fight the only way you can—and that is by continuing to give proof of your success. Do not give up. Promise me that. You are in the right place, doing the right thing. Your clinic, that we have built up, will bring results for those who have been labelled incurable. That is the important thing: that you will get results where so many have given up.

On the day Gischler died, December 6, 1951, his wife sent Issels a note reaffirming what her husband said.

By 1952 the Ringberg Klinik became more widely known as patients and relatives spread the word. In the first three months of that year, thirty-six new patients, suffering from eleven different types of cancer, were admitted. In each case the diagnosis had been made by the referring surgeon or physician; often they wrote on the case-notes that a patient was classified as beyond further conventional help.

Issels began to write medical papers, expounding his theories and arguing for a wider acceptance of them. He sent them to the leading German medical journals and they were returned as unacceptable to their referees. Angered, Issels sent them to medical periodicals, which had a lesser medical reputation. His ideas did not fit the thinking of his day. Nor did his terminology help: he used words culled from the nineteenth century. Two decades later those same words came into vogue among his colleagues. By advancing his views he struck out at the medical establishment's thinking, and suffered growing disdain and rejection among his peers: there were some critics who also believed he used his own literary ability to disguise the fact that his premises were not always as firmly rooted as he passionately asserted them to be; sometimes they said his written work amounted to something approaching a cavalier rejection of long held views.

But his published work brought him growing attention. He began to lecture throughout southern Germany. A few doctors who heard him were impressed enough to refer patients.

In February, 1952, Dr. Otto Walter, consultant physician to *Deutsche Bundesbahn*, German Railways arrived at the clinic. He explained he was touring the country to inspect a variety of hospitals which might be suitable treatment centres for railwaymen suffering with progressive cancer. At the end of his visit, the consultant said he had been impressed by what he saw. Issels explained the problems he faced: mounting opposition in medical circles, the need to have patients referred to him before they became moribund. Walter said the only way to resolve the situation was to gain official recognition: that could be done by a properly appointed medical commission examining the clinic. Walter said he could arrange for the German Department of Labour to organise such a visit. Issels eagerly accepted the offer, and on May 24, three doctors arrived to investigate his methods. They were led by Professor M. Bauer, consultant physician to the Department of Labour; his colleagues were Professor K. Bingold, professor of physical medicine at Munich University, and Professor H. Siegmund, director of the pathological institute at Münster University. To Issels:

> They were icy cold. From their first question it was clear what they felt. I was asked to justify my claim to have found a cure for cancer. I strongly denied such a claim. Bauer said that was the general impression they had about my work, that I made impossible claims. I replied that they had been misled. I claimed to do no more than try and help those who had gone beyond the stage of surgery and radiotherapy.
>
> For the next two hours they questioned me as hard as

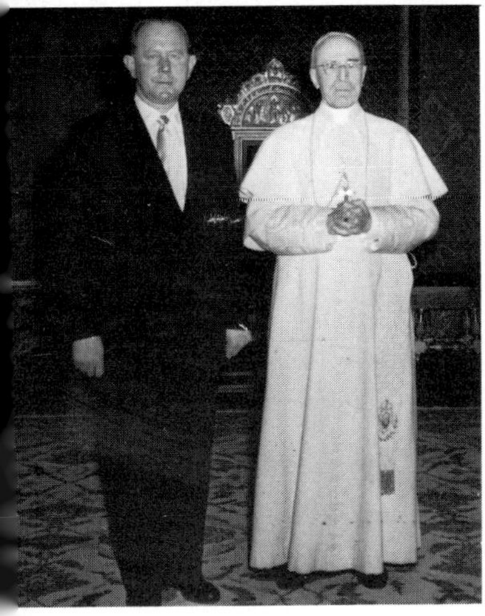

Issels with the Pope
at their Private Audience

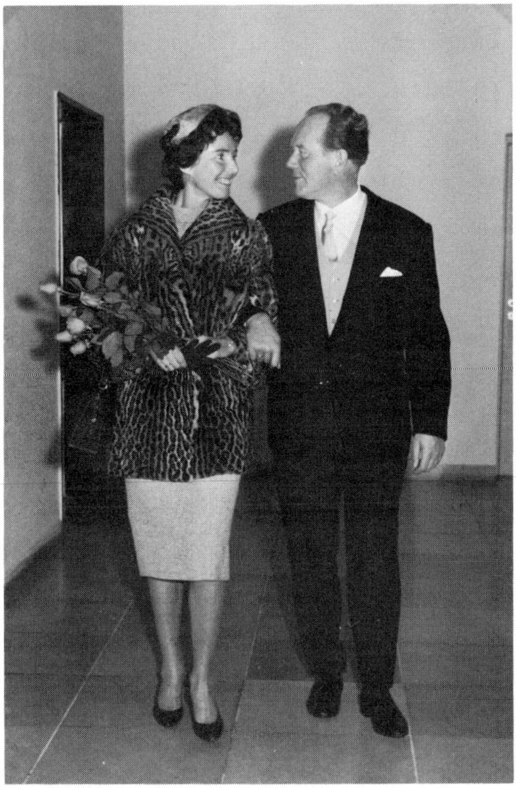

Isa and Issels
on their wedding day

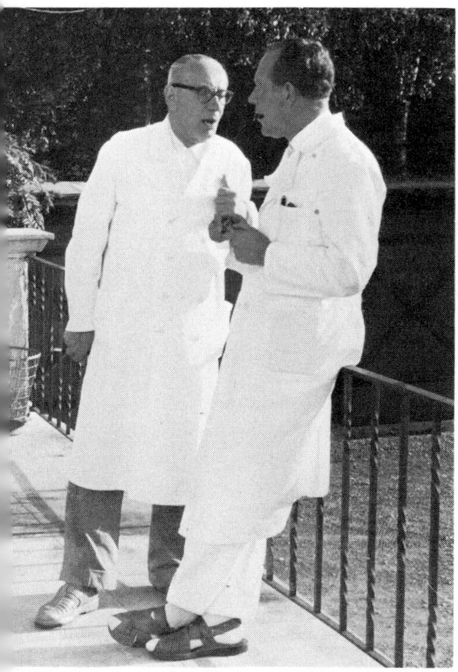

Issels with Professor Gerlach,
1959

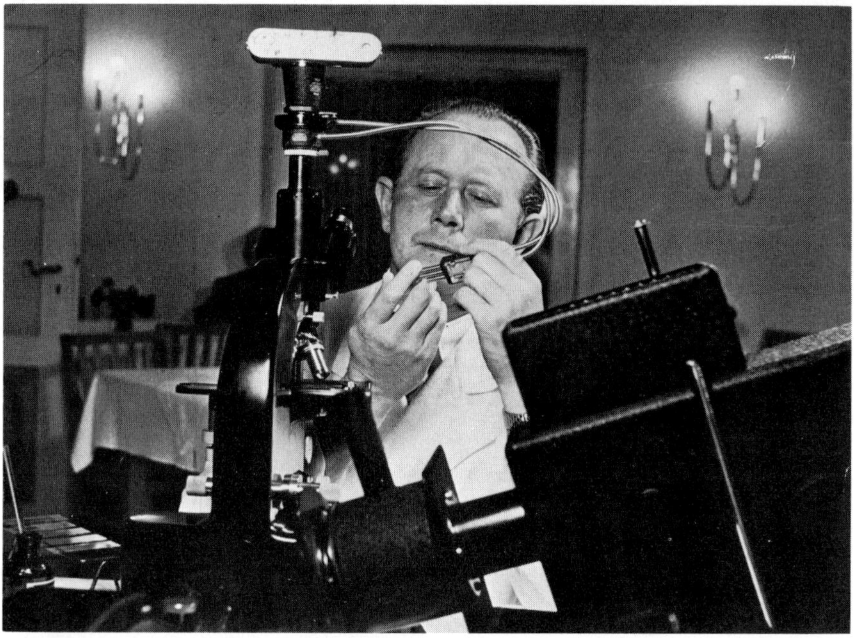

Issels—the researcher

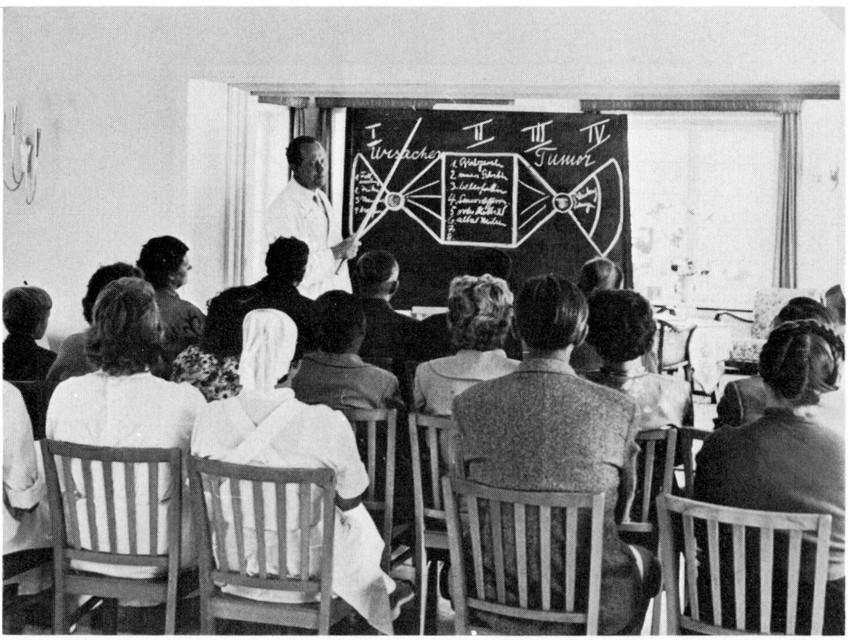

Issels—the lecturer

they could, determined to force me into an admission that I claimed for my methods more than I actually did. There was no let-up. When one paused, another took over. When I suggested a break for coffee, the coffee was ignored. My whole concept was stripped down and laid out in a series of blocks which they turned over and over, attacking from one angle after another. At the end they asked to tour the clinic. They examined patients, case histories, and treatment facilities. They had the air of an execution squad. I felt increasingly depressed that they had not, could not, or would not grasp what I was doing.

Next day they resumed their inquisition. Once more my beliefs were dissected. But this time I detected a glimmer of friendliness. At 5 p.m. Siegmund asked for a coffee. Sipping it, he said: 'What I have seen here is so new. You have pioneered something.' I couldn't believe my ears. Then the other two echoed it. Bauer added that they were so impressed that they were going to recommend the Department of Labour to make me a payment of DM 10,000 as, in his words 'an indication of positive support for your work'.

That night Issels invited the three doctors to dine with him and Irmengard. After dinner Siegmund turned to Irmengard. She remembered:

> I thought at first he was just going to make some polite reference to our hospitality. Instead he said: 'Frau Issels. I feel you and your husband should know we had been sent here to find evidence that your husband is a charlatan and his clinic should be closed down. I am happy that we failed. But he has more enemies than he realises.'

Irmengard felt a new premonition of danger. For months she had been aware of criticism in medical circles: Siegmund had revealed the full extent of the opposition. He also reinforced her belief that Issels had been wrong to give up the security of an established practice for the specialised, and understandably depressing world for her of the fatally ill. It was undoubtedly hard for Irmengard, a woman raised to comfort, to have exchanged her antiques, her Persian rugs, her expensive porcelain and her gilt mirrors for a small room adjoining a number of others filled with terminal cases.

Issels received his cheque from the Department of Labour. But it did not bring him official recognition. In later years Issels grimly held the view that was the time when the medical opposition against him totally solidified. It is impossible so long after the event to unravel the exact circumstances; but what emerged indicated a somewhat odd business. The commission's report ended up on the desk of the Department's Secretary of State, then Dr. Klaus Sauerborn; questioned later he had no recall of it. But investigators later uncovered some evidence which showed that the report had been passed on to the German Ministry of Health for comment. What followed was not clear. Health Department officials later said there was no record of the report—though one of them conceded in 1969 that it 'was highly possible that if the report was favourable to Issels it was dumped'. The three doctors who inspected the clinic are dead—and they left behind no copies of their assessment.

In July 1952 Irmengard's mother, Fanny, was admitted to the Marien Hospital, Stuttgart. Her doctor believed she had liver cancer. A biopsy was taken. It was examined by Professor A. Dietrich, who was then the President of the German Cancer Society. He diagnosed an advanced state of liver cirrhosis. The family were told their mother could be helped no further by conventional treatment. She was given a life expectancy of a 'few weeks'. She became a patient in the Ringberg Klinik. On the day Issels admitted her, Professor Erich Reichl, the professor of surgery at the Marien Hospital told him: 'Maybe you can improve cancer patients with your treatment. But you will find it impossible to treat progressive liver cirrhosis. The patient will assuredly die.'

In spite of that considered prognosis by a most experienced surgeon, Issels felt he must still try and help his mother-in-law. Irmengard did her best to give supportive companionship to her mother, and managed most of the time to hide her apprehension. From the outset Issels realised his treatment would be enhanced by Fanny Linder's positive desire to live. She accepted everything as being important for her chance of recovery. After five months she was discharged with no signs of cirrhosis. She was examined again at the Marien Hospital and that diagnosis was confirmed. Fanny Linder lived for another ten years, and died of a heart attack at the age of seventy-two years.

But the strain of spending every day with the fatally ill showed in Issels. He felt every death to the point of tears. On more than one occasion he doubted if he could, or should, go on. In those moments he escaped to the *weinstuben* around the lake to find distraction from brooding about those he failed to help. But he only had to see a patient improving to regain his sense of purpose.

Nineteen fifty-two was marked by a private visit, in August, by Professor A. Dietrich, President of the German Cancer Society. Dietrich was impressed with the nursing care, and the positive thinking underlying the treatment regime. But he warned Issels to expect opposition for some of his methods. It was friendly enough, but the implication was clear; the tolerance of the medical establishment was running out. After Dietrich left, Issels recalled the words of a previous visitor, Professor Robert Kollath, an apostle of the unorthodox: '*ganzheitstherapie* is to orthodox medicine what the law book is to the Ten Commandments.'

On October 29, 1952, Issels broke yet again an unwritten tenet of medicine which said no doctor should claim to treat with success a patient his colleagues gave up after administering every known conventional treatment.

When Thea Döhn was admitted to the Ringberg Klinik she had certainly been given up for dead. The day before she journeyed south from Mönchen-Gladbach a priest gave her the last rites, and expressed the opinion to her distraught parents that he doubted whether nineteen-year-old Thea would survive the six-hundred-mile journey. It was an opinion her distinguished doctors shared. Professor Eduard Dormanns had diagnosed a fibro-blastic sarcoma and referred Thea for immediate surgery. On September 26, 1952 she was operated on in the Maria Hilfe Hospital at Mönchen-Gladbach. During surgery several secondary tumours were found in the diaphragm. The surgeon's post-operative report stated: 'The major part of the tumour was removed, but total removal was impossible.' On October 11, she received radiotherapy: nine treatments of 3,000 roentgen, a relatively high dosage. At the end of treatment, the hospital's chief surgeon, Dr. William Gross informed her parents that the treatment had appeared 'largely unsuccessful'. Twelve days later Thea developed a haemato pneumonothorax. Further treatment was impossible. Dr. Gross suggested the parents called a priest. On October 28, Thea received the last rites.

She had withstood surprisingly well the long journey to the Ringberg Klinik. She listened calmly as Issels outlined the treatment he proposed. She felt a 'ray of hope' that he believed something could still be done. X-rays were taken and a large haemotoma revealed on the left side following her surgery. The surgeon's report offered Issels even less comfort: it showed part of the sarcoma still attached to the spine, between the ninth and tenth ribs; in the opinion of Dr. Gross, 'it cannot be totally removed as the tumour has grown completely around the spine'.

Issels accepted that diagnosis by one of Germany's foremost clinicians as being accurate.

In the case of Thea Döhm the clinical signs of cancer were clear enough. Issels began treatment on November 1. Along with the combined 'whole body' treatment Thea Döhm received daily doses of the Toxinal vaccine. After sixteen days her case-notes recorded: 'indications of strong reaction by patient to the therapy. Patient very well, gets up, eats, performs normal body functions.' As with every patient, Issels explained the stages of the therapy to Thea. It was one more way to instil a necessary psychological belief in the benefits of his treatment: it helped remove in Thea a fear, almost universally held, that cancer was a terrible and implacable disease. Within a month she talked about her sarcoma free of all the emotional distress she showed on admission.

In January, 1953, she was X-rayed again. The plates revealed a considerable reduction in the tumour, though it still encircled her spine. A month later she was well enough to travel home. On the day she was discharged, the case notes stated: 'Patient free of pain, has gained weight and colour. Follow up treatment through her family doctor. She is to return for a check-up in December.' In December that examination indicated: 'the tumour is dormant. Every indication she can return to a normal life.'

Issels closed the case file and turned to help new patients. A year later he made a brief visit to Mönchen-Gladbach to see his brother, Reinold, and learned that Thea was in hospital with a secondary fibro-sarcoma. Issels was surprised she or her family had not been in touch with him. The reason emerged under his questioning. In August, 1954, Thea fell in love. With the wedding date set, her fiancé changed his mind. Within two months she developed symptoms of her old cancer. She was admitted to the Maria Hilfe Hospital and received an intensive course of radiotherapy; she did not respond. Though nobody said as much, Issels felt her cancer had been psychologically triggered. Thea had lost her physical and moral strength and showed signs of giving up the will to live. There was a degree of acceptance and composure over her fate which was at total variance with her previous attitude at the clinic.

Issels knew that in some cases, an acceptance of approaching death could be helpful; he had seen enough fatally ill patients to know there was certain value to be gained from such an attitude.

He did not believe Thea Döhm was in that category. After discussion with her family she was re-admitted to the Ringberg Klinik on November 11, 1954. X-rays taken that day showed a large tumour on the left lung. Treatment began, using a different immunotherapy vaccine. It was Novacarcin, a preparation developed by a Russian doctor, Boris Pawlotzky, that had been tested, and condemned, by researchers of the American Cancer Society Incorporated. The Society had circulated all the national cancer organisations in the world the results of its findings. In Germany, the national cancer society warned all state hospitals not to prescribe the drug. But no details were sent to the Ringberg Klinik, though it was the only one of its kind in the world treating terminal cancer patients. Unaware of the official attitude, Issels prescribed daily doses of the vaccine. Her case-notes recorded progress which may have astonished the clinicians at the American Cancer Society: X-rays taken in January, 1955 showed a definite reduction in the tumour.

But Thea's psychological condition remained unchanged.

Issels knew it stemmed from her broken romance. After carefully considering the move, he decided to talk to her former fiancé. He found a pleasant young man who listened gravely as he heard the clinical story of Thea's condition. He readily agreed to help. He started to visit Thea at the clinic. Within weeks they were in love again, and the effect on Thea was astonishing. Psychologically and physically she progressed. Finally she was able to go home. In Mönchen-Gladbach a doctor at the Maria Hilfe Hospital examined her and reported, 'her tumour shows marked signs of diminishing'. Two later check-ups at the hospital showed continuing good progress. On August 20, 1957—five years to the day the original cancer was diagnosed—Thea married. Six months later she returned with her husband for a routine check at the Ringberg Klinik. The final entry in her case file stated: 'There has been a complete disappearance of the secondary tumour. The original one remains dormant. Patient is entirely free of any active cancer.'

In 1968, Thea's family doctor, Dr. Philipp Wirtz, added a postscript to the case: 'I have examined the patient. Sixteen years after being dismissed as incurable she is alive and cured. The latest X-rays show her lung free of any malignant tumour. Her original spinal tumour is still dormant. She leads the usual busy life of a mother of three children, and has every reason to expect a full life span.'

That year the American Cancer Society Incorporated placed Issels on its 'Index of Unproven Methods'. On page 35 of a document circulated to cancer specialists the world over was the entry:

> One of the best known European exponents of Novacarcin is Dr. Issels, chief of the Ringberg Klinik for Chronic Diseases and Tumours, Rottach-Egern, who has lectured to many groups and published many articles on his experience with Novacarcin.

To a layman the words were innocuous, but to cancer specialists they were a clear condemnation of Issels and his work. But the American Cancer Society Incorporated had never sent a representative, qualified or otherwise, to investigate the clinic; to this day it will not reveal the process of deduction which allowed it to come to a conclusion based, it would seem, at best on second-hand information.

But for every successful case such as Thea Döhm's, there were many more in those first years who did not recover. In 1952, two hundred and twenty patients were admitted. All but a few died either during, or shortly after their stay in the clinic. It was the same in the early part of 1953: the death rate was appalling.

Issels reviewed his whole method of treatment. He knew that *somewhere* in the regime was a flaw. In March, 1953, he found it: it was so obvious that he had overlooked it several times:

> I had not been removing infected tonsils. My reason had been a simple one. I had not felt that terminal cases, many in a moribund state, could have withstood the strain. But I saw that after one or two patients had tonsillectomy they showed considerable overall improvement: their bodies were better able to cope with the toxic effects of the cancer. The laboratory analysis confirmed my belief this was an indirect, but important measure for raising the body's natural resistance because it eliminated endogenous damage to the body. The tonsils showed an excessive degree of atrophy and they contained hidden abscesses in a high percentage.

From then on patients had their tonsils removed. Issels said he saw a definite improvement in their physical condition after such surgery.

Visitors came steadily to the clinic; among them were a number of professors who privately expressed what they felt unable to state publicly: that the clinic deserved official support. Issels gained national fame when a popular weekly magazine included him in a series devoted to German cancer specialists. He was given the same space as the views of Professor Karl Bauer, professor of surgery at Heidelberg University, and Germany's outstanding cancerologist. After the articles, Issels was warned about the ethical dangers of appearing in the lay press: Bauer received no such stricture.

Issels continued writing and lecturing, preparing both his

papers and talks with great care. He was fluent with pen and on the platform. His name became firmly established in the public mind as the man offering a positive alternative to usual cancer treatments. He published a book in 1953, *Grundlagen und Richtlinien für eine Interne Krebstherapie,* Fundamentals and Instructions for an Internal Treatment of Cancer, a restatement of his whole philosophy. The book enjoyed success.

That year Issels was invited by Professor Werner Zabel, the oldest living exponent of *ganzheitstherapie*, to address a medical conference at Berchtesgaden. Zabel's personal influence brought together distinguished members of the German Cancer Society and practitioners of the unorthodox. The conventional delegates were led by the tiny Professor Karl Bauer, *altvater* of the German cancer world, and author of *Das Krebsproblem*, his newly published work which vied for space in the bookshops with Issels' slimmer volumes. Issels eagerly read Bauer's book, and spotted discrepancies in the professor's explanation of cell changes in cancer. Having delivered the final lecture to the conference—the transcript showed his views were well received—Issels pressed Bauer to explain the contradictions in his books. The professor's answer was short and angry: though the book carried his name, parts of it had been written by his assistants—and in a book of such length contradictions could happen.

Over the years Bauer became a hardened opponent of all Issels represented: for him Issels anthologised all the sins of arrogance, obstinacy and ignorance of unorthodox medicine.

Among those who read Issels' book was Albert Schweitzer. He wrote from Lamborene on February 11, 1954:

> Your study about carcinoma was an experience for me . . . I can imagine that many doctors are reading your statements with the same surprise and satisfaction as I do . . . and with the same gratitude. How good and right that you have been able to create a hospital where you can research your own ideas. I know how much effort this takes. In my circle of family and friends I have experienced much sadness with cancer. Maybe one day I will ask you to admit some person close to me at your hospital. Please grant me this.

A correspondence began that climaxed when the two met at Lindau, in southern Germany. Schweitzer had travelled from the Congo to attend a Nobel Prize Winners' Conference. He was a world citizen—and the world paid homage to him in Lindau. Issels found the old doctor's bedroom thronged with people. But when he had identified himself Schweitzer locked the door, straddled a luggage-rack and invited Issels to sit opposite him, a few inches away. For long minutes the philosopher peered into the eyes of Issels, satisfied, he said: 'Now I know you.'

Both found an immediate rapport. Schweitzer shared Issels' views on the limitations of conventional cancer treatment; they discussed at length the concept Issels had developed. Issels found what others discovered on meeting Schweitzer: that he was a complex and thoughtful man, a man of immense depth. He had one other quality which especially attracted Issels; all his life Schweitzer had stirred controversy by his unwillingness to accept generally held truths. Other letters followed that meeting; they encouraged Josef Issels to continue speaking and acting for himself, without being influenced by what Schweitzer termed was 'expected' of a doctor. It bolstered the individualistic perspective which had always been strong in Issels.

But increasingly another, and darker, facet of his personality came to the fore. The cause was the sheer strain of struggling for the lives of his patients. In addition there was increasing tension at home. The result was havoc in his private life.

Irmengard and the children had moved into a small house near the clinic. She had furnished it with her usual good taste, but did not help the situation. Outbursts at his wife, Rolf and Uti became frequent. All three retained memories of Issels becoming enraged over small matters. Rolf later saw: 'The tension was so great in him that he just had to explode. Anything could make him angry. It was only later that I realised the pressures he suffered. I don't know if my mother ever fully appreciated that.'

Irmengard's recollection was that the rows could be traced back to money. It was as short as ever for domestic use. An adjoining property had been obtained to meet the expanding demands of the clinic, but fees from patients barely met the substantial bills for their care. Salaries of the medical and nursing staff were high because of the special strain their work carried; a doctor received twenty-five per cent more money than he would in a State hospital. Sometimes, this attracted the wrong kind of person to work in the clinic. Even with a generous pay scale and excellent fringe benefits—food and accommodation provided by the clinic at cost, long holidays—the staff found the constant effort needed with the dying was often too great a demand and left. In spite of the pleasing location, new staff were never easy to recruit. Some doctors hesitated to accept posts because they feared their future in orthodox medicine would be endangered. In many doctors and nurses there was also a genuine doubt whether they were simply capable of handling nothing but dying people every day. They found they had to constantly give spiritual as well as bodily help; and in the end it often proved of no avail. Death intervened. Many a doctor and nurse found death hard to bear, because in their relationship with the mortally ill they found it impossible to remain impersonal. The strain in the nursing staff also showed in other ways: many a nurse or clerical worker became convinced she had cancer and constantly sought medical confirmation that they were free of the disease. In moments of particular tension, the *Chefarzt* took out his doctors and nurses. For Issels it was a chance:

> To forget the tensions of work. All the staff felt it to one degree or another. So we went out together and tried to jolly ourselves out of the depression we felt when a patient died. But no matter how late we stayed out, we were all bright and fresh for work the next day. That was one rule I absolutely insisted upon. Nobody had to be late, or out of condition for the patients. We all—and that included the patients—benefited from those very necessary nights out. All the staff worked far better afterwards. We had relaxed. The burden of our tension had gone.

Issels became a familiar figure in the bars around the Tegernsee. He sometimes preferred to be alone, sipping Rhine wine and brooding. His thoughts often centered on the importance for him, as indeed for any doctor to keep a proper balance between continuing treatment and accepting that some patients were beyond it. That called for sound judgment, not only in dealing with a patient, but also with relatives. Issels became familiar with families who left no possibility unturned, even though a case was hopeless. Juggling, as it were, with the niceties of death, was a burden he increasingly felt.

Then the extraordinary amount of research he undertook imposed additional penalties on his mind and body. Apart from his conventional laboratory work with blood—blood counts, including thrombocytes, sedimentation rates and Weltmann tests—he also performed other experimental work in blood chemistry that was highly unusual. He set out to show that also in cancer patients the *quality* of blood corpuscles was as important as the *quantity*. It was an avenue of exploration which took him further away from conventional medical thinking. His papers were published in magazines whose medical status was repeatedly questioned by the German Cancer Society. Issels also maintained a tremendous in-flow of information from professional journals and reprinted articles.

The accumulated strain of doctoring, philosophising, researching and reading became too great. One autumn afternoon Issels collapsed. His chief assistant diagnosed double pneumonia. Issels grew rapidly worse. The registrar told Irmengard he expected her husband to die. Irmengard was terrified not only at the prospect of impending widowhood, but also at a future which seemed bleak. She knew the clinic was barely showing a profit and that their private bank balance showed a debit. At Issels' request she sent for the family lawyer so that her husband could make his will. On his sick bed, Issels signed a testament bequeathing the entire clinic to the German Red Cross, having stipulated Irmengard and the children should receive an 'adequate' sum of money each month to live on.

Back at work, after a gradual recovery, he found the pressures mounting again on all fronts. Hints began to appear in some of the more sensational continental magazines that Issels was a dangerous experimentalist, who, in the words of an Italian magazine, 'believed he has some Divine right to play around with sick people'.

Issels answered that charge, and others like it:

> I work empirically—yes. Dangerously—no. All the patients receive the same basic treatment. I do not use any of them as control groups. They are terminal patients, no-hopers. But that does not give me the right to do anything to shorten their lives still further. If I see there is nothing I can do, I will do nothing. But if there is a chance, and I judge that chance by my own accumulated clinical experience with the whole therapy, then I will begin treatment. I do not know how successful it will be, or how long a patient will live. But if a patient, who has, say, a month's life expectancy under normal prognosis, is given a lease of life, free of pain, for a year, or even two years, then I can honestly say I have done good. At the most, conventional medicine could only expect about 1 per cent to 2 per cent 'spontaneous regression' with similar cases. I know that some of my drugs are not yet recognised by the profession. But that does not mean they are not useful drugs. The whole history of drug development is studded with men who were accused of dangerous experiments, and were later praised for their work. I inject myself with all the drugs developed for immunotherapy before my patients receive them. Then they are given to patients. If that is experimenting, then I experiment. But I do not call that experimenting. And most people working in conventional medicine would be also guilty of experimenting by that standard. The fact is that I have conclusive proof my approach works. How many others working with terminal patients can say that?

In Munich another file had also been opened on Josef Issels. Since 1953 a group of German doctors began to secretly gather information against a colleague many medical men attacked with growing ferocity.

By 1956, 1,473 patients had been treated at the Ringberg Klinik. That year Dr. Arie Audier of the University of Leiden, Holland, visited the clinic to make a preliminary statistical study of success and failure. Audier was not a recognised statistician, though he had considerable experience in tabulating clinical work of one kind or another. He felt competent to evaluate the case histories of the Ringberg Klinik. With his experience as a psychiatrist he was especially interested in the repeated references to mental upset in those histories. But in the end he decided it was: 'too early to make any worthwhile conclusion, not one of the patients had then survived the required five years'.

Audier was impressed by the clinic's definition of 'terminal cases' as those who underwent all available conventional treatment, and had independent medical evidence to support that; those who had metastasising carcinoma; those who had a strictly limited life expectancy because of progressive cancer. Audier said he would return in two years to conduct a detailed survey. Issels accepted the offer: he accepted anything which might properly promote his aims in medical circles.

There were already a number of striking successes in the clinic's case files. There was the case of Alice Mann, diagnosed with inoperable cancer at Frankfurt-Main Hospital in May, 1952. After a course of treatment at the clinic she was pronounced in August, 1953 as 'free of active cancer'. Her family doctor confirmed that verdict. There was the story of Hedda Kurz, diagnosed with a glioma brain tumour at Mannheim General Hospital in 1951. She had two brain operations. But the tumour grew anew. She received radiotherapy. In March, 1952 she was diagnosed as beyond further treatment. That month she came to the Ringberg Klinik. After five months she was discharged with a diagnosis that 'the tumour is arrested'. Four years later, in 1956, she still remained untroubled by further symptoms. A whole procession of men and women, according to the case notes, had survived far longer than their own doctors had ever expected.

Many, of course, did not survive. In one month Issels saw fifteen patients die. On another occasion a woman was discharged after a fairly long spell of treatment. As she walked out of the clinic on her husband's arm, she collapsed and died of haemorrhage.

Issels found such incidents harrowing. He tried to relax.

One night he took some of his staff and Irmengard for a night out in Munich. The party travelled in two cars. On the way back Issels and the second car became separated. Shortly after he arrived home the police telephoned with the news that the car had been in an accident: two of the occupants, his secretary and his niece were dead; their companions, two clinic doctors, had suffered severe head injuries.

The shock ended Issels' social life for a time. At home the question of divorce was openly mentioned. Irmengard refused. The tension between them increased. In the end Issels threatened to close down the clinic unless Irmengard gave him a divorce. She divorced him in November, 1956. For a while they still shared the same house until Issels found an apartment of his own.

The divorce left a lasting impression on Irmengard. In 1972 she tried to rationalise the cause as she saw it:

> Jupp said he had to be independent. He loved his freedom. He was fanatical about his work. That was one factor. Then my honesty in certain matters upset him. That was another factor. Then there was his behaviour. He felt it was all right to go off with other girls and expect me to put up with it. But I think the biggest mistake I made was not to make him jealous. If I had made him jealous things might have ended differently. But I had my work in the clinic, the children, a home to run. I had no time to even think of creating a situation where he could be jealous. Besides, I am not very good at that sort of thing. Another mistake I made was that I accepted everything, and he took advantage of that. He did not mean to do it. It is just the way he is made. He said to me after the divorce that the children and myself would never suffer any financial hardship, but that he must live for his therapy. He has done both things. I have no complaints there: he has been fair and generous. And I suppose the special quality of the man is that I still love him. I have no bitterness about the divorce. It had to happen.

Issels buried himself in his work. After an initial period of coolness, his relationship with Irmengard became easier than it had ever been for the last few years of marriage. It was one more paradox of many in the character of Josef Issels that he retained the friendship of his former wife who was always ready to advise him—even on whether he should remarry again.

8

Mounting Opposition

THE DIVORCE PRODUCED A MARKED CHANGE IN JOSEF ISSELS. Though sad at the automatic excommunication from the Church which followed the annulment of the marriage, he saw it was a small price for the relief of being freed from a relationship weakened by years of incompatibility. His stress disappeared. Patients and staff found him considerably more relaxed.

In December he travelled to Rome for a private audience with Pope Pius XII. The Pope had an abiding interest in cancer research, and had read of Issels' work. Vatican staff made it clear to Issels that even though he was an ex-communicant, the meeting would still take place. On December 14, 1956 the two men met. The Pope questioned Issels thoroughly on all aspects of his treatment, particularly about the ethical problems arising with continually assisting those termed incurable. Pius had earlier told an international medical conference that more should be done to eliminate the words *incurable* or *inoperable* from conventional thinking, and he was deeply interested to learn how Issels tried to do that. The Pope told Issels he was impressed by his methods, which coincided with Papal thinking on the problems of managing progressive cancer. The Audience ended with Pius blessing Issels' work and promising continued interest.

That meeting was another watershed in Issels' religious life. It was particularly significant for him in its timing: it came after a great personal crisis and with attitudes within the medical profession growing more barbed. He looked upon the Audience as symbolic of a greater force guiding him. Like Denis Burkitt, one of the world's outstanding cancerologists, Issels felt a religious influence in his work. In other ways the similarity between the two men was strikingly close: they shared the same dedication, the same ideals, and often, the same frustrations. When they eventually met, Burkitt identified another quality common to both of them:

> I am a religious man, and I am not at all surprised to learn that Dr. Issels believes at times that he, too, can be guided by God when it comes to making what conventional cancer researchers would dismiss as no more than an intuitive guess at how to handle a patient.

It was a quality Albert Schweitzer also detected in Josef Issels. The letters between the two men reflected a common attitude towards their life and work. Issels, apart from reading medical literature, delved deep into metaphysics, philosophy and religion. Like Schweitzer, he found existentialism offered no answer to the philosophical reflections filling his mind. Issels found himself unable to identify with the mainstream of current ethical and religious thoughts; he believed it was a poor substitute for individual thinking. Time and again he parted company from the modern dogma of what was acceptable to relive the experiences of Kant and Nietzsche, who called for a super-dictator to govern society. In other ways Josef Issels turned his back on the crowd. Mysticism held an increasing fascination for him. He believed on more than one occasion he contacted his mother. The belief that she was at peace gave him great comfort.

> I had no doubt that another life existed beyond this one on earth. I began to feel a real affinity with the spirit world. Then one day I experienced a remarkable happening. I was doing my morning round on Ward One, the ward reserved for the acutely ill. I went into the room of an elderly woman patient close to death. She looked at me and said: 'Doctor, do you know that I can leave my body?'

I knew approaching death often produced the most unusual phenomena.

'I'll give you proof,' said the woman. 'Here and now.'

There was a moment's silence. Then she spoke again: 'Doctor, if you go to Room 12, you will find a woman writing a letter to her husband. She has just completed the first page. I've just seen her do it.' She went on to describe in minute detail what she had just 'seen'. I hurried to Room 12, at the end of the ward. The scene inside was exactly the same as the woman described it, even down to the contents of the letter. I went back to the elderly woman to seek an explanation. In the time I had gone she had died. It was the first, though not the last, time I experienced unusual happenings with seriously ill patients.

He believed such phenomena was directly linked with working constantly in the shadow of death. Perhaps that was also an explanation for the influence the supernatural had on his later life. Certainly, it rationalised his own attitude towards death: he did not fear it. For him death was only a momentary pause in a greater life beyond that on earth. But he understood precisely the fears those in his care had about dying. In trying to assuage them, he discovered not all patients who held deep religious convictions found reassurance in the last stages of their life through faith; a proper belief in Eternal Life did not remove anxiety about death. On the other hand, genuinely non-religious persons had less fear at the terminal stage.

By 1957 the clinic had doubled its original capacity of thirty-two beds. Much of the expansion followed Issels' outright purchase of the freehold. It cost him DM 160,000 for 17,000 square metres containing four substantial buildings housing three wards and laboratories. Eighty staff cared for the patients. Issels constantly introduced a personal touch to the wards which created a feeling of peace. There were fresh flowers daily and gay prints in each ward. He consciously produced an atmosphere of intimacy which relaxed patients.

He recognised that for the majority the worst moment was

probably on arrival when they learnt, generally for the first time, the full clinical extent of their illness. He tried, whenever possible, to reveal the truth himself. If he could not, then a trusted deputy had the task. Nearly all adult patients welcomed the truth. Children were not told the exact prognosis; rather 'that they must do everything they can to help the doctors make them better again'. It was a blanket statement which the boys and girls who came to the clinic accepted.

From the foundation of the Ringberg Klinik Issels recognised a fundamental problem, and for him a real danger, in treating the so-called untreatable. It was the matter of hope in relation to a cure. Many dying people, especially those with money, try to escape death by going from one clinic to another, accepting treatment from anybody who promises cure. It is a journey which can take them completely outside the medical profession to the world of other 'healers' with their assured but baseless claims; particularly so with cancer sufferers.

Early on medical opponents dismissed the Ringberg Klinik as such a place. They said it was a clinic for the gullible, the wealthy and always the desperate. They added that Issels was a medical heretic, preaching false hope.

Issels claimed that from the outset no promise was ever made to any patient of a cure. Issels' whole attitude was summarised in a memo he wrote to staff in 1956:

> I would remind everybody that it has been the firm policy in dealing with questions relating to prognosis to tell a patient or his responsible relatives that the first step is to arrest the tumour. That will prolong life. The next step is to make the tumour smaller. That will bring a further prolonging of life. The patient should be told that the eventual medical aim is to try and reach the stage where the tumour disappears completely. Finally, time itself is a factor: patients should be told that cure *is* a matter of time—in their case five years free of disease. Our aim is to try and achieve that situation. But we can make no promises. And we never talk of a 'cure' but 'remission'. And we also talk with the knowledge that positive treatment can be offered. That is much more precise and beneficial.

It was a timely reminder, for by 1957 grateful patients expressed through numerous Continental magazines their belief that Issels was a 'miracle doctor' who had 'cured' them. They gave the interviews without his consent. They meant well: they could not know those articles were being collected by other doctors as evidence that Issels was a charlatan.

The stories made lurid reading. They contained scant information about how the treatment evolved: the emphasis was on sensational recovery when all seemed lost. A popular Press view of Issels rooted him in the public mind as rather a dictatorial man with a missionary fervour towards his work. It founded a legend which finally turned Issels into a mythical character. He allowed the fables to go largely unchecked, such as the widely reported story that he climbed the 6,000 feet Wallberg Alp every day. Even in Issels' excellent physical condition the climb would have meant taking about five hours away from his working day—something he never did for personal pleasure. Yet that story, like many others, became accepted through repetition: it was a good example of historicity at face value.

Rarely given attention by the media were Issels' rules for speaking to the dying which were later followed in many countries. In 1971 Dame Alertine Winner, deputy medical director of St. Christopher's Hospice, London, an excellent home for the dying, publicly recognised the value of Issels' frank approach. She felt it was:

> Very remarkable. Dr. Issels promises the patient nothing, but undertakes to do his best and he and the patient co-operate in a fight to save the patient's life. The patients are full of gratitude: something active is constantly being done, hope and encouragement are well given and devotion between Dr. Issels and his patients is marked.

Issels reduced formality wherever possible without sacrificing medical care or nursing. His ward rounds were long and leisurely. Nurses were encouraged not only to know a patient but also his relatives. Issels always believed moral support to a family was important in the context of recovery of a loved one.

Away from the clinic the problems of the ill pursued him. Relatives frequently stopped him in the streets around the Tegernsee for advice and reassurance. He was realistic with both. Rottach-Egern is a small town which increasingly profited from the clinic's presence. Relatives stayed in the numerous pensions and guest houses; those who could afford it put up in the two de-luxe hotels. In time many of the visitors to Rottach-Egern came because of the clinic. It was a situation the town's burghers viewed with mixed feelings: a cancer clinic was a poor image for an exclusive holiday resort—but it brought in money.

Issels himself spent generously, especially at *fasching.* Carnival time, January 1957, found Issels dressed as a Spanish matador, cutting a rakish figure among the costumed Arabs and clowns filling the Tegernsee Valley taverns. Issels, a bachelor again at the age of fifty, kept the fun going at a tremendous pace. More than one young girl found she was no match for the sheer stamina which kept him dancing into the small hours: there was a magnetism about him that dazzled many a local belle. If they entertained ideas of pursuing the affair beyond an amusing dalliance, they must first circumvent Issels' sister, Charlotte, who had moved into the clinic as administrator after the divorce. She and her sister, Margot, suspected many women had designs on their brother. On his side, he demonstrated unusual dutifulness in listening to them.

Invariably Issels drew his social life from those he worked with. The doctors, nurses and laboratory technicians became friends he relaxed with. They enjoyed themselves to the full in his company. But each one had to be punctual for work. Physically, Issels had never been in better shape. He played an excellent game of tennis: those who knew about such things believed he could make the national team with a little more effort. Off-court, he climbed every one of the peaks around Rottach-Egern. In the spring of 1957 he gave up smoking—like Mark Twain he did so with some regularity—ate sensibly, and emerged as a man tolerant of his friends, a generous host and a jovial social companion.

By the middle of the year Issels was much in demand as a lecturer. He took every opportunity, and sometimes created them, to explain his ideas to a public beyond the medical societies. He was a skilled exponent of that still-young profession: public relations. He travelled far to present his ideas to a variety of audiences. He was a gifted speaker in German—though in later years he found it a strain using English to address the Royal Society in Edinburgh or a group of scientists in Japan. His choice of subject matter, with appropriate adaptation, served for any audience. In 1957 he produced a standard lecture containing all the elements of his beliefs. It included the following passages:

> Cancer has a language all its own among medical men. They talk of the anti-metabolities and the nucleotides. But one word you will rarely hear mentioned is 'incurable'. It makes most doctors quite uncomfortable to even think about it, leave alone speak over it. For it is a word which makes it tragically clear how limiting surgery, radiotherapy and drugs can be in cancer treatment. The patients I treat have all progressed beyond such treatments. And, and it is a big 'and', only about twenty per cent of all patients suffering from cancer, including cancer of the skin, live for five years or more after surgery, irradiation or chemotherapy. Despite improvements in technique, a decisive increase in this percentage cannot be expected in the present state of knowledge. For the remaining eighty per cent of all other cancer patients, present methods cannot even offer a five-year remission. In 1953 I showed the need for a new approach to these cases. I argued for a concept that cancer must be understood and treated primarily as a chronic systemic illness of the whole body. Therefore, we cannot expect to solve the cancer problem by surgery or radiotherapy.
>
> Nor is it enough to do just research work with mice and other animals. Only by research on cancer patients in their sick-beds can we develop a new therapy. In that sense the Ringberg Klinik is a total experiment because, until now, the so-called 'incurable' patient has never been treated. He has been sent home to die with a few pain-killers. *That is not treatment*. At the Ringberg Klinik we treat such patients in the belief that it is a normal thing to do. There are some simple rules in that treatment. Seeing that the

body can eliminate toxic substances is as important as the immunotherapy, biological drugs, used to attack the actual tumour. Unless the body functions properly to eliminate the toxics, it is impossible to continue treating the localised tumour. Active immunotherapy sometimes does not work if focal points of infection are still present. They affect the immunotherapy. Experience shows this is especially so before tonsils are removed. Afterwards, the growth rate of the tumour is generally slowed in all kinds of cancer. This gives more time for the immunotherapy to work. This prepares the way for the body to eliminate toxics more easily. Tonsils are the great curse of the body. They can appear normal. But on laboratory examination they are found to be grossly infected in all cancer patients. Many cancer patients have a high pulse rate—120, 140, even 160—caused by intoxication of the heart. I believe poisons from the tonsils make their way into the blood stream and eventually poison the heart. One thing I do know. That high pulse rate caused forty per cent of deaths in the clinic through heart attacks. When tonsilectomy became obligatory, the figure dropped to under five per cent.

How does the body evacuate toxic substances? Partly through the urine. There are various other systems, such as the kidneys and the sweat glands. But the main, and most important, organ to evacuate the toxic protein is, I believe, the mucosa of the big intestine, which I call the 'filter'. For every patient I have one hope—to open this 'filter'. No scientist can easily explain the process of how the 'filter' becomes blocked and unblocked. But in the opinion of doctors of another age—and why should we still not listen to them?—the end of the big intestine, or colon, is the organ which evacuates toxic substances. There is no way of proving it by clinical examination in a living patient—and autopsy shows nothing. But we do have one guide as to the state of the 'filter', and that is the tongue. It is a mirror of the intestines. A normal tongue is rosa-coloured, always wet, covered with mucous. In chronic disease, and cancer patients the tongue is dry, white, grey, steel-blue or black. The 'filter' is blocked—and the tongue mirrors that blockage. The poison remains in the body, eventually bringing death. The signs of a blocked 'filter' are clear: a high temperature, high blood sedimentation, a reduction of red blood cells. It is a constant battle cry at the Ringberg Klinik to 'open the filter'.

British and American doctors continually resisted his insistence that tonsilectomy had any significant part in affecting the body's defences. But by 1971 German doctors were not so sceptical. Published work in West Germany showed that in tonsilectomies 85 per cent of the organs were infected to a measurable degree, and the abscesses had frequently drained into the blood stream, undoubtedly affecting body resistance.

Along with tonsilectomy, other treatments had been added to the combined *ganzheitstherapie*. Auto vaccine from diseased teeth and tonsils were given in the belief they 'desensitised' a body. A mixture of oxygen and ozone—100 c.c. oxygen to 3 c.c. ozone—was administered through the rectum. It was supposed to help with cellular regeneration, and was not an unpleasant experience. Another treatment had a more alarming effect on the patient. It began with an injection of a drug called *Pyrifer*, an ethical preparation available to all doctors. Made from mixed bacteria which had been specially treated, it irritated the fever control mechanism in the brain. Within four hours a patient had a high temperature. Until it reached a peak of 105°F. patients kept their own careful temperature chart. Then, at 105°F. blankets and hot-water bottles were packed around 'fever' patients to help maintain that level as long as possible. Some patients remained at that level for five or six hours. In that time the fever stimulated the body's natural resistance and mobilised the toxicity so that it could be more easily evacuated. The weekly fever treatment was one more way to open the 'filter' of every patient.

For years Issels' claims for that particular treatment were rejected. But, in the late 1960s, research work began, independently, at the Sloan-Kettering Institute for Cancer Research, New York and at King's College Hospital, London, on the effects of such treatment on cancer cells. It was found, in the opinion of Professor John Anderson of King's to be:

Beneficial. At a temperature of around 105°F. the malignant cells in the body can be adversely damaged. Healthy cells are not damaged because the temperature is not allowed to reach the point where they would suffer, 109·5°F.

Four hundred and twenty-one patients received such treatments in 1957. Among them were a number of women with breast cancer. Rather than undergo surgery they went to the Ringberg Klinik. Like Issels they found it no answer to be told by such experts as Dr. Maurice Sutton, consultant radiotherapist at the North Middlesex Hospital, in *Cancer Explained* that:

> The operation of removing the breast is perhaps, one of the commonest cancer operations performed today. It might be thought that the removal of a structure that contributes so much to the female contour would be very disfiguring. In actual fact, this is not so: brassieres designed for women who have this operation are available and make the asymmetry quite undetectable when wearing clothes.

Filled though the clinic was with a sad selection of all kinds of cancers, a number of beds were still reserved for patients unable to pay. In 1957 Issels gave DM 70,000 worth of free treatment.

By the end of the year his tenth paper had been published. It contained the usual number of words taken from a bygone age: 'canalisation', 'blocked systems' and 'resistance'—references to the elimination in the body of toxic substances, or a patient's inability to induce fever. They were a standard part of his repertoire.

In August he addressed a medical conference in Düsseldorf. It was not the first time the audience heard the Issels' *Hypothesis of Pathogenesis of Cancer*, which he had formulated in 1952. He had now refined it to a single diagram. On it, he listed the causes of diseases and their effects on the organs. He called it the 'secondary damage' stage, which affected the body's resistance and at the same time produced complex metabolic disturbance. He said that was the

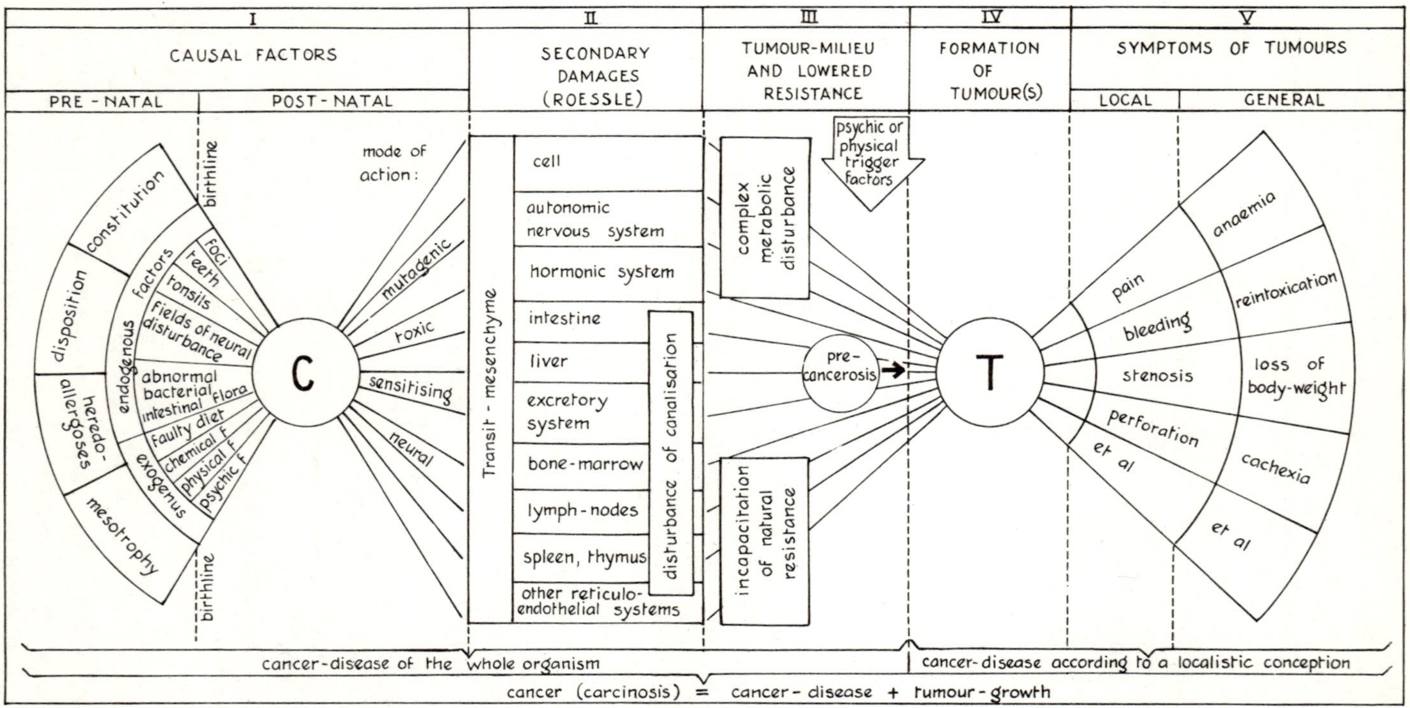

Hypothesis of Pathogenesis of Cancer

Pre- and post-natal endogenous and exogenous causal factors (I), by mutation, toxicity or neural effects, via the 'transit mesenchyme', produce secondary damage (II), in cells in control mechanisms (nervous and hormonal systems), in the detoxifying, excretory and defence systems.

Effects on excretory canalisation lead to complex metabolic disturbances which lower natural resistance and produce an imbalanced condition gradually developing into a 'tumour milieu' (III).

From such primary, pre-cancerous condition (III), a secondary pre-cancerous condition may develop at a place of least resistance, and when defence potency is lowered further an oncogenous condition may result in a malignant growth developing at the site of least resistance.

'Localistic conception' with respect to malignant disease means the tumour and its local and general symptoms, the tumour being regarded as the *cause* of the disease. 'Holistic conception' means latent oncogenic disease. Complete malignant disease, therefore, includes latent malignancy of the whole organism (I, II and III) and the cancerous growth (IV) with its symptoms (V). This conception regards the tumour as the *symptom* of the disease.

cause for all chronic disease. But, in certain conditions, that stage also created a 'tumour milieu'. He identified that as the 'primary, humoral, pre-cancer state'. He argued that his 'primary' state was a pre-condition for the 'secondary pre-cancer state' of orthodox medicine when doctors recognised a patient was generally at risk. He claimed that removing the tumour itself by surgery or other means did not remove the 'primary' state. He labelled that 'primary' state as the cause for all secondary cancer.

He found support for his ideas among such men as Professor H. Siegmund, director of the Pathological Institute at Münster University. Late in 1957 Issels had an opportunity to show his treatment could also be a prophylactic when he admitted Elsa Stein.

She was a twenty-four-year-old woman with a long history of a recurring growth on the left breast nipple. Between 1949 and June 1957 it had been removed six times by surgeons at the University of Cologne Hospital. The growth was always found to be benign. But the intervals between surgery were increasingly shorter. Finally, in June 1957, Professor A. Cellen, director of the Pathological Institute at Cologne University performed a biopsy on the latest growth. He concluded the lump was in 'a pre-cancer state', that would soon turn to total malignancy. Elsa Stein was advised to undergo radical mastectomy that would include not only total removal of the left breast but also the lymph glands in the armpit of that side as well.

Her family physician, Dr. Werner Geiger, feared the psychological effect would be great for a woman still young and planning to marry soon. Geiger referred Elsa to the Ringberg Klinik in October, 1957.

Issels found the growth had returned yet again. He removed it in the clinic's operating theatre and sent separate sections to four pathological laboratories, including those attached to the University of Munich and Würzburg. Two biopsy findings showed particular sections to be benign. The third section was diagnosed: 'the presence of cancer is possible'. The fourth section, sent to Munich University, showed the growth to be malignant.

Issels began basic treatment and immunotherapy. Two months later there were no clinical signs of the tumour returning. Elsa Stein was discharged. Her family doctor continued follow-up treatment under direction from the clinic. She was seen at regular intervals by hospital specialists in Cologne. They also reported no further signs of abnormal growth. Fourteen years later she was still free of any growth, living a full life of wife and mother of two equally healthy children she had breast-fed.

Her case did not find its way into the file a group of German doctors continued to assemble in the belief that eventually enough evidence would be obtained to convict Issels in the criminal courts of malpractice, remove his name from the medical register and close down the Ringberg Klinik.

They had opened their file after Issels clashed with Professor Karl Bauer at the cancer conference in Berchtesgaden in 1953. There was no suggestion that Bauer was involved in the early gathering of information, though his opposition to Issels, sincerely enough held, lent authority to the group. The basic questions of who formed the group and exactly why will never be known, but by the end of 1953 it was actively probing into every aspect of Issels' life and beliefs.

For him the cancer congress at Berchtesgaden had also been a turning point. It brought him into direct contact with many of Germany's leading cancerologists. Some found what he said interesting. Others, led by Karl Bauer, totally rejected Issels' concepts.

His opponents increasingly saw him in another light: for them he was simply a pedlar of false hopes—and making money out of it. Yet such accusations ignored certain important factors. There was mounting, independently, and medically verified, evidence that Issels achieved success with his methods. Insurance companies sent patients to the clinic. The powerful *Knappschaft*, a society responsible for the welfare of Ruhr miners, ordered its medical adviser to inspect the clinic. Professor Carl Blumensatt concluded:

> I am of the opinion that in the interest of cancer patients we cannot take the responsibility for ignoring Issels' work. He has shown a way to improve the destiny of so-called incurable patients. I am of the opinion there is a responsi-

bility to examine the methods of Issels. This can be done by referring histologically verified inoperable cancer patients to the Ringberg Klinik and to use its treatments in our wards.

He did refer patients who had been histologically verified as beyond further conventional treatment. A number of them survived considerably longer than they had been expected to. The *Bundesministerium für Arbeit,* the government welfare agency, also sent patients until the medical opposition intervened in 1954.

That year his opponents found a new way of stopping Issels. On May 28, 1954, Professor A. Dietrich of the German Cancer Society, wrote to the organisers of a cancer congress in Saõ Paulo, in South America, that it would be 'inappropriate' for them to allow Issels on the platform. Dietrich's letter contained the passage: 'One reason for refusing him is that his opinions create confusion. To talk about cancer disease without a tumour is nonsense.'

Issels was refused permission to speak. The same happened at other medical conferences where the influence of the then President of the national cancer society was felt. Issels saw Dietrich's opposition as evidence of a growing 'conspiracy' against him. By early 1955 he saw the situation as: 'Dietrich and the rest believe the tumour makes the sickness, while I argue that the sickness makes the tumour. Result: conflict.'

In March, 1955, Dr. H. Weiler, the President of the Bavarian Medical Association visited the clinic. He told Issels there were rumours that he over-charged, promised a cure, and when patients could not pay, they were thrown out to die. Issels believed he satisfied Weiler that the accusations were untrue.

The surreptitious collection of evidence continued. The number of doctors involved remained inexact, but by March 7, 1956, a cabal of a dozen medical men emerged from a weekend meeting at Hinterzarten in the Black Forest determined, in the words of one, Dr. Hans Schubert, to 'put an end to the charlatan Issels'. The group pressed ahead with that aim. On May 5, 1956, one of its members, Dr. Gunther Barth, director of the Radiotherapy Institute at Erlangen wrote to Anni Wiesinger, whose husband, Karl, had just died in the Ringberg Klinik. Barth explained he was: 'One of twelve doctors interested in your husband's illness and we would like to use his case-notes for a scientific society interested in the cancer question.'

Barth specifically wanted the case file because he genuinely believed it contained evidence against Issels. Mrs. Wiesinger agreed her husband's file could be used. It became a prized exhibit. But still more proof was needed. Professor Walter Büngeler, secretary-general of the *Deutscher Zentralausschuss für Krebsbekämpfung und Krebsforschung*, the German National Cancer Society, another member of the group, wrote to Professor E. Schwarz, director of the ears-nose-throat clinic at the University of Tübingen, near Stuttgart, that the problem was finding material offering: 'Perhaps a medium to stop the peculiar way of treatment in the Ringberg Klinik.'

In 1957 the hunt took a new turn. A doctor in the Ringberg Klinik was approached by the local medical association, to obtain evidence within the clinic against Issels. In a later affidavit he swore that: 'Anything was acceptable. Case notes, X-rays, files, private letters. Anything I could get my hands on.'

The doctor refused to do that and left the clinic.

In 1958 Dr. Helmut Spohr, general administrator of the National Cancer Society, travelled to Munich to attend two meetings. Spohr later testified that: 'Members felt it is high time that we got rid of Issels because his principles do not fit the concept of conventional medicine.'

In August 1958 his opponents found an ally in Dr. Helgo Teicher, who joined the clinic staff that month. He had gone to the clinic at the recommendation of the Bavarian Medical Association. They told him it was 'a good and interesting clinic'. Later, according to Teicher's sworn testimony, 'I got an order from the Association to collect material in the clinic'. Teicher saw nothing reprehensible in his behaviour; like many others, he felt his methods were acceptable when it came to dealing with Josef Issels.

As the first snow of the winter of 1958 fell, the hunt for anything incriminating took on a more definite shape. Somewhere in the higher echelons of German medicine the 'order' was given to concentrate on obtaining anything 'which might point to Issels using the clinic as a means of furthering his own financial ends'.

The hope of uncovering proof to substantiate the charge was doomed—because it did not exist. On the contrary, Issels had compiled a list of patients who, over the years, had bilked him of payments. It was a sad catalogue of men and women, who, in some cases having received months of treatment, had left the clinic, often improved in health, and then blandly refused to pay for their medical care.

At first Issels had shrugged such behaviour aside. But when journalists began to question him about fees, and wrote articles hinting at fat profits from treating the seriously ill, Issels felt forced to counter by revealing details to other reporters of patients who had diddled him. The list also served his justification that patients must pay a month's fees in advance. Newsmen from Britain who expressed surprise at this were told, correctly, that this was common practice in Germany.

Yet the whole question of money nagged Issels to the point where he wrote a diary note in December, 1958:

> Over forty percent of my patients are fully insured under policies for their treatment. I only wish all my beds were free like State hospitals. After all, ninety-five percent of my patients are referred to me from State hospitals. But we don't get a penny of official support to maintain them or to continue treatment. Nor will such support come until the day dawns when the medical establishment finally recognises, as it must, that this is a valid way to treat the so-called 'incurable'.

Issels continued to devote himself to treating those cases other doctors had given up. In doing so he finally became vaguely aware that all was not well. Some patients told him that they had been solicited to make statements complaining about their treatment at the clinic. Not one did. Issels was reassured by such loyalty.

There were also other things to think over. By 1958 scientists from a dozen countries had visited the clinic. With one exception they asked that Issels made no public reference to such visits, they quite properly feared cancer societies in their own countries would terminate vital research grants if it became known they had actually called on a man blacklisted by the powerful American Cancer Society Incorporated. The exception was Dr. Josef Eller, director of the department of dermatology at New York Hospital, and author of a textbook, *Tumours of the Skin*. Eller was impressed enough by what he saw and said so. Eller was a powerful single voice, but even he could not overcome the implacable rejection of Issels by the medical establishment.

Yet in spite of all the opposition, Issels still maintained some access to medical conference platforms. In August, 1958, he addressed his biggest audience, 1,000 doctors, at the important 'Therapy Week' Conference at Karlsruhe. He explained his views. At the end he received a standing ovation. In that moment he actually believed a breakthrough for his ideas was imminent. It was, perhaps, a symptom of the increasing exhaustion he felt that he believed such a thing. His sister, Charlotte, had noticed for some weeks that once more strain had accumulated in her brother. As he left the conference, she resolved the situation in characteristic fashion: she walked him to Karlsruhe station, thrust a ticket into his hand for Borkum, a North Sea resort, and sent him off to relax for two weeks on the holiday island.

9

Arrested

AFTER A WEEK AT BORKUM ISSELS LOST HIS PALLOR AND HIS tension. He swam, sun-bathed and found ready companionship among the girls. One day he came out of the sea and walked to a beach hut where a pretty, slimly-built woman sat in the shade. He was struck by her green eyes and soft smile; she noted the sheer vitality of his movements. Both later recalled exactly the exchanges which followed:

'Excuse me,' he said. 'I've left my sunglasses somewhere around here.' He found them and smiled at the woman. 'Why don't you swim? The conditions are ideal.'

'I have some heart trouble,' she said.

'Heart trouble? But you are too young to have heart trouble. Tell me, have you had your tonsils out?'

'No.'

'Then you should have them out. Have you any dead teeth?'

'Yes.'

'Then take them out as well.'

He smiled pleasantly, put on his sunglasses and walked away.

Ilse Maria Klos, Isa to her friends, was intrigued by such advice. In her thirty years nobody had ever spoken to her like that. She wondered whether the holiday might after all turn out to be exciting.

A few days later Issels came hand-springing down the beach to her tent. It was a typical gesture towards a woman who had continually intrigued him since their first encounter. Soon they were in deep conversation, leap-frogging naturally from one topic to another. He was impressed by the maturity of her views; she was constantly astonished that a man well into middle-age had such a youthful outlook. Frequently the talk veered towards medical matters, and Issels restated his belief that a visit to a dentist and tonsilectomy would help Isa's heart condition.

'Are you a doctor,' she said.

'Yes. I have a clinic on the Tegernsee.'

'You're not Dr. Issels?'

Issels admitted he was and Isa explained that for some years she had collected his medical papers.

'You see, I thought if any of my family had cancer I would bring them to you,' she added.

Issels gently drew out the details of her background. She had a brother, Walter. Both benefited from an excellent formal education supplemented by parental encouragement in the arts. Isa grew up in a cultured, loving home. Then Ernst and Hilda Klos fled with their children from Sudetenland in 1945 when Czechoslovakia regained the territory. Her father lost his entire fortune in the move. A gentle, philosophical man, he had slowly built up a new life in West Germany as an importer of raw textile materials. Isa, a gifted linguist, worked as a secretary-translator for her father until the age of twenty-five. Then she studied French and political science in Geneva and Paris. She had travelled widely in Europe. On holiday in Zermatt, Switzerland, in 1958, she had a heart attack following a severe bout of influenza. Borkum was a convalescence.

In the course of a full life Isa had received several proposals of marriage. She had rejected them all after careful consideration because no man matched the special criteria she wanted for a life partner: he had to be somebody she could make real sacrifices for.

That afternoon, early in September 1958, on the sands at Borkum, Isa felt she had at last met such a man. By the end of his fortnight's holiday, she knew she loved Issels deeply and selflessly. He had also overcome initial doubts that she was 'a little bit too thin', and had fallen in love with her mind, the liveliest he had met in a life-time of escorting beautiful and intelligent women. He invited her to come to the clinic to have her teeth and tonsils removed. She accepted and the romance was sealed. On their final afternoon together at Borkum Isa took Issels' arm and he felt: 'An electric shock which ran through my body. No other woman before had ever produced such an effect. It lasted for a long, long time. I knew then that I was truly in love.'

Isa came to the Ringberg Klinik and shared a room with the only other woman who retained a lasting place in Issels' affection—his sister, Margot, also was recovering from a minor illness. Isa had her tonsils out and a couple of teeth pulled, made an excellent recovery and stayed on to help Issels with translations work. The clinic's postbag brought letters from all over the world. After Isa answered them she lectured the foreign-language patients on Issels' concepts. When she was not lecturing she helped plan diet meals and comforted the sick. It was against such a background their romance developed. Both were in no hurry to commit themselves to marriage; Isa recognised that he needed time to adjust to any relationship which would be lasting. She was content to wait and not force the situation. On his side was a deep conviction that a second marriage must last forever. In those first months they carefully explored each other's attitudes on everything important to a lasting relationship. They increasingly discovered a great deal in common among other things about religion and philosophy.

He told her stories of his childhood that he had never before revealed. He talked about the war, God, dying, reincarnation and much that he told no one else. He was a man in love again. And, as many another man argued his suit by showing-off before his girl his prowess as a swimmer or his skill at the wheel, Josef Issels set before Isa his concept of what cancer was and how it should be treated.

Isa demonstrated time and again her complete mastery of his ideas. She also showed herself as a woman with the gift of control without the dullness usually associated with it. Never would her talents be better displayed than during those winter months of 1958 when Issels took every opportunity to impart his theories. Dinners took on a special quality of their own as Issels used the backs of menus, napkins and even the tablecloth as an impromptu blackboard.

She, in turn, brought a new feeling of vitality into his life. For months his sense of humour had been marked by its absence; under her gentle teasing it returned.

Emotionally in other ways it was a joyous period of his life. The patients showed a general improvement and the death rate dropped to three or four a month. He was filled with new ideas for expansion, taking more patients, assuming more responsibilities. Though he worked extraordinarily hard, an average twelve hours a day, seven days a week, he found time for the physical tests he so much enjoyed: mountain climbing, long walks, tennis and swimming. In January, 1959 he and Isa snatched a few days ski-ing in the Austrian Tyrol. He was thrilled by her ability on the slopes; nothing gave him greater pleasure than to be in the company of good athletes.

When he returned from holiday he finally did what he had previously put off. He confronted Dr. Helgo Teicher, not because he learnt of his assistant doctor's theft of clinical material; rather he felt Teicher undermined patients' confidence in the treatment regime. Issels respected the right of any doctor to sincerely challenge his concepts. Teicher went further: he preached rebellion to patients about the treatment. He did so in the hope he might obtain further information which would place Issels in the dock. On January 9, 1959, Teicher was sacked on the spot after a patient complained about his attitude to Issels.

Teicher immediately left the clinic, but did not give up his apartment in the clinic's grounds. From that house, he later confessed, he directed his efforts, collecting anything for the Bavarian Medical Association which remotely suggested Issels was guilty of malpractice.

Teicher was not alone in such behaviour. In Heidelberg. Bonn, Frankfurt and Munich medical men, eminent in their profession, expressed growing concern. They steadfastly denied any but the highest motives for their behaviour. Men like Professor A. Dietrich, former President of the national cancer society, carried to their graves a belief that Issels was a quack. It is difficult to understand Dietrich's particular opposition because he had positive proof that, in at least one case, Issels' treatment was effective. Fanny Linder,

Issels former mother-in-law had survived a diagnosis of fatal liver cirrhosis that Dietrich himself had confirmed; later the cancerologist had visited the clinic and expressed astonishment at the improvement he saw in clearly terminal cases.

By the spring of 1959 the front-runners of the opponents were the Bavarian Medical Association, closely followed by the German Cancer Society. There was a regular exchange of information between both organisations. Much of it was oral: it was felt too dangerous to actually commit to paper evidence of what could be considered outlandish behaviour by doctors.

In May, 1959, Issels believed that he was the object of something approaching active hatred among his peers. On the twenty-third of that month he wrote to the German Cancer Society offering them full freedom to inspect the Ringberg Klinik. He extended a similar invitation to the Bavarian Medical Association. Both offers were rejected. Issels felt he could do no more than allow events to take their course. He hoped that eventually the rumours would die away in the face of growing proof that he was getting meaningful results.

Earlier that year independent statistical evidence relating to the Ringberg Klinik was produced. It had been collated by Dr. Arie Audier, a psychiatrist from the University of Leiden. Audier had returned to the clinic late in 1958. He took a properly selected random sample of two hundred and fifty-two case histories. They included cases of cancer of the lung, liver, stomach, breast, cervix, jaw, pancreas: in all twenty-two different types of cancer were included in Audier's selection. Next, he verified that all the patients had actually suffered cancer that could be properly termed as beyond surgery, irradiation or chemotherapy.

He interviewed doctors all over Europe who had been involved in the cases at one time or another. He checked the histology, the cell study, of every patient in his sample. He correlated the various treatments they had received in other hospitals with the declining condition, and the remaining life expectancy, of the patients at various stages in their illness before and after treatment at the Ringberg Klinik. Each patient met the following criteria:

All had independently proven histological and clinical results from other hospitals proving a conclusive diagnosis of malignant cancer that was no longer treatable by conventional means.

All had secondaries.

All had entered the clinic before May, 1954, to meet the criteria of the accepted five-year cure period for cancer.

All had received two months of the combined therapy.

Comparative numbers of cases had to be sufficient to allow statistical evaluation. Comparative numbers of patients from other hospitals, treated normally, had to be available for analysis.

It took Audier weeks of careful research to meet such exacting standards. He received assistance from members of the Leiden University faculty. Finally, Audier found that forty-two of the patients, all 'terminal' cases with a life expectancy of under one year, had survived for five years and led 'a normal life'. That gave, on his sampling, a statistical cure rate of 16·6 per cent for patients written-off as beyond further treatment by some of the most famous hospitals in Europe. Statistically, such patients, according to the figures of the World Health Organisation and the International Union Against Cancer, would have experienced 'spontaneous regression' in under 2 per cent. Issels had obtained eight times better results with his treatment. It was a highly significant conclusion. Even the dry, objective and noncommittal style of Audier's paper failed to hide his assertion that the treatment methods at the Ringberg Klinik deserved acceptance:

> On the basis of the above figures and our interpretations, we are convinced that there exists a necessity for immunological treatment after operative and radiation treatment. All patients should after operation and deep-ray treatment, as a matter of course, be given immunological after-treatment to reduce the danger of metastases and to increase the number of complete cures. The above results have confirmed the awareness that only close co-operation between surgical, radiological and internal ther-

apy for cancer will bring about an improvement in the chances of complete cure.

Audier's reputation as a serious scientific investigator was respected in European medical circles. Yet one German medical journal after another rejected his paper. No official reason was given. But Audier later claimed one medical editor told him:

> Highly interesting though my findings were, he could not publish them for one basic reason: they applied to Issels and the Ringberg Klinik. The editor explained that for some years it had been a policy among the leading journals to publish nothing relating to either Issels or his clinic. To publish my paper would have meant seriously upsetting some powerful men in the German cancer world.

Audier was a resourceful man. He expanded his paper to include a more general approach to 'The Problems of Immunological Cancer Therapy'. References to Issels were buried in the text, though the importance of his work remained clear to scientists used to picking their way through the arid wastes of such reports. The paper was finally accepted for publication by *Die Medizinische,* a German medical journal of high repute, with, according to its editor, no prescribed policy for contributors; the Audier paper was accepted 'because it was of interest'.

Its appearance in medical circles caused a flurry of excitement. Doctors all over Europe wrote to the clinic for further information; some travelled from Sweden, Belgium and England to investigate at first-hand the remarkable evidence of full cures that Audier reported. Later those doctors heard another, and more sinister story: that the Audier report was untrue. Exactly who started that story will never be known.

Members of the German Cancer Society had passed the paper around German statisticians, who found no fault with the methods Audier used to conduct the survey. Audier's findings were now ridiculed on the grounds that in each case he had selected, the original diagnosis had been wrong. Audier later recounted how:

> The word was spread from one medical meeting to another. By sheer repetition it gained credence that none of the cases had ever suffered from cancer. It was a classic example of how the medical establishment will fight to preserve what it believes the *status quo* should be.

The paper dropped out of sight.

The cure rate Audier reported had been achieved without the help of a new drug hailed in 1958 by science reporters as a major discovery in cancer treatment. While cyclophosphamide, popularly known as Endoxana, fell short of the hopes of some newspapers, it nevertheless was an important addition to the conventional means of treating the illness.

It had been developed by a German company, Asta Pharmaceuticals. Endoxana was unusual among cytotoxic drugs in that the side-effects associated with its use were predictable and in almost all cases reversible; all the same they were drastic: alopecia, haemorrhagic cystitis, nausea and vomiting, diarrhoea, mental depression, impotence and dermatitis were listed as possible after-effects from injections of Endoxana. But the manufacturers claimed it had no toxic effects on the liver or kidneys, two important organs for evacuating body poisons in the combined *ganzheitstherapie*. Issels began using the drug. Later he made an important clinical observation that a few other doctors also noticed:

> Giving small doses over a lengthy period did in fact lower the body's resistance, and gave limited success. I decided to change the dosage. Patients received one or two massive doses of cyclophosphamide spaced at an interval of two or three weeks. In that way I believed the immunological mechanism would not be severely impaired as they were by regular smaller doses of the drug.

The recommended dose of Endoxana was 50 to 300 milligrams daily. At the Ringberg Klinik from then on doses of up to 6,000 mg. were given dependent on the patient's weight. The drug was mixed with distilled water and transfused intravenously over a five-minute period. The after-effects were dramatic: white and red cell blood count dropped from 6,000 to around the zero mark. Blood transfusions and standard medicaments restored the situation. Patients became bald overnight under the influence of the drug; the clinic provided women with wigs. Such massive doses produced a spectacular arrest and regression in many types of cancer. It was by no means the complete answer to the disease, but it gave Issels more time to call into the play his immunotherapy and general combined treatment.

He was one of the pioneers of massive infusions of Endoxana. He wrote and lectured on his clinical findings whenever he found an audience. But such high doses were frowned upon by many cancer specialists as reckless experimenting.

Early in 1969 British specialists began to give similar doses to their patients. The results were as beneficial as Issels had seen earlier. One of those specialists—a respected physician in a London teaching hospital who specifically asked that his name be withheld because he feared possible repercussions to his research grants—said in 1970:

> When we heard about Issels' approach to cyclophosphamide many of my colleagues dismissed it as another example of the esoteric. We didn't stop and consider whether he might just be right. As one consultant said to me: 'How can Issels be right, tucked away in the Bavarian mountains?' One of the problems with medicine today is that unless the report comes from one of the big cancer institutes, it is brushed aside. And there is a sort of unwritten law which says 'the more you spend, and tell the world you have spent, the more impressive your claims are bound to be'. Everything is geared to the big cancer institutes. When a man like Issels comes along and says, as he did, 'I have experience with 1,000 patients to prove my point,' he is shrugged off. He didn't have a grant, from say, the Imperial Cancer Research Fund, so how can he possibly be right? That's the sort of thinking which abounds today. In that climate men like Issels haven't a snowball in hell's chance.

Dr. Helgo Teicher had spent a busy summer in 1959 gathering material. He waylaid patients outside the clinic and collected any item of gossip, however unfounded, which would be useful to the Bavarian Medical Association or Professor Walter Büngeler, secretary-general of the national cancer society. Teicher found his activities so demanding that he recruited his wife to help him. Together they flitted among the clinic's patients snatching at anything which sounded remotely incriminating. Teicher had also recruited a contact inside the clinic. Dental surgeon Dr. Rudolf Glaeser handed over case histories and X-rays.

Even with the success he saw with Endoxana, Issels still believed the real answer was immunotherapy. From 1958, his mind was filled with a new and tremendously exciting possibility. Professor Franz Gerlach had accepted the post of Director of Research at the clinic, a position which Issels previously filled himself. Issels saw the arrival of Gerlach as a major advance in his search for an immunological answer to cancer.

Gerlach's reputation was known to cancerologists all over the world for decades. A graduate of the University of Vienna, he remained on the campus as a professor until he retired. He became the Austrian Government's delegate to the League of Nations Committee on infectious diseases in 1937. He worked at the Pasteur Institute in Paris, continuing his life time's research into effective immunological agents. The war years saw him working in a cancer institute in Berlin. In 1946 he returned to Government service, representing Austria at the International Conference of Micro-Biology of Cancer. Three years later he received a prize from the Austrian Cancer Society for yet another paper on immunology. His work in that field brought him further honours; he became a Fellow of the Academy of Medicine in Paris; his papers were read in research centres all over the world. In 1953, eager to study the effects of cancer in sub-tropical conditions, he worked in Government research institutes in Turkey and Chile. Then the Portuguese Department of Health appointed him director of the Central Laboratory for Veterinary Pathology in Angola.

When Gerlach arrived he instituted a series of research programmes which made it familiar to cancer specialists everywhere. He found the work exciting, but both he and his chief assistant, Dr. Irma Heikkilä, whom he married later, increasingly suffered from years in the tropics. They looked for a suitable institute in Europe. A number of research centres offered them posts. But Gerlach, approaching his seventieth birthday, had little enthusiasm for life in a big laboratory in some huge town. He wanted:

> A quiet life. I wanted to live in the country, to enjoy peace as I worked on my studies. That was what attracted me to the Ringberg Klinik. Not only were the research facilities adequate, there was also a firm promise from Dr. Issels that nothing would hamper me in my research into mycoplasma.

He first published his theory about mycoplasma in 1937, showing all human and animal tumours contained a virus-like substance. He was ahead of his time; few cancer-ologists could follow his theory on how mycoplasma could be bred from tumour ascites and turned into a non-pathogenic organism by passing the original culture through culture media. Later, in the post-war years, researchers followed, and expanded, the trail Gerlach had pioneered twenty years earlier. By then Gerlach had produced a bio-logical vaccine against cancer which he had tested first on animals and then on himself. He regularly published proof of its effectiveness in serious scientific journals. He was care-ful in his claims—and modest about the success he achieved. It was an attitude which gained him further respect.

He had brought to the clinic a supply of his vaccine which Issels prescribed to selected patients. Gerlach said it should be administered by intravenous or intramuscular injections. Issels noticed that this method often produced too strong a response in some patients when used in con-junction with whole body treatment. He switched to the homoeopathic way of giving medicine: the vaccine was rubbed on the skin or trickled on to a patient's tongue.

After cancer patients received the drops, many felt a reaction or pain in their tumours; others saw their growths swelled before reducing in size. During the thirty years of intensive research Gerlach observed these occurrences in animals and men but was unable to say precisely why, or, how, the vaccine worked. For him it was:

> Perhaps these occurrences could be considered as immune reactions belonging to the field of allergy. The vaccine follows a path to the tumour, or secondaries, damaging any healthy cell or healthy organ. It attacks only specific tumour tissue which might allow us to suppose the presence of a specific antigen. Such antigen-antibody reactions are well known. I believe this line of research could indicate a way for further development of immunotherapy.

It was a piece of deduction which many clinicians who came to the clinic failed completely to understand: men of the status of Professor John Anderson of King's College Hospital, London, were baffled by how the vaccine worked. On one occasion Gerlach is said to have told Anderson: 'Professor, you shouldn't be too worried about *how* it works, you can *see* it works. In any case, nobody has quite been able to explain exactly how smallpox vaccine works—but we have all *seen* the results.'

Issels found the vaccine had an unexpected side-effect. After receiving drops, a patient sometimes complained of pain in another part of the body where no cancer had previously been diagnosed. X-rays were taken. They showed metastases where the pain occurred that had not been suspected before. The vaccine became an extra aid to diagnosing.

In the clinic wards it was a period of some remarkable remissions. There was Georg Hohner, a twenty-three-year-old lorry driver from Berlin, who shortly before getting married, was diagnosed with cancer of the testes. He postponed his wedding and went into hospital. The right testes was surgically removed early in 1959. Unwilling to undergo follow-up radiotherapy he entered the Ringberg Klinik in April that year. Three months later he was discharged and got married. Ten years later his family doctor, with Hohner's permission, reported to the B.B.C.: 'The patient is still free of all cancer and has produced children.'

That case was one of thirty that the B.B.C. followed up for the year 1959 during its lengthy enquiry into the Ringberg Klinik. In each case, the Corporation's investigators followed similar rules to those Audier laid down for investigating the clinic's claims; in addition the B.B.C. acquired the services of Professor John Anderson, who verified the original diagnosis, is such cases as:

> Case No: 117/58. Mrs. B.S. had a brain tumour which was operated on at the beginning of 1958. It was partially removed. No more could be done for the patient and she went with 'a o per cent survival chance' to the Ringberg Klinik on 3/4/58. She was under 'whole therapy' there until 26/7/58 when she was discharged with the verdict that: 'the growth or the tumour had been stopped.' Dr. Hertel, her physician, said on the 29/1/69 that: 'the patient is well and totally free of cancer.'
>
> Case No: 330/58. Dr. Peter R. Diagnosed carcinoma of the stomach and a metastasis in the liver in 1958. On the 2/3/58 a resection of the stomach was performed and Dr. R. advised his son to attend the Ringberg Klinik. He was admitted on the 16/9/58 and finally discharged on the 6/8/59. In 1969 Dr. R. stated that his son was free of any form of carcinoma. On the 29/1/69 the father rang from U.S.A. to confirm that his son was totally alright, could not be better.
>
> Case No: 270/59. H. Vom S. An inoperable carcinoma of the colon ascendens was diagnosed in 1958. A biopsy was performed by Dr. Derra in Düsseldorf, but due to the condition of the patient no further operative measure was taken. The patient arrived with a 'o per cent survival chance' on the 4/8/58 at the Ringberg Klinik and was finally discharged on the 16/9/59 with a verdict that: 'the tumour had reduced in size.' Dr. Faulenbach states that she last heard of the patient on the 21/1/67 when he was well.
>
> Case No: 326/58. T.U. A sigmoidal carcinoma was diagnosed. The patient did not undergo an operation, but was

> admitted to the Ringberg Klinik with a 'o per cent survival chance' on the 15/3/58. He was under 'whole therapy' and was also advised to undergo an operation to remove the tumour. This operation was performed locally at the Tegernsee Hospital and the patient survived until 26/4/63 when he died. According to Dr. Rothardt the patient died as a result of a road accident. Dr. Rothardt also stated that he was well until that time, and totally free of cancer.

By August, 1959 Issels had personally treated some 2,500 men, women and children who had all been adjudged by other doctors as being beyond further treatment. The majority had gained worthwhile extensions to their lives, amounting to several years in many cases.

By August, Charlotte, Issels' sister who administered the clinic, insisted he took a holiday—alone, away from Isa. Charlotte said she did that because she felt her brother needed a complete rest from everybody. Isa later claimed the holiday was her idea: she hoped that it would: 'Give Jupp a chance to finally make up his mind about whether we would marry. I had known him a year. I knew my mind was made up. I wanted to marry him. But I did not want to force matters.'

Whoever suggested it, Issels packed his bags and left the clinic. But after six days of sunning himself at Kampen, a North Sea resort, the separation from Isa became too much. He telephoned her to join him. When they met he proposed.

The wedding date was set for November 6, 1959. Before that day Issels called on his first wife, Irmengard:

> He came to me [she later said] and after some small talk, came right out with it: *did I want to re-marry him?* I said that was out of the question. He asked me if I was quite sure and I said that I was. Though I still loved him I could not go back to a life that had been impossible. Then he calmly announced that he was going to marry Isa. I never understood why he had asked me if I would re-marry him. Afterwards I wondered what would have happened if I had said, 'yes, let's try again.' I also had a feeling that maybe he wanted me to approve of his choice of a second

wife. Isa was a very nice woman, and I told him I hoped they would be very happy together.

Issels maintained he had only discussed the question of his re-marrying with Irmengard because of the children: he insisted his proposal to his first wife had been no more than a wish to 'establish the exact situation'—though exactly what that meant he never made clear.

After he married Isa he remained friendly with Irmengard. She returned to the clinic once to assist with administrative work when Isa was ill. Irmengard admitted a feeling of satisfaction that the clinic retained a visible mark of the years she spent working there; a building was named *Haus Irmengard*. Only one other woman received such a public accolade. There was a *Haus Adelheid*, in memory of Issels' mother.

Isa Klos was thirty years old when she married. Her husband was over twenty years older. She never felt any age gap. If there was such a thing as a typical marriage, then theirs was far from that. Apart from her wifely duties, Isa played many other parts in a way few have recognised. She was listener, adviser and mentor, and she managed all her roles without losing her own identity. She was an intelligent and vivacious woman, married to a man who already had experienced the fruits of a broken union, whose emotional involvement was frequently linked with the memory of his mother, and who was utterly involved with his work. In many ways Isa was a friend, audience and critic. But she never assumed the role of a second mother to him. As the children came—Hellmut in 1960, Christian in 1965—she played in some ways the role of father to them. Though Issels was a concerned parent in moments of crisis, the daily existence of children was seldom allowed to interrupt work; nor did he always find it easy to accept the changes which came to a household when a new generation claimed its rightful place. Yet, with a growing family, Isa still maintained a close interest in her husband's work. It was that quality, above all others, which nourished the marriage.

By the summer of 1960 Isa had created a home which reflected her own quiet good taste. It was a place Issels relaxed in fully: in the evenings, when Hellmut was asleep, he and Isa sat and talked about literally everything. From the outset she saw that:

> The important thing is to maintain a sense of perspective with Jupp. He can be difficult, tempestuous and sometimes totally undiplomatic. But I believe that all men of genius are like that and the important thing is not to be blinded by his brilliance.

Sensibly, she never allowed that to happen. Time and again she spotted the weakness in an argument he advanced, an attitude he adopted, a belief he clung to. Then she challenged him with rare honesty—yet never sacrificed an iota of her loyalty to him and what he represented. She once said: 'Nobody can ever suspect his motives because they are so utterly honest. But often his ways of explaining things have not been those most likely to encourage their easy acceptance.'

Her role, though she disliked the word, was to see that he explained his motives to the world in a way everybody understood.

In that first year of marriage Issels clearly established his own standing within the relationship. While he was the unchallenged head of the household, he rarely became involved with the details of its running. It was enough that he paid the bills; he had no interest in the trivialities of existence.

Isa accepted the situation and the summer of 1960 passed pleasantly. Issels began work on a second medical book about his theories. Isa took over responsibility for purchasing the clinic's needs, organised soirées for patients, supervised their diets and paid regular social calls on foreign patients who came from all over Europe, the Americas and South Africa. They were referred by specialists who confirmed no further treatment was possible in their hospitals. Over 300 patients had been admitted that year and less than a score had died. Professor Gerlach produced a new batch of vaccine in July, and the first indications suggested it gave even better results. By early September Isa was regularly discussing with the clinic's housekeeper, details of the ninth anniversary party for the staff, scheduled for the evening of September 15.

That day dawned unusually fine. The sun was already warm by the time Issels rose and showered at 7 a.m. He drank a coffee for breakfast, kissed Isa goodbye, and drove the seven minutes to the clinic. He wore newly pressed white trousers, a white shirt and white tie. At the clinic he slipped on a white coat. Sharp at 7.30 a.m. he began visiting the more seriously ill patients. There were only four that morning. By 8 a.m. he had seen them all. He made his way to Ward One. There Dr. Gally Galiatsatos, the ward doctor, and the ward sister, joined him for the regular morning round.

By 9 a.m. they reached Room 18, knocked on the door and entered. So far the round had given Issels great personal pleasure: almost every patient showed signs of improvement. That happy situation continued in Room 18, where a man with stomach cancer had lain for weeks showing little sign of getting better. But that morning he was definitely improved. There was colour in his cheeks and a lift to his voice which had not been there before. Issels looked at the treatment chart. It confirmed definite clinical progress. As he put down the chart a nurse knocked and entered.

'Chief, can I please have a word with you outside?'

Issels went into the corridor. The nurse told him two men were waiting in his office demanding to see him immediately.

'Now? But I am in the middle of a ward round.'

'I told them that. But they insisted,' said the nurse.

'Who are they?'

'I don't know. But they said it was very important.'

Issels grunted. In nine years at the clinic his ward rounds had never been interrupted. Clearly it was some sort of emergency that relatives felt he only could deal with.

'Very well. I'll see them.'

He walked to his office on the ground floor. Standing by his desk was one man. The other stood by the office door studying a photograph of Issels and Pope Pius XII at the Vatican meeting. Both moved towards him as he entered.

'Dr. Josef Issels?' one man asked.

'Yes.'

'We are police officers. We have a warrant for your arrest.'

One of the policemen produced a typewritten document and handed it to Issels. It was the formal warrant ordering his arrest. The officers watched impassively as Issels read Warrant No: 1 GS 300/60, five pages of accusation which stunned him.

The document's opening preamble stated:

> The accused claims to treat the cancer disease and even to cure the so-called incurable cancer patients by means of the so-called tumour therapy. In fact the accused has neither reliable diagnostic methods nor a method to treat cancer successfully. It is contended from his behaviour that he is aware of the complete ineffectiveness of the so-called internal tumour treatment. The accused must be held in custody because he might flee or conceal information. Further, the accused has patients from abroad. For some time those patients were asked by him to deposit their fees with foreign bankers. The accused is not bound to the Federal Republic and he has to count the fact that he will be unable to practise at least to the same extent as he has until now, which has involved him in an extremely high income. Therefore the assumption is justified that he would try in future to work abroad.

The document listed a number of specific and non-specific charges. The specific accusations charged Issels with defrauding four patients and 'manslaughter by negligence' of two of them. The patients were:

Karl Wiesinger, from Coburg. He had been at the clinic from July until September, 1954 and for a further period in January and February, 1955. He had died at home on September 23, 1955.

Richard Vogel, from Tübingen, near Stuttgart. He had been a patient from November, 1958 until January, 1959. He died at home on July 6, 1959.

Rudolf Schönek from Detroit, U.S.A. He came to the clinic in April, 1958 and stayed there until the day he died, July 9, 1958.

Friedrich Dehm who was admitted in November, 1959 and stayed until January, 1960. He died on March 11, 1960.

The manslaughter charges referred to Wiesinger and

Vogel. Issels was accused of preventing them undergoing surgery for their cancer. The fraud charges accused him of taking money from all four patients 'knowing there was no hope of the promised cure'.

The non-specific allegations said that Issels had deliberately faked case-histories showing he had urged surgery when the opposite was true, and 'knowingly presenting photographs at his lectures to patients of cases which failed to reflect a true clinical condition'.

Issels was shattered by the enormity of the charges. He denied them to the two policemen. They looked as impassive as ever. The next minutes remained in his mind forever:

> I asked them what was to happen. They said they would take me to prison. I protested that I had sick patients. Surely I could complete my rounds first.
>
> 'No.'
>
> I asked if I could tell the ward doctor to continue with the round.
>
> 'No. Send somebody else.'
>
> I buzzed my secretary and told her to do that. I looked at my clothes. They were highly unsuitable for prison. One of the men said I could go home and change. Outside I walked to my car. A policeman came with me. That was the moment I really felt my freedom going. Isa was in the kitchen when I reached home. I remember her face: a smile of surprised welcome, then a sudden fear as she saw the two men. I explained what had happened. She just shook her head and kept saying: 'It's a mistake, all a mistake.' A policeman said we had to hurry. He came upstairs with me and watched me change. I skimmed through my wardrobe wondering what would be suitable for prison. I chose a grey suit, packed my toilet bag and went downstairs. Isa was very calm. She said: 'It will only be a few days at the most. Then they'll discover it's all a mistake. Look upon it as a rest. There'll be no telephone there to bring you problems.' I kissed her goodbye and walked out of the house.

Exactly nine years from the day he drove into the Tegernsee Valley to open the Ringberg Klinik Josef Issels was escorted out again like a common felon. He increasingly felt that behind the warrant lay, not so much a prosecution, but more a persecution. As the police car travelled around the lake he fancied he saw more than one familiar face looking curiously at him. He did not care about that; what concerned him were his patients. He felt they would die without his help.

10

Imprisoned

By mid-morning Issels found himself locked in cell number six in Miesbach County Jail. After the initial shock of the arrest wore off, he sat on the edge of the cell's iron cot staring blankly into his memories.

The warning signs had always been there. In Mönchen-Gladbach the hospital's administration had banned him from treating cancer patients. A colleague had warned him the night before he left the town of the dangers involved in pursuing his beliefs. In Rottach-Egern, the local medical association disbelieved his advertised claim of offering positive treatment for the conventionally untreatable. He had openly clashed with one of the most powerful figures in German medicine, Professor Karl Bauer. His papers had been rejected by the leading medical journals. He had been denied the right to express his views at cancer congresses through the intervention among others, of Professor Dietrich of the German Cancer Society. His appeals to have the Ringberg Klinik assessed by independent medical experts had fallen on deaf ears. Yet, until that morning in Miesbach prison, he had no real concept of how deep-rooted the opposition was. The arrest warrant dispelled any doubts, not only that he faced a grave personal crisis, but also about his very philosophy that treatment was medically possible outside that prescribed. That much was clear from the cases in the indictment.

Friedrich Dehm, a director of a Munich savings bank, had been close to his sixty-first birthday when he had been admitted to the Rechts-der-Isar Hospital in Munich and swiftly diagnosed, in July, 1956, with cancer of the left lung. The lung was removed by surgery. He made a normal recovery and was discharged. For two years he showed no further symptoms of cancer. Then, in November, 1958, he became suddenly paralysed in the left larnyx. For months he coped, with increasing difficulty, with a worsening condition. In the spring of 1959 he consulted his family doctor who arranged for a biopsy of the larynx to be taken. It was found to be inconclusive. But Dehm's condition steadily worsened. Further tests were carried out; Dehm was found to have cancer of the bronchus advanced beyond conventional treatment. He volunteered to go to the Ringberg Klinik, and was admitted on November 14, 1959.

Early on at the clinic his wife, Emilie, complained that her husband's food was cold, that a nurse was impolite, that things were not exactly as she would have ordered them. The allegations were carefully investigated by Issels and found to have no substance. It emerged that Emilie Dehm had a past history of complaining about those who had looked after her husband.

Dehm's medical treatment included the extraction of three teeth, tonsilectomy, infusions of the chemotherapy drug, Endoxana, and drops of the Gerlach vaccine. By January, 1960, his condition showed no response to treatment.

Emilie Dehm continued to complain about the food and nursing attention. Investigation again showed the charges were baseless.

On January 23, Dehm discharged himself, complaining of vague dissatisfaction with the treatment. His stay at the clinic had incurred charges of DM 5,000 to cover his medical treatment and accommodation for his wife and himself during the nine weeks they stayed at the Ringberg Klinik. Dehm paid DM 4,000, but his wife refused to pay the outstanding DM 1,000 because she believed there had been no 'positive treatment'. She felt sure of her grounds, not only legally, but also medically, after Dr. Helgo Teicher and

Dr. Rudolf Glaser called on her when her husband had returned home.

Precisely what occurred at that meeting is not known. What is clear is that the two doctors tendered their medical opinion that Dehm had received improper treatment. Afterwards, on February 19, 1960, her son, Gunther Scheibeck, a Munich lawyer, took down an affidavit from his dying step-father. It listed a string of trivial complaints that had already been investigated, and rejected, by the clinic. But there were other, more serious, allegations in the eight-page document. Dehm had returned home with a series of X-rays taken at the clinic. But, due to an administrative error in the clinic's X-ray department, Dehm received *one* plate of another patient. It was an unfortunate mistake, but one which could happen in any busy hospital. It was an error that Scheibeck seized upon as an example of fraud. For the plate showed a clinical picture of improvement in a patient—but that patient had not been Dehm. In his affidavit Dehm claimed a deliberate attempt had been made to trick him, to make him 'part with about DM 3,000 to DM 4,000'. He had spent the money 'because Dr. Issels promised a cure knowing it was impossible, and had done so just to receive my money'. Doctors and lawyer worked on the affidavit, injecting medical terms into the dry legal paragraphs, giving a sinister interpretation to an error that the clinic's radiographer openly admitted to later as a genuine mistake. By then the affidavit had long been lodged with the Public Prosecutor in Munich. In Dehm's name it called for the prosecution of Josef Issels. On March 11, 1960, Friedrich Dehm died.

The Public Prosecutor added Dehm's case to that of commercial traveller Karl Wiesinger. He had been fifty-nine years old when his family doctor in Coburg diagnosed cancer of the penis. Wiesinger received injections of Iseador, a biological preparation derived from mistletoe. In 1952 the Dermatology Clinic at Würzburg University confirmed the continued presence of cancer and recommended surgery. Wiesinger refused. He had a deep-rooted fear of any operation.

In January, 1954 Wiesinger was seen by Dr. Helmut Schmidt, medical director of the *Landeskrankenhaus* in

Coburg. Schmidt urged a biopsy to establish the state of malignancy. Wiesinger refused that simple surgical procedure. He looked around for a kind of treatment which would not involve him in an operation.

On July 7, 1954 he arrived at the Ringberg Klinik. Issels' examination revealed a nut-like lump on the penis. He suggested to Wiesinger that surgery, after all, was the answer; Wiesinger could return to the clinic for post-operative treatment. Wiesinger refused to even consider that suggestion. Issels then began his normal treatment.

On September 10, 1954, Wiesinger was discharged from the clinic. His physical condition had markedly improved. But the growth remained unchanged. Issels again suggested that Wiesinger consider an operation—and met with another flat refusal. In November Wiesinger wrote to Issels, 'my tumour is growing again'. He returned to the clinic on January 11, 1955. The growth was bigger and there was swelling in the groin. Issels again urged surgery. Wiesinger stubbornly resisted the advice. Normal combined treatment began.

Shortly afterwards Wiesinger travelled, without the knowledge of anybody in the Ringberg Klinik, to Munich University Hospital. He was seen by a consultant. Wiesinger did not reveal to that doctor that he was a patient at the clinic. He received familiar advice: surgery was the answer. He refused and returned to the clinic. After a month's further treatment he left, with the original clinical picture unchanged. The following May his family doctor in Coburg gave him a course of injections, never specified, and the tumour mushroomed to the size of a plum. On June 24, 1955 Wiesinger finally overcame his fear of surgery and his penis was amputated at the University of Erlangen hospital. A month later he underwent further surgery to remove a gland in the groin, received follow-up radiotherapy, but died on September 23, 1955.

Seven full months had passed since he had been treated at the Ringberg Klinik. In that time he had received injections, surgery and radiotherapy.

On May 5, 1956, one of the doctors who had unsuccessfully treated him, Dr. Gunther Barth, director of the Radiotherapy Institute at Erlangen, wrote to Mrs. Wiesinger explaining he was one of a dozen doctors: 'Interested in your husband's illness and we would like to use his case-notes for a scientific society interested in the cancer question.'

The scientific interest of that society was never revealed—though it became clear an organisation of sorts existed for the express purpose of ending the career of Josef Issels. It also remained a close secret just how case-notes allegedly obtained for a serious medical purpose ended up in the hands of the Public Prosecutor. Somewhere along the line medical and legal opinion fused to produce in the warrant a picture far different to the clinical notes held by the Ringberg Klinik:

> The accused, against his duty, kept the patient from surgery. When the patient asked the accused about surgery that had been recommended elsewhere, Issels omitted, again against his duty, to insist on the necessity of an operation. He even actually opposed it. The patient paid between DM 3,000 and DM 4,000 for treatment only because he had confidence in the treatment methods of the accused.

It is hardly likely that Wiesinger would have paid if he had *not* retained confidence in the treatment. Nevertheless, the warrant felt it necessary to hammer home the point to sustain fraud.

Wiesinger's case was further reinforced in the warrant by that of Richard Vogel's, a fifty-three-year-old janitor from Tübingen, near Stuttgart. In October, 1958, the E.N.T. Clinic at Tübingen University confirmed by biopsy that Vogel suffered from advanced larynx carcinoma with metastases in the lower jaw, the size of a plum. Vogel refused surgery, and on November 5, 1958, Professor E. Schwarz, the clinic's director, reported in his case-notes: 'the prognosis is very dubious'. That day Vogel entered the Ringberg Klinik—a verified case of progressive cancer.

After examination Issels decided that surgery could still offer a solution—with the clinic providing follow-up treatment. Vogel refused the suggestion. A week later his wife, Frieda, wrote to Issels that her husband was 'unhappy with the diet and would like to go home. Please use your influence to make him stay'. After talking to Issels, Vogel agreed to remain at the clinic.

On December 27, 1958, Dr. Helgo Teicher, then employed at the clinic, wrote to Vogel's insurance company AOK-Tübingen:

> As you know we have to deal with a very extensive larynx carcinoma. The present situation now indicates the success of surgery to be dubious. Therefore the patient has come here to undergo intense biological treatment which, according to our experience, has the highest chances of stopping such a process and obtaining improvement.

In that December, a further incident occurred which Teicher observed. Issels again discussed with Vogel the need for surgery. He ordered Teicher, Vogel's ward doctor, to officially record in the case-notes the statement: 'patient still refuses surgery'. Later, Issels checked and found the entry had not been made. Teicher said he had delegated the job to a junior doctor. Issels confronted her. She said she refused to make the entry on the grounds that Vogel was too deaf to have understood Issels. He ordered her to make the entry claiming Vogel had understood him. Teicher included the incident in his regular reports to the Bavarian Medical Association. The incident was passed on to the Public Prosecutor—and it formed the basis of the warrant's reference to falsifying case-notes.

Vogel continued to worsen. Issels, as he had done with other acute cases, called upon outside help, referring Vogel, in January 1957, to Professor A. Hermann at the E.N.T. Clinic at Munich University. He recommended radiotherapy. It was carried out at Vogel's home town clinic at Tübingen University Hospital under the supervision of Professor E. Schwarz. The treatment produced measurable relief, but by June Vogel needed further irradiation. He died on July 6, 1959.

Afterwards Professor Walter Büngeler, then secretary-general of the national cancer society wrote to Schwarz that Vogel's case might be used to stop the 'peculiar' treatment at the Ringberg Klinik. It was only a step for Vogel's file to end up with the Public Prosecutor, Dr. Parsch, who contended in the warrant:

> The accused was opposed to surgical intervention. He decided he could cure the case by other means and surgery was not performed. When Dr. Teicher succeeded in getting Vogel presented to Professor Hermann in Munich, who, together with Professor Schwarz from Tübingen, both saw it was too late for surgery. Vogel, as a janitor, could only afford the costs of DM 3,000 with the help of others, and he spent the money because of the promises of the accused that his methods alone would be successful.

The prosecution alleged a similar promise—amounting to a cruel fraud—had been made in the case of Rudolf Schönek, a thirty-two-year-old draughtsman from Detroit, U.S.A.

In January, 1952, a pigmented naevus of the forehead was removed by surgery at the Memorial Hospital in Van Dyke, Michigan. The pathological report on the tissue was Melanomablastoma. The report showed the lesion had not been 'adequately excised'. At the end of January further surgery was performed, including removing the frontalis muscle of the forehead. A split thickness graft was taken from the thigh and applied to the defect. The pathological tissue failed to reveal further signs of malignancy.

Two months later Schönek underwent further surgery to secure the skin graft. During a post-operative check enlarged lymph nodes were noted in his neck. In September, 1957, a 2 cm.-sized lymph node was excised from the posterior triangle of the neck. The pathologist's report was Metastatic Malignant Melanoma. Schönek was wheeled into the operating theatre again, this time for a 'right radical neck dissection including the pariaricular area and paratoid area'—major surgery which left him permanently scarred. The pathological reports revealed no signs of malignancy.

Schönek made a normal recovery, But in March, 1958, he returned to the Memorial Hospital with new and alarming symptoms. His clinical notes revealed:

> Patient complained of pain about the right hip and near

the tip of the spine, increasing constipation, urinary symptoms of frequency, urgency, nocturia and burning sensation on voiding. An X-ray of the lumbosacral spine showed slight compression of the body of the 11th thoraxic vertebra with loss of anterior cortical detail. The possibility of beginning metastatic involvement of the 11th thoraxic vertebral body is to be considered. Severe pain in the area of the right hip and parasthesia in the left groin and perineal area. He has received large doses of Chlorpromazine and Meparidine HC1 but with little relief. It is felt that these pains are probably secondary and metastatic involvement of the cord or nerve roots. A lumbar puncture was performed, and a catheter inserted to take over normal functions.

At that point, March, 1958, Schönek's brother, Gabriel, a Detroit businessman, telephoned the Ringberg Klinik but Issels was not given a full clinical picture. If he had been, he claimed he would have advised against the journey. Instead, the telephone call left Issels with the impression that Rudolf Schönek was in a relatively good physical state, able to walk and in control of his bodily functions.

He arrived at the Ringberg Klinik on April 6, 1958, partially paralysed in the lower half of his body. With him came his wife, Magdalene and Gabriel, who paid for their trip and stay at the clinic. Examination revealed that Rudolf Schönek was in a critical condition. Issels began to treat him, using chemotherapy as well as the combined regime. Schönek steadily worsened. By June he received regular heavy doses of morphine; a month later, on July 7, 1958, he died at the clinic.

The warrant indicted Issels of fraud because:

According to all doctors who had treated this patient, he was a hopeless case. Yet in spite of the complete hopeless state of the patient the accused promised to the patient and his wife on their arrival at the clinic that after four weeks there would be an improvement. Only because of this they made financial efforts to pay for the treatment. The costs for Schönek and his wife amounted to DM 10,000.

By the end of the morning in his cell at Miesbach Jail, Issels was convinced the accusations against him were totally unfounded. Later that day he penned six pages of calm rebuttal: Wiesinger and Vogel, whose deaths formed the manslaughter charges, had been repeatedly urged by him to undergo surgery and both refused. No promises had ever been made to the patients or their relations about a cure. In a crisp paragraph he rejected the non-specific allegations in the warrant:

> It is impossible to falsify X-ray plates because they are completely outside my control from the moment they are exposed. The allegations of banking money outside the Federal Republic are a travesty of the truth. There was only one case, a French patient, who experienced difficulty in his own country with currency exchange regulations. I told him he could open an account for me in Paris to cover a balance-of-treatment payment of about DM 300, a trifling sum.

Issels was convinced when the Public Prosecutor read his statement the whole case would collapse.

Isa also came to the same conclusion by the end of a full day. It began when she called a meeting of the clinic's doctors and enlisted their support in keeping the news of Issels' arrest from patients and staff. Some of the staff had to be told—they were members of the family. Isa's sisters-in-law, Charlotte and Maria, and Maria's husband, Paul Lamerz, worked in the clinic's administration. That first family council was united by shock and disbelief. Later, when Isa emerged as the natural link between defence lawyers, the family took time to accept that this should be so. But after their first deliberations all were convinced that Issels would be soon freed—especially as they planned to retain Dr. Alfred Seidl to defend him. Seidl was one of a handful of German lawyers whose name was widely known as a skilled courtroom tactician.

Next day, September 16, the world knew of the arrest. The German press, rarely slow to miss a sensation, especially a medical one, bannered across front pages the words FRAUD CLINIC and MANSLAUGHTER.

The police then made a move which gave the Issels family a lasting impression that, in the words of Isa, 'the warrant was little more than a device to close the clinic and wreck the whole concept of combined treatment for cancer'. A detective sealed the clinic archives after removing twenty-two cases. In all the police took away some four hundred case files.

When she saw the newspapers, Isa drove to Miesbach Jail and persuaded the chief warder to keep them away from her husband.

Unaware that he was the topic of speculation over breakfast tables everywhere, Issels had slept soundly, awakened early, and used his time doing physical exercises in his cell. Later, during outside exercise, he played football and chopped fire wood. Later, he met Seidl, who accepted the case. A mood emerged in which Issels believed he would be soon released on bail, or even possibly allowed out of prison during daylight hours to treat his patients. Eighteen of them had delivered a petition to the Public Prosecutor in Munich urging a similar course of action.

Isa and Issels met in Miesbach Jail late on September 16. It set a pattern for later encounters: it was brisk and businesslike:

> I was afraid to make him sad [Isa said later]. Nor would that help matters. Time was always short for essentials, leave alone personal matters. Jupp used me as a messenger service to the clinic doctors. I relayed advice, instructions on doses, and the general management of patients. They were always foremost in his mind.

Immediately he accepted the case Alfred Seidl set his legal sails to catch a faint breeze. He demanded before a judge in chambers that Issels be freed on the grounds there was no evidence to suggest he would flee the country. The motion was denied. Seidl, a lawyer of considerable legal acumen was not dismayed. Five days later he again challenged the validity of Issels' imprisonment on the grounds that the prosecution proceeded in an unusual manner. No attempt had been made to interview Issels or his clinic doctors and staff. Again he was refused.

Early in October Issels was moved to the fortress-like Stadelheim Prison in Munich. He found himself in solitary confinement in a wing filled with hardened criminals. Even though he was a remand prisoner he was forced to wear striped convict garb. On October 3, Seidl put on another dazzling display of legal fireworks. He urged Issels should be bailed because 'patients are in danger of their very lives because they have been deprived of their doctor'. He had fifteen expert witnesses, including Professor Werner Zabel and clinic doctors, to testify that it was safe to free Issels to continue his work. The witnesses stated that Issels sincerely believed in his methods, that he often gave free treatment and that the fees were within the scale of private clinics in Germany. Clinic doctors and nurses swore that Issels never made any promise of a cure. Seidl offered bail of DM 250,000, raised through mortgaging the clinic. It was refused.

Seidl was baffled. Issels was being treated as a dangerous criminal. Yet the charges barely supported such an attitude. There was no suggestion of deliberate murder in the deaths of Wiesinger and Vogel. It was 'manslaughter by negligence', serious enough, but by no means a capital charge: it was the sort of charge a drunken driver could face. The sums involved in the alleged frauds were small. The other charges in the warrant in no way justified, in Seidl's opinion, the denial of his client's liberty. The lawyer came to the conclusion that Issels was being held in custody not because of what he was alleged to have done, but for what he represented. If Issels was held for long enough it was likely that his clinic and his beliefs would suffer such serious set-backs that he would never recover.

The defence felt that was what lay behind the whole prosecution. The first evidence had been lodged with the Public Prosecutor early in 1959. Since then a mass of material, much of it turning on expert medical interpretation, had been collated. From the warrant it was clear that the material had been poorly interpreted. Teicher and Glaeser had made statements, though the police could not have felt entirely happy about their two key witnesses. Nor had the police interviewed any other medical staff at the clinic, if only to establish how widespread the accusations against Issels might be. Nor had Issels been interviewed before his sudden arrest.

Seidl made another attempt on October 11 to have Issels bailed. He failed again. A few days later he flew to the Far East feeling there was no more he could do until the trial.

Issels looked upon the rigours of Stadelheim Prison as a purgatory to be combated by his own harsh demands of himself. As a remand prisoner he could order food from outside. He chose a staple diet of black bread and garlic, washed down with six pints of water every day. He told his fellow prisoners he was 'building up my body and garlic cleanses the blood'. A number of convicts joined him in this spartan regime, and the cell block reeked like an authentic bistro.

Issels was allowed books. As well as those on philosophy and religion, he ordered Professor Bauer's tome, *Das Krebsproblem*. He recognised, correctly, that the prosecution would lean heavily on this standard work on cancer to bolster the medical charges. He gutted Bauer's theories and felt able to contest them should the need arise. When he was not reading he worked on the draft of his own book on cancer treatment; within a short time he had written 300 pages. He also wrote daily to Isa. After a week in prison, he rationalised for her his captivity:

> All is Fate, including my own will. What happens now must be. I cannot escape. It is written down in my inner brain. Believing that, I cannot be destroyed by my destiny. I have no hate of those who accuse me. Fate will find them out, so that my Fate can be fulfilled. That is why I am not bitter. I have no self-pity. It is my Fate, and knowing that gives me strength to continue the way Fate has directed me.

On their first wedding anniversary he wrote:

> My beloved Isa,
>
> How much I regret that this should happen to you, more so because we have been married for such a little

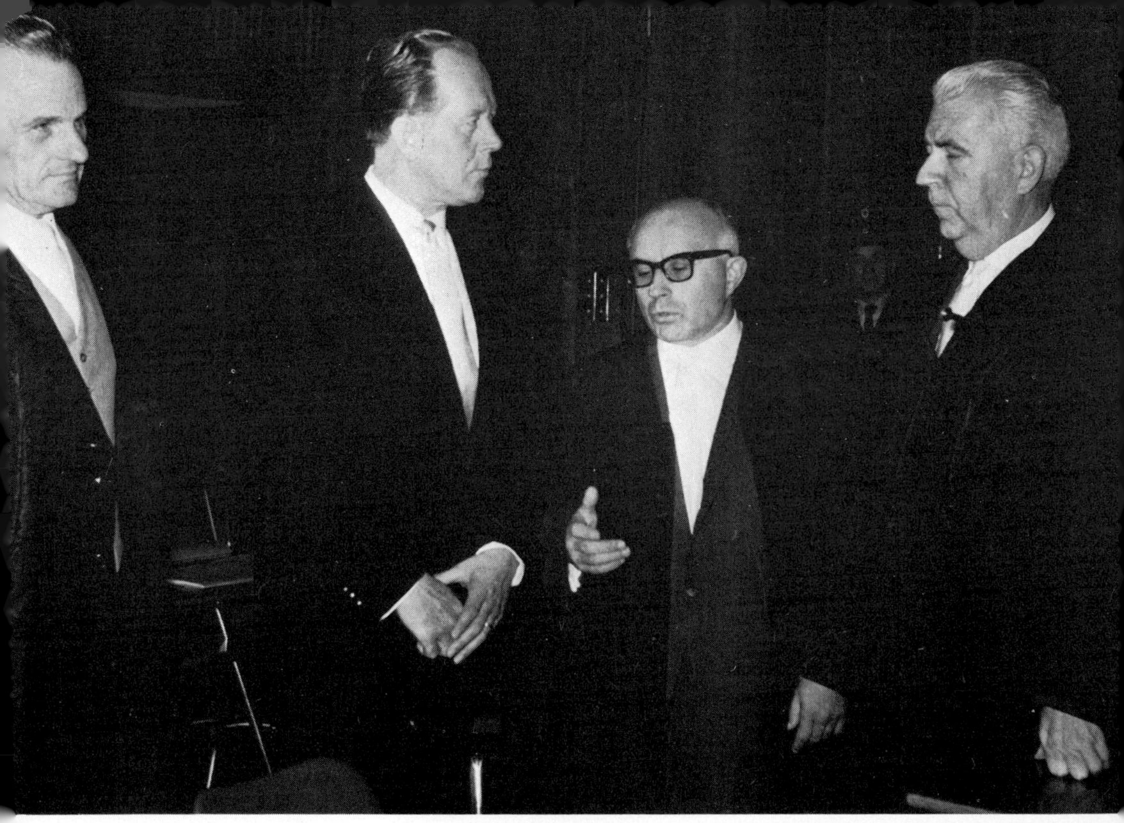

The first trial: (*left to right*) Fock, Issels, Seidl, Kirstein

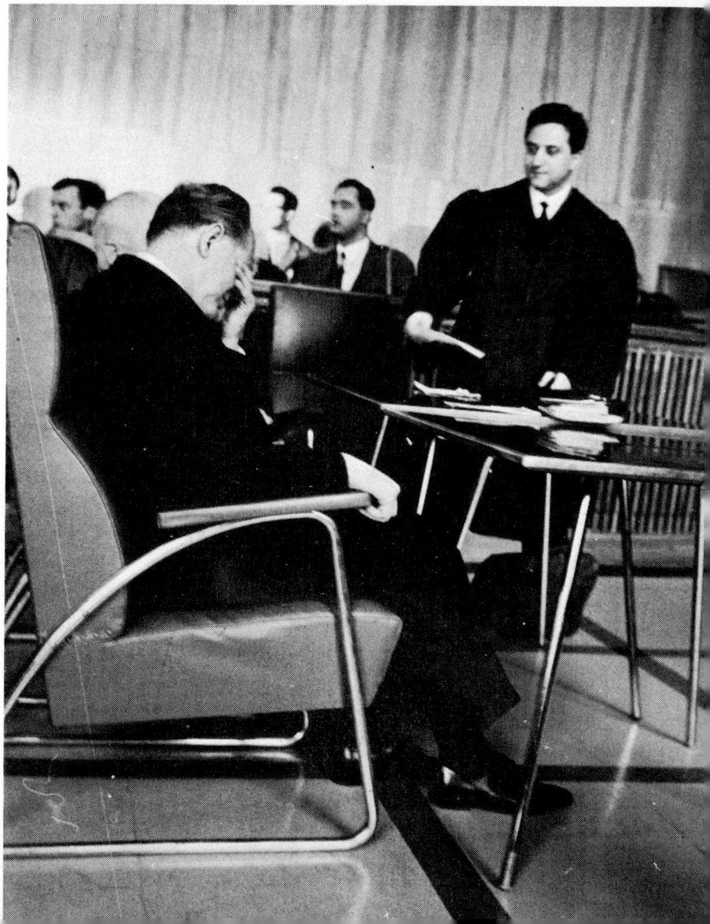

Issels, close to exhaustion, ponders a question by efence lawyer Kückelmann

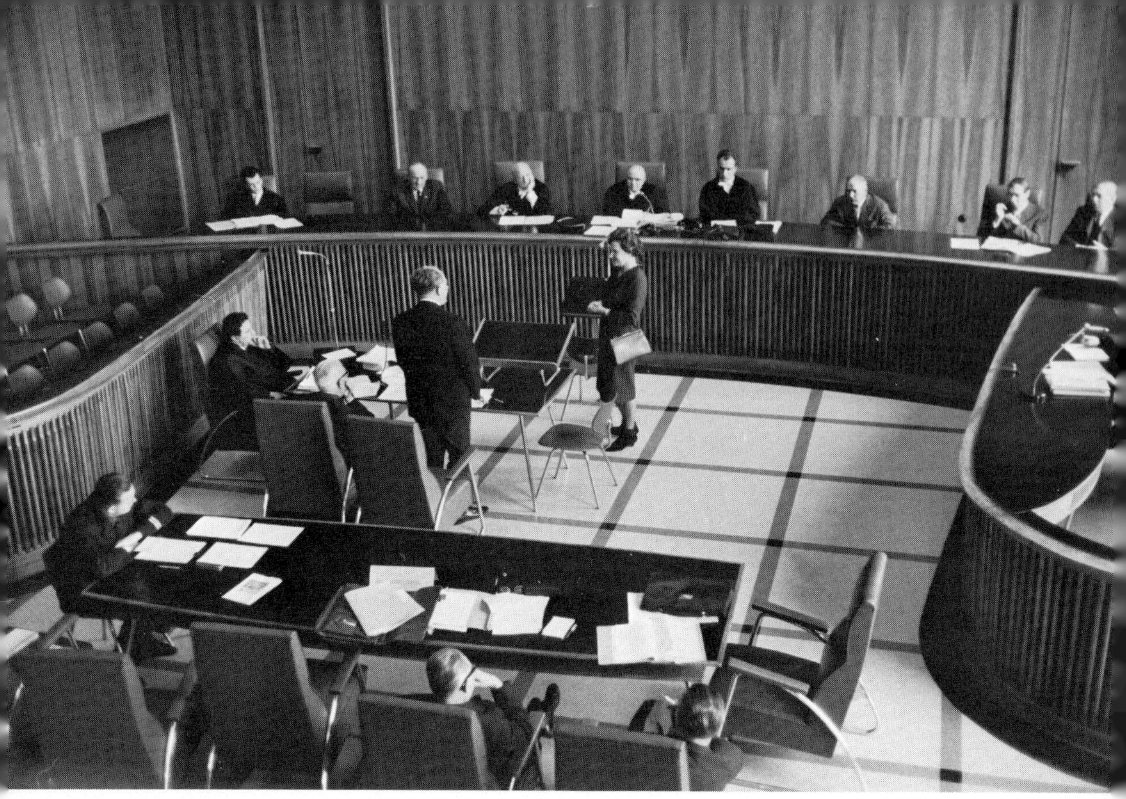

The second trial in session

The day of the experts for the prosecution. First row behind Issels: (*left to right*) Becker, Bauer, Bock and Haplerl

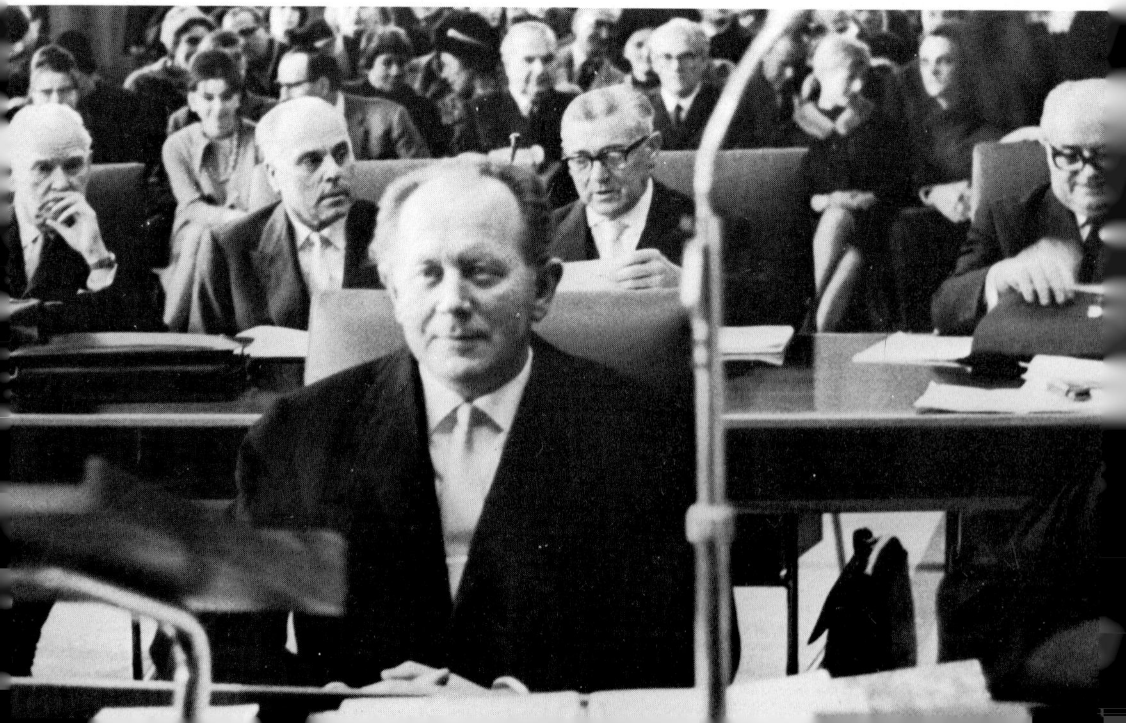

time. I know you do everything to maintain the clinic and yet you cannot prevent its steady decline. I have the impression that the aim of the prosecution is to destroy forever the internal cancer therapy, my clinic, and which is not so important, myself. I do not lose courage, but we have to be realistic. No surgeon or radiotherapist should be free now because they *do* promise cures to their curable patients which I have never done with incurable patients. They often cannot fulfill their promises. All I have done is to try and help those that orthodox methods have failed. That is all. You remember how happy we were and that we used to both be afraid that something could destroy our happiness. Well, they have tried to do that. But they will not succeed. All my love, my confidence, my feelings are with you, my beloved one, and nothing can change that.

Such words helped sustain Isa in an increasingly difficult time. The clinic was in 'steady decline'. By October only a handful of patients remained and the staff were under notice. Among them were doctors who had asked for, and received, five-year contracts shortly before Issels' arrest. Some of them began legal proceedings against the clinic for breach of contract. In the end Issels settled with them. A legal formality also meant that members of the family received notice from positions they looked upon as life-time jobs. Issels later adequately compensated them.

By November, 1960 money increasingly concerned Issels: money for the defence lawyers, money to pay for the expert witnesses needed to rebut the prosecution charges, money to meet clinic debts already standing at DM 60,000. He instructed Isa: 'Sell as much as possible of the clinic grounds to meet the more pressing debts. Make every economy possible. We must now both face the possibility that I will be kept here for months. Talk to Father.'

Isa did, and Ernst Klos, provided all told, DM 90,000 free of interest or security. His wife, Hilda, took over caring for Hellmut. Isa was freed to battle for her husband's freedom. That night she wrote in her daily letter to him:

I am convinced that you are totally innocent. Never forget

> that. All your actions were guided by the highest motives to help your patients. I am proud to be your wife. We have to go through this terrible test, which only later will show both of us why it had been necessary. I pray every day that God will give you the strength to endure this terrible time. I know you have more strength than most others—and I hope that I will also have enough strength to meet the many demands, and to make the right decision. You are a pioneer, so you have to face the tribulations of those who are not. You have been selected to meet these tests. You will overcome all opposition, and I will always be there to offer all my love and strength in this fearful time.

In prison Issels was a popular and respected man among his fellow prisoners and warders. To them he was polite and obliging. But the strain built up; days and weeks had passed and he was still incarcerated for crimes he passionately denied. Nor did the Public Prosecutor seem in any great hurry to bring matters to trial. For Issels, a man used to a full life, his world had shrunk to a few square feet. One night he found himself trembling violently in his cell in a state of acute depression. Next morning he felt little better. During an exercise period he found himself next to a murderer, sentenced to life imprisonment. The man had already served thirteen years. He looked squarely at Issels and said: 'To be here for thirteen years is no reason to lose your personality.'

Issels felt his depression lift. It never returned.

He felt the prison authorities were bent on breaking his spirit. After four weeks in Stadelheim he was transferred to a wing housing only convicted killers, a move for which there is no contingency in the German Penal Code. He found himself harassed and bullied by warders. After three weeks he was transferred back to his old cell block.

Shortly afterwards the Public Prosecutor, Dr. Leo Parsch, began his interrogation of Issels. The sessions were spread over seven hours a day for ten days. Every word was recorded. In the end Issels' statement ran for 178 pages; on every page he denied his guilt and rebutted such hectoring as:

Q: Name the patients from whom you have taken DM 100,000 for treatment.
A: There are no such patients.
Q: Name the patients you have taken DM 50,000 from.
A: There are none. I have already told you that I only have taken DM 7 to DM 10 a day for myself for each patient. No more.
Q: Name the patients who you took DM 20,000 from.
A: There are no such patients. I will stay here all my life if you can prove one case in which I have taken more than DM 7 to DM 10 marks a day.
Q: Do you know we have witnesses to prove otherwise?
A: Have you seen the patients' exact account cards showing exactly what they have paid?

Dr. Parsch later examined the clinic records. He found Issels had only taken up to DM 10 a day for his own services.

By the end of the interrogations, Issels was convinced:

> It will be a show trial. The judge has told my lawyer this. 'If we can convict Issels of fraud we have a list of over 100 other doctors we can also arrest—and then the internal cancer therapy is finished!' My case is the first move to completely close down the internal combined therapy. If they can discredit me they can ensure no other concept outside orthodox belief will ever again have a chance.

On November 26, 1960 the Ringberg Klinik closed. The doctors and nurses dispersed. Professor Gerlach returned to Vienna with his vaccines. The administrative staff found other jobs. Only Isa and housekeeper Annalisa Lipp remained to walk through the deserted corridors. By December 1, the clinic's audited debts stood at DM 1,000,040.

The legal moves continued to try and free Issels. Bail was finally posted at DM 200,000. It was guaranteed by an old school friend of Issels, industrialist Ernst Weller. The two men had not seen each other for ten years. But Weller immediately posted the money. On December 16, Issels was released, pending trial, with a warning he faced immediate re-arrest if he practised medicine while on bail.

11

Waiting for Justice

Many of the patients who had been in the clinic the day he was arrested had died during the three months Issels spent in prison. He always maintained some of their deaths were directly attributable to his not being granted bail at the outset.

Three patients, like ghosts at a wake, waited for him in the reception area when he completed his tour of the clinic buildings the morning after his release from Stadelheim. He found the walk through the deserted clinic a distressing experience. The encounter with those three patients hurt him further. They explained they had stayed at a nearby pension when the clinic closed. News of his return brought them shuffling into the clinic grounds seeking treatment. There were tears in their eyes as they pleaded with him for help. Close to crying himself, Issels gently explained he was legally barred from treating them. They said they would go to the Public Prosecutor in Munich to have the ban lifted. They went—but their pleading failed. Soon afterwards all three died.

The clinic, as an entity, had survived through the efforts of Isa. When financial problems threatened to engulf everything she recognised the only solution was to rent-off the property to avoid it being auctioned over their heads through the demands of the most pressing creditors. She approached every insurance company in West Germany with the proposition they leased the clinic as a sanatorium or a convalescent home. She received curt refusals: the press publicity had turned the Ringberg Klinik into a Brunhilde edifice where only the trolls and warlocks were missing.

Isa next tried to find a private buyer to avoid an auction. Again, there was only one buyer. Through an intermediary, Dr. Julius Ries, director of the Radiotherapy Institute in Munich University, tendered an offer to buy the clinic as a cancer centre offering conventional treatment. Ries had been one of the medical cabal opposed to Issels. Isa refused to entertain his bid. Instead she looked around for any organisation in need of a convalescent home.

Finally, she heard that the *Arbeitsgemeinschaft Für Krebsbekämpfung*, a welfare agency with a special interest in helping cancer patients, needed a sanatorium. She travelled to the agency's head office in Bochum. They agreed to lease the Ringberg Klinik.

Isa and Issels signed a formal agreement with the agency late in December, 1960. The contract specified that the clinic be renamed Sanatorium Bergfrieden, literally 'peace in the mountains'. It would have 150 beds. In return for a weekly income of DM 9,800, Issels provided food, heating, lighting, and all staff, except the doctors. There was one clause which was unusual: 'Dr. Issels has no right to interfere with medical and technical matters.'

A director of the agency bluntly told Issels it meant that if he spoke one word about cancer to any patient or doctor the contract would be immediately cancelled. In practice, the income left Issels with DM 1,500 a week, about £200 sterling. Out of that he had agreed to pay off all his creditors, with interest, in eighteen months. To survive he needed an immediate injection of capital. Twenty banks turned down his attempt to raise a DM 200,000 mortgage on property valued at several times that amount. The twenty-first bank loaned the money because 'it was good business'.

There were people determined not only to destroy Issels in the courts—but also by other means. They used innuendo, smears in the press and scandal-mongering about his professional and social life. The B.B.C. later collated the stories as part of their inquiry. In a document titled *Myths And Rumours Analysed,* the Corporation's investigators stated:

Many rumours circulated about Issels in the period after his arrest. Some of the rumours achieved the status of myths or near-myths. They were even repeated by some honest members of the medical profession as being true. However, when questioned as to the authenticity or source of the rumours, not one doctor gave a convincing answer. In Munich, Bonn, Frankfurt and Heidelberg we met with: 'Professor A, B, or C told the story so it must be true.' When we approached those professors, they passed us on to another source, always vouched as 'thoroughly reliable'. After considerable research it was difficult to escape the conclusion that the rumours were an attempt to blacken Issels' entire reputation.

There was a story which said he had performed abortions on nurses in the clinic. No nurse was ever remotely identified to us as having had a termination at the clinic, or elsewhere, at the instigation of Issels.

There was another story that Issels had been a mental patient during the last war, and that his illness had permanently affected him to the point where he was unable to evaluate any form of medical treatment. We traced that story to an eminent doctor. He denied being the source, though he admitted he believed it true. A thorough examination of Issels' war record failed to reveal any truth in the story. It is reasonable to infer that such lies were promoted to further the medical opposition to Issels.

The nature of the medical opposition can be gauged from an incident on February 24, 1961, when the executive committee of the National Cancer Society met in closed session in Frankfurt-Main. They passed this resolution:

The executive committee has dealt thoroughly in today's session with the take-over of the Issels clinic by the *Arbeitsgemeinschaft für Krebsbekämpfung*. The D.Z.A. (the national cancer society), which had not been consulted before the contract was made, has serious objections to the continuation of the Issels clinic by the *Arbeitsgemeinschaft*. The executive asks the *Arbeitsgemeinschaft* to consider whether the contract made with the Issels couple can be cancelled.

The executive of the national cancer society did more than merely 'ask': it exerted every ounce of its considerable muscle-power to force the agency to change its mind. But the contract was legally binding. Issels, when he discovered what had happened, looked upon it as yet another attempt to ruin him—and it is difficult to find another interpretation for the cancer society's behaviour.

He also felt that the prosecution was at least propped-up, if not actively egged-on, by whole sections of the medical profession in Germany. Dr. Leo Parsch was a competent public prosecutor. But neither he, or his legal assistants, could have hoped to interpret alone the medical evidence. By late 1960, it ran to millions of words (estimates varied between seven to ten million words). There were the four hundred case files the police removed from the clinic: each filed numbered some hundred pages of often technical medical jargon. There were reports from hospitals and clinics all over Germany about patients referred to the Ringberg Klinik. Parsch did not, and could not be expected to, understand much of what he read.

But early on, the prosecution realised it needed more than covert medical opinion to obtain a conviction. So, throughout the icy winter of 1960, a stream of men and women made their way to Dr. Parsch's office in Munich. They were doctors and nurses and relatives of patients who had died in the clinic. The medical staff had all left the clinic for one reason or another; the relations had refused to pay for what they regarded as unsuccessful treatment.

On December 28, 1960, Dr. Parsch lodged with the Munich Criminal Court the *Anklageschrift*, a formal statement of the accusations against Issels, who received a copy.

There were some surprising omissions from the original warrant. Gone were all the allegations that he would flee the country, had secret bank accounts outside Germany, and was a charlatan who switched photographs at his weekly lectures to patients. The prosecution also modified its opinion about his treatment. In the arrest warrant of September it had flatly stated: 'The accused has neither reliable diagnostic methods nor a method to treat cancer successfully . . . he is aware of the complete ineffectiveness of the so-called tumour treatment.'

The *Anklageschrift* asserted: 'The prosecution will not attempt to discuss scientific principles. It is the task of this trial to judge the behaviour of the accused in specific single cases, and how a doctor with a sense of duty should have behaved.'

Three other cases had been added to the original four. They had been drawn from a stock-pile of files removed from the clinic's archives and dissected by medical experts. Fraud was alleged in the case of Hermann Lang. Accusations of 'manslaughter by negligence' were made about the deaths of Albert Matzeit and Else Warnken.

The defence felt the new cases clearly indicated the difficulty the prosecution had found in obtaining enough evidence to convict. Issels' view hardened that the trial was simply a device to remove him forever from practice; that the real prosecutors were the medical establishment.

Hermann Lang was an architect who lived with his wife, Magdalene, in Munich. His work brought him a modest income. In 1960 Lang was diagnosed in the Maria-Theresia Clinic in Munich with a 'suspicion of a right lung tumour'. He was seventy-nine years old—an age that precluded surgery. The clinic decided against even a minor exploratory operation to establish how widespread the malignancy was. He was sent home to die.

Magdalene Lang decided to make one last try to save her husband. She went to the Ringberg Klinik with X-rays taken at the Maria-Theresia Clinic.

Issels studied them and agreed to accept Lang for treatment on the strict understanding that no promise could be made as to the outcome.

Magdalene Lang did not inform the clinic's administration that, due to reduced circumstances, she and her husband drew social welfare—and they had no money to pay for private medical treatment. Nor did she reveal to Issels the true medical condition of her husband.

Hermann Lang arrived in a comatose state in the clinic on April 20, 1960. Examination revealed a large tumour in the right lung, and a second growth in the abdomen. Treatment began to redress a poor prognosis, and gradually an improvement occurred in his general condition. Later, in May, a series of X-rays showed a local reduction in the tumours.

Sometime in May Issels learnt through the Lang's family doctor that they were on welfare. Issels suggested that Hermann Lang moved from his private room into a double room to reduce costs. It was meant as a helpful gesture. The Langs rejected it. For them it was important to have the status of a private patient.

The late spring of 1960 showed a steady improvement in Lang's condition. He had some teeth and tonsils removed. From bedrest he became a sprightly old man, able to rough-out blue-prints on a drawing board, and quip with doctors and nurses. He looked as if he might be another success story for the clinic. Then, on July 28, 1960, he had a sudden dizzy spell, slipped and bruised his hand. Two days later he left the clinic—announcing he was taking his wife on holiday. His case-notes recorded: 'Patient thanked staff for their help. Overall improvement of general condition. Significant reduction in his local carcinoma.'

The Langs left the clinic owing bills amounting to DM 3,123. They went on holiday in Switzerland. On August 8, 1960, Lang suddenly collapsed and died in a Berne hospital ten days later without regaining consciousness.

His widow returned home to find a number of bills waiting to be paid. Among them was a polite reminder from the Ringberg Klinik about the DM 3,123. Mrs. Lang put aside the bill. There were apparently more pressing accounts to settle. In September, 1960, she read of Issels' arrest. She went to the Public Prosecutor and claimed Issels had promised a cure for her husband—and that she had not paid the outstanding bill because she believed Issels was a fraud.

The story of Albert Matzeit was the sadly familiar one of a man frightened of surgery. The fifty-six-year-old printer had been diagnosed in June, 1956 at the E.N.T. Clinic at Düsseldorf's Medical Academy as a suspected case of cancer of the left larynx. He refused a biopsy to confirm the diagnosis. Twice that year—in late June and October—the clinic wrote to Matzeit insisting on a biopsy.

He refused until November, 1958, when he suffered a sudden choking fit. Recovered, but fearful, he went to the clinic. An immediate biopsy was performed. It confirmed the presence of cancer. An operation was urgently recommended. Matzeit refused and discharged himself.

His search for a solution outside surgery took him from one doctor's waiting room to another. In each case he was told an operation was the only answer. Finally, in February, 1959, a homoeopathic doctor suggested he went to the Ringberg Klinik, where he was admitted on February 21. He was immediately seen by an outside consultant, Dr. Hermann Tross, an E.N.T. specialist, who did weekly sessions at the clinic. Tross recommended surgery. It was a view Issels endorsed. Matzeit refused.

He received a course of combined treatment. It improved his overall situation, but there was no change in the growth. By April 6, 1959, his condition changed; the case-notes recorded: 'patient has *inward* growing tumour on the left larynx.' April 27: 'on the last *Chef*'s round patient was again informed about the limits of the internal tumour therapy. It was pointed out to him that surgery was still possible. Patient in spite of that, wishes to continue treatment without surgery.'

Issels continued to press the need for an operation. On May 8, Matzeit finally agreed. He discharged himself, saying he would go to the Medical Academy in Düsseldorf for an operation. Somewhere on the six-hundred-mile journey to Düsseldorf he changed his mind; possibly his old fears returned. He turned up in Bonn seeking yet another medical opinion. It was the same as all the others: immediate surgery was the only hope. In June another choking fit nearly killed him. He survived and went to the Medical Academy where an immediate operation removed the malignant larynx. He had a course of follow-up radiotherapy. On July 1, he was discharged and told to return for a second course of irradiation in October. He failed to keep the appointment for unknown reasons. But, by March, 1960, he was back in hospital with a relapse of his cancer of the throat. He had a month's course of radiotherapy. On May 25, 1960, Albert Matzeit died.

A full year had passed since he left the Ringberg Klinik

vowing to undergo immediate surgery. He had finally been operated upon, and received supportive radiotherapy. It seemed that was unimportant in the prosecution's opinion. They pinned their hopes on the premise that 'the accused recommended an operation too late'. Later it emerged that the prosecution's medical advisers felt such a charge could be substantiated—though it also became clear they had no real belief it would succeed.

It is impossible to know exactly who advised that the case of Else Warnken be included in the bill of accusal.

The story of the young Bremen housewife was a particularly tragic one. Married, with an eight-year-old daughter, thirty-three-year-old Else had been diagnosed with cancer in the left breast at the St. Josef Stift Hospital in Bremen in December, 1954. During the biopsy a lump, the size of a pea, had been excised. But further drastic surgery was recommended: it entailed the amputation of both breasts and ovarectomy. Else was deeply distressed at the news. She was young and pretty, and feared such surgery could wreck her marriage. Her husband, Artur, had read about Issels and wrote to him on December 28, 1954: 'I know that you cannot promise a cure of 100 per cent. But I have the confidence that you can help. How soon can my wife come to your clinic? We take the responsibility for this step—just let me know the costs.'

On January 3, 1955, Else was admitted to the clinic. She stayed until March 18, showing considerable improvement of her general condition, and was discharged into the care of her family doctor, with instructions about follow-up treatment prescribed by the clinic. For an unknown reason Else did not carry out that treatment; a likely explanation is that she felt well enough to risk ignoring the somewhat rigid demands of the follow-up regime. In July, 1955, the family doctor noted a hardening of the original biopsy scar. In October, Else returned to the clinic where minor surgery removed a small hard nodule in the scar. The pathologist's report showed it to be malignant. A full course of combined treatment was given. By December 7, Else was discharged with no detectable signs of cancer. Once more she received instructions about follow-up treatment at home. Again she failed to carry out Issels' instructions. In March, 1956, the family doctor detected a new nodule in the biopsy scar. Issels wrote for further details and received no reply. In April, Issels wrote to Else's husband, who finally replied in July, 1956: 'After thinking things over, my wife does not wish to have further treatment at your clinic. I assume that in the meantime you have received my family doctor's report.'

It came in August, 1956. It was short: 'My patient has decided against further treatment at your clinic because in spite of intensive treatment there was a metastasis.'

Issels ignored what many doctors would have accepted. He was interested to know what Else felt about the situation. He wrote her a number of letters. He received no reply. Then, in March, 1957, her family doctor wrote to Issels about: 'A plum-sized tumour in the original biopsy scar. Above are two smaller tumours the size of cherry pips. Plum-sized nodules in the lymph glands.'

The letter added that Else had been on a vegetarian diet for a year, and now wanted to fast in the belief it would help her condition. Issels wrote back that dieting alone had no part to play in helping her situation: he felt only surgery was clearly indicated.

He heard no more for a year. In April, 1958, he wrote Else a routine letter he sent annually to all former patients: it inquired after her condition. In May, her family doctor wrote: 'My patient underwent surgery on August 27, 1957. Her present condition shows progressive metastases.'

In the next year Else Warnken received follow-up chemotherapy and deep-ray treatment. In July, 1960, she died—five years after being treated in the Ringberg Klinik. The prosecution contended her death could be directly traced to Issels not insisting on surgery immediately he had examined her all those years before.

By February 1961, Issels and his lawyers—Alfred Seidl and Kurt Kirstein—had mapped out a defence to all the charges. Seidl, sun-tanned from his Far East trip, was a direct contrast to the quiet, soberly-dressed Kirstein. Both complemented each other as they shaped legal strategy. Both felt that in the trial medical politics would play a very important part. Therefore, the defence set about destroying the medical opposition, knowing that was the only way to ensure an acquittal. Further, the defence relied on proving three premises:

That the combined treatment worked.

That no patient had ever been kept from surgery at any time.

That no promise of a cure had been made.

Seidl and Kirstein had stripped the defence to bare essentials. It would be fleshed-out by the testimony of patients who had been cured and by Issels' own account of events. Seidl felt it unnecessary to call expert medical witnesses as rebuttal: he intended to attack those called by the prosecution on the simple, but effective, ground that however learned they were, they had no first-hand knowledge of the treatment methods at the Ringberg Klinik, and, more important, they had publicly declared themselves to be opposed to it.

Even without expert witnesses, the defence became an increasingly costly business. Each lawyer received a retainer of DM 20,000. Isa's father helped find the money. Issels sold his car; Isa dismissed her housemaid. Unable to afford a secretary, Isa worked long into the night typing up medical documents for the defence.

Socially, it was a barren time. Old friends shunned them. In Isa's later words:

> They were probably embarrassed meeting us. So we stayed more and more at home, not because we were afraid to show our faces, but only because we did not wish to become a further source of embarrassment to those we had been friendly with.

The Issels house drew patients from far afield. They came seeking treatment. To everyone Issels explained he was unable to practise until he established his innocence. He spent his days working in a lay capacity in the clinic, filled now with sanatorium patients.

By March, 1961, Issels at last realised how widespread the prosecution's inquiries had been. The Public Prosecutor made available not only lengthy affidavits by Teicher and Glaeser, but also sworn statements by other former employees of the clinic; they all claimed, in one way or another, that Issels was unfit to practise medicine.

The accusations deeply wounded him. But over the weeks he drew comfort from hundreds of letters from all over Europe pledging support for his cause. The publicity had tapped a vast fund of goodwill among the public. Soon newspapers, always sensitive to their readers' wishes, ran articles favourable to Issels. He never sought the publicity. But he recognised it had a certain value in so far as it brought the problems associated with cancer before a wide audience.

On March 3, *the Eröffnungsbeschluss*—a formality peculiar to German law—was announced by the judges of the Second Criminal Chamber of the Court of Munich. It repeated all the charges in somewhat more elegant language than previously used and set the trial date for June 7, 1961.

Issels wrote a personal letter to the Court—another device peculiar to the German legal code—asking for a postponement to give him more time to prepare his defence. The request was denied.

He spent the next three months assembling patients and their doctors who would all swear that his combined treatment had produced lasting benefit.

Early in June he and Isa moved into a modest hotel near the court in Munich ready to take part in what one newspaper billed as the medical trial of the century.

12

Trials and Tribulations

As often occurs in a trial where chief counsel were virtuosos, the case had begun some weeks earlier with a joust in chambers. Alfred Seidl lodged a petition demanding two of the prosecution's medical experts be barred: Professor Walter Büngeler and Professor Max Eder had 'expressed opinions indicating clear prejudice towards the defendant'. Both men had either written or spoken out against Issels' combined treatment. Büngeler had also played a significant part in harnessing the prosecution: Helgo Teicher, the key prosecution witness, had sent material from the clinic to Büngeler, then secretary-general of the National Cancer Society—though there was no suggestion that Büngeler knew how the case files had been obtained. Public Prosecutor Leo Parsch still denied bias on the part of the experts. The Court promised a decision when the trial began. Both Seidl and Parsch fully recognised the legal by-play behind the petition: it cast Issels as a victim of the medical establishment—a role he never relinquished.

For 'administrative reasons' the case was postponed for a week. It gave the defence invaluable time to run through strategy. Seidl felt the all-important thing was unseating Büngeler and Eder; he believed it would establish a defence superiority from which the prosecution would find it hard to recover. A third lawyer had joined the defence team: Ernst Fock was retained, at a fee of DM 15,000, to handle medico-legal questions arising in the manslaughter cases. Thin-faced and intense he would share the bulk of the cross-examination with Seidl. Kurt Kirstein was the defence anchor-man: his task was selecting, sifting and constantly evaluating the material presented in court.

Issels would be allowed an uninterrupted opening statement broadly outlining his answer to the charges. Next, the prosecution and defence would call witnesses to describe the clinic's environment. The court President would then begin examination of each specific charge; afterwards prosecution and defence would pick up the questioning. Issels could himself question witnesses or address the court on specific medical issues. Witnesses could be constantly recalled as new evidence involving them demanded testing. Compared with Anglo-Saxon law it was a complicated procedure.

Sharp at nine o'clock on the morning of June 14, 1961, the black-gowned judges took their places in courtroom number twenty-eight in Munich's Palace of Justice. The President, Judge Claus Seibert, was flanked by two other senior members of the Munich judicary, Judge Wehohsky and Judge Stenglein, in their tri-cornered hats and robes. Near the bench sat two lay assessors, whose role was roughly equivalent to an English jury.

The courtroom was newly painted and shiny, and looked much like an American police court; there was no pageantry or ornate trappings. Yet, despite its barren props, the setting generated that special ambiance which marks every great criminal trial. A German reporter setting the scene wrote:

> It was a stage for high theatre. The judges looked stern and uncompromising. The President had the unfortunate look of a man whose face expressed a mind made up. There was an angry sparkle—*Augen blitzen von Angriffslust*—to his eyes, and his mouth was thin as a razor-blade, *Mund ist messerscharf*. Issels was distinguished in striped pants and black coat. With his silver tie and white shirt he looked like a diplomat about to present his credentials. He sat between his trial lawyers. Prosecutor Parsch, young, tall, bespectacled, had the air of an elegant sphinx, in which nothing made a discernible impression.

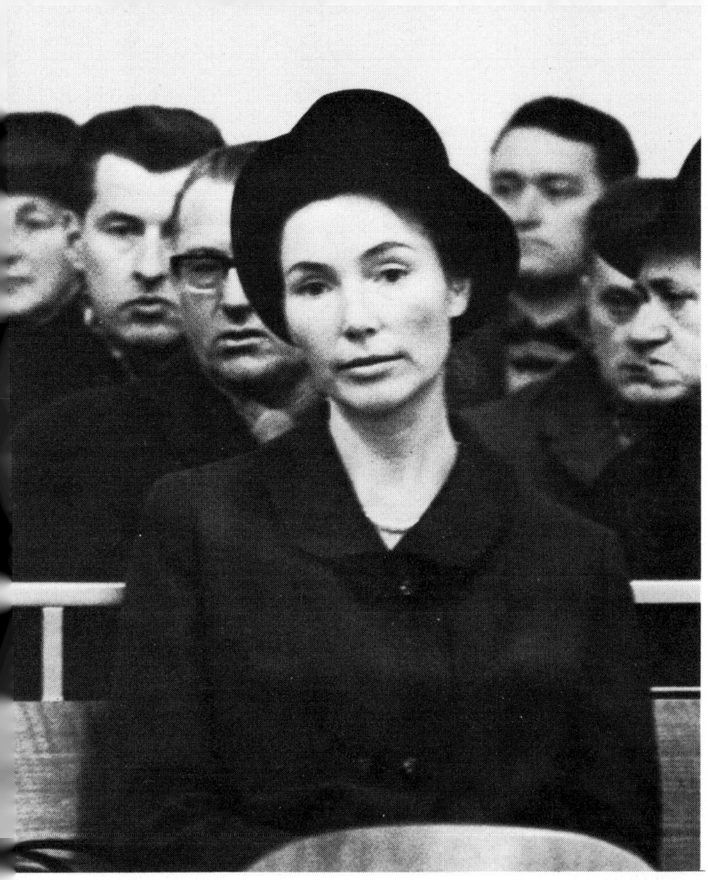

A pensive Isa waits for judgment on her husband

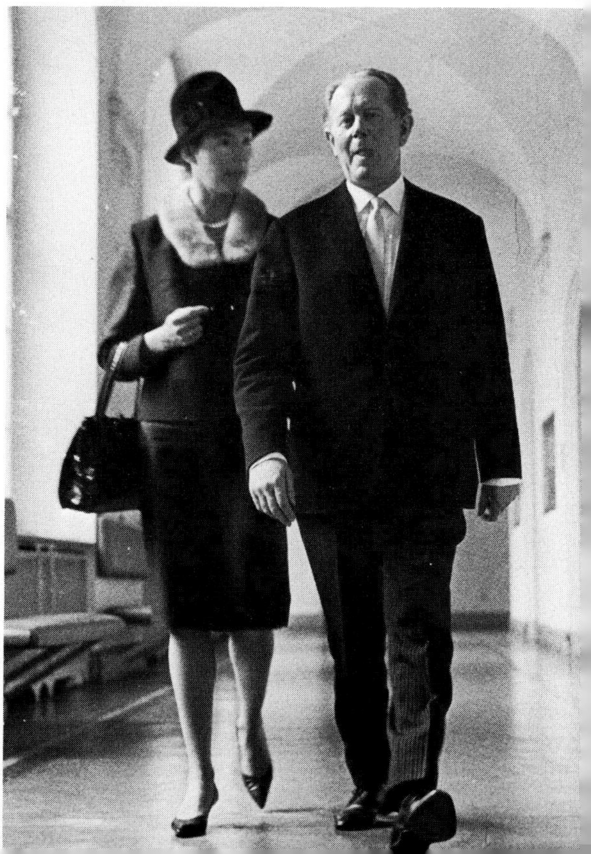

Waiting for the verdict of the second trial.

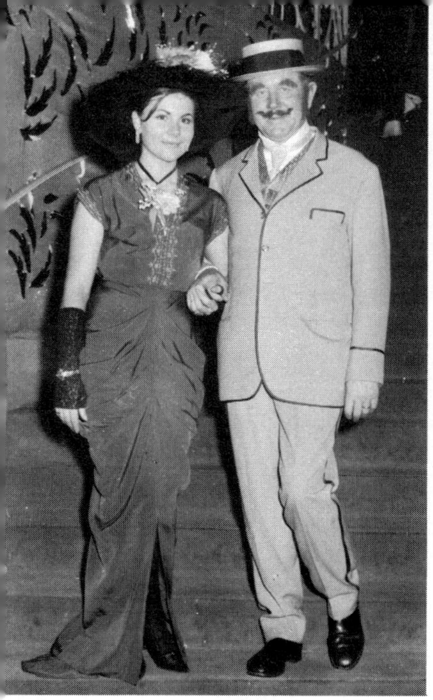

Issels at a carnival
with his daughter, Uti, 1964

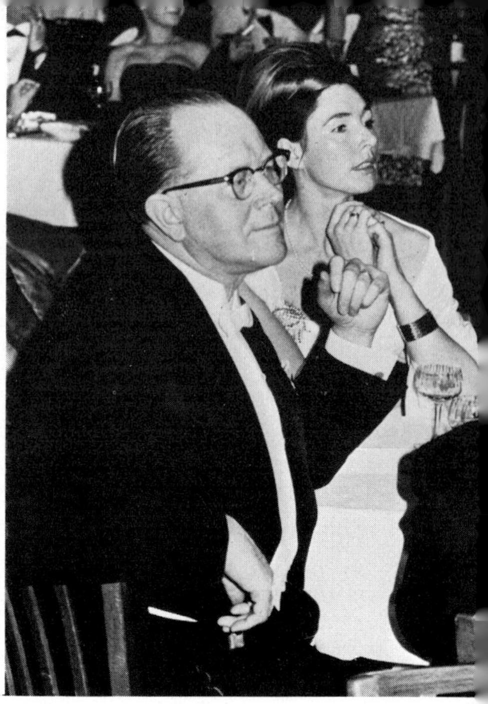

Issels and his wife
at a gala ball in Munich

Tea time at the Issels family residence includes their dog, Nick

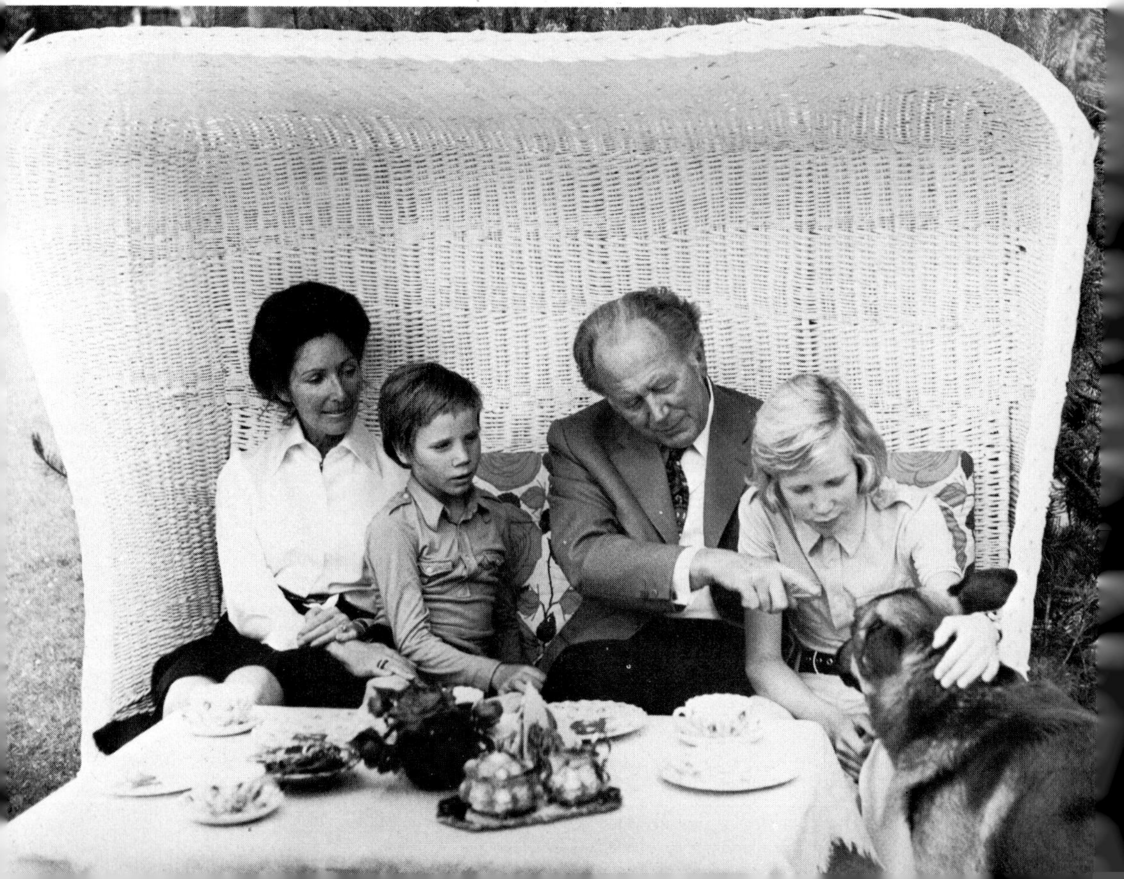

Seidl immediately established himself as a personality when he opened his bulging black brief-case and revealed it contained only his silk black robe—the one he wore at Nuremberg when he defended Rudolf Hess in the War Crimes Trials. Gowned, Seidl looked what he was—the quicksilver genius of the German bar. Kirstein resembled a dignified bank manager: well hidden was the fact that he had a brilliant mind with extraordinary dedication. Fock had the air of a mortician—a cultivated aura which unnerved many a witness.

Isa sat in the front row of the packed public seats. More than one reporter commented on her quiet elegance and confidence. She had a note-book on her lap. During the trial it filled with notes which she passed to the defence table; they contained astute observations about witnesses' evidence—and frequently formed the basis of a blistering counter-attack by defence lawyers.

Beside Parsch sat the prosecution's expert medical witnesses. Büngeler and Eder were joined by Professor Hans Schulten, medical director of the University of Cologne Hospital and Professor Hermann Eyer, professor of microbiology at Munich University. Büngeler had been retained in his capacity as director of the pathological institute at Munich University; Eder was lecturer in pathology at the same institute. All four would buttress the prosecution whenever it needed medical support. The quartet looked bleakly as Seidl rose to his feet a few minutes after nine o'clock.

He reminded the court of the objection he had lodged weeks before of the presence of Büngeler and Eder: 'They are prejudiced, and their attitude towards the accused is well known. I submit both should take no part in the trial.'

After a brief deliberation, President Seibert announced the court would postpone a decision.

Seidl, watching developments through a larger prism, was well satisfied. He had publicly introduced the question of bias—and scored a psychological victory.

The indictment was read, and the clerk of the court stated there were no previous recorded convictions against Issels.

Shortly before ten o'clock, Issels began to address the

court. He spoke steadily, showing no signs of emotion. He traced his career as a surgeon and family doctor, and the emergence of his belief that cancer could be treated by means other than surgery or radiotherapy—though he stressed he never refused a patient any form of conventional treatment. Quite the reverse was true:

'In my published work I have always emphasised the importance of surgery and other conventional measures. But equally I believe that not just the local symptoms, the tumour, must be treated, but also the body as a whole which has produced the tumour.'

Nor had he ever promised a cure. He always talked of no more than: 'a chance, the same as any other doctor would do if faced with a gravely ill patient for whom treatment is still possible.'

The judges listened intently in their high-backed chairs as Issels explained the principles of his combined treatment, immunotherapy and homoeotherapy. He dwelt on his struggle to help those who were the 'so-called incurables'. He believed they were not incurable—and in the course of the trial planned to demonstrate the truth of that conviction. In all, he talked for two full days. When he finally sat down, the defence lawyers felt their client's long-range position had improved even further.

Eager to press the advantage, Seidl raised again the question of the continuing presence of Büngeler and Eder in court. A recess was ordered.

There followed a complicated piece of legal manoeuvring between Seidl and Parsch. The Public Prosecutor conceded to 'temporarily' remove his two experts in return for Seidl's agreement to 'temporarily' not call patients who claimed they had been cured by Issels. Seidl felt he had got the best of the bargain: the removal of Büngeler and Eder was worth all the patients who could testify favourably.

Seidl recognised what few others in court sensed: the lay defence witnesses could be attacked by the prosecution's medical experts whose job it was to cast doubt on Issels' 'cures'. Seidl had deliberately decided against calling experts to rebut such doubts: he planned to strip bare the motives of the prosecution doctors. He did not want 'to be cluttered up with our own experts who would come under Parsch's fire.'

Seidl also saw what was behind the prosecution's revised indictment. The defence had already submitted to the court all Issels' published work, and introduced literature from all over the world supporting their client's beliefs. Faced with such evidence—it included research reports from New York's Sloan-Kettering Institute for Cancer Research and other world-famous cancer centres—the prosecution realised it could make little headway in its hope of discrediting the combined treatment. Parsch intended to deal only with specific cases.

It meant the trial might still become a clash of experts. Unseating two of them at an early stage was the sort of legal move which made Seidl a feared lawyer. The trial continued without Büngeler and Eder.

Procedural arguments were presented. Both sides had submitted a list of witnesses to the court. Parsch intended to call sixty; twenty-seven would give evidence for Issels. The court announced it would decide in which order to hear them.

On the fifth day Parsch launched his first counter-ploy. He blandly asked the court to recognise three new medical experts: Professor Alexander Herrmann, director of the E.N.T. Clinic at Munich University; Professor Rudolf Zenker, director of surgery, Munich University Hospital; Professor Hans von Braunbehrens, director of the Radiotherapy Clinic, Munich University.

All three had international reputations. Seidl decided not to challenge them. He sensed the prosecution could call still more distinguished doctors, and eventually the court's patience would be exhausted by defence objections. Besides, he planned to make use of the old legal stratagem—*tu quoque*—a retort charging the prosecution with having behaved no differently to the accused—when cross-examining the experts.

Parsch, for all his studied politeness, had shown he was an avenger. On the eighth day he revealed the basic strategy for a conviction. He called witness after witness to throw 'a flashlight on the Ringberg Klinik'. Gradually, the trial assumed an ugly, explosive character; at times the courtroom sounded like a Nazi *Volksgerichtshof*, a People's Court, as former clinic staff testified. A Dr. Gudrun Guilino who had worked at the clinic for six months, stated she 'had not seen remission or cures'. Seidl's sharp cross-examination elicted the admission that six months was not long enough to pass judgment on Issels' methods—when in fact the accepted definition of a cure was a mandatory five-year period free of the disease.

A Dr. Karl-Heinz Grözinger took the stand and talked of 'wrong X-ray diagnosis', and 'no effectiveness of the Gerlach vaccine'.

Seidl asked one question: 'How long were you at the clinic?'

'Three months.'

'Thank you. No further questions.'

Next Dr. Wolfgang Mueller-Hepburn gave evidence. He was a slow, ponderous man, and it took him a long time to come to the point of his evidence: he had been at the clinic when Rudolf Schönek had flown in from America. Mueller-Hepburn said he had heard Issels promise the dying man a cure.

Seidl fixed the doctor with a piercing look of contempt. Mueller-Hepburn waited uneasily in the hushed courtroom.

'Doctor,' said Seidl softly. 'Did you leave the clinic on your own initiative?'

The silence stretched.

'Well—doctor.' Seidl whiplashed the words to Mueller-Hepburn. 'What is your answer?'

'No.'

'Why did you leave the clinic?'

'I was dismissed.'

'Thank you. I have no further questions.'

Deliberately Seidl turned his back on the discomfited witness and sat down. He had succeeded in what he planned: Mueller-Hepburn was discredited; his testimony over an alleged cure would be weighed by the court against the fact that he had been sacked.

Early on the defence established an attitude towards cross-examination. Where the allegations were plainly fanciful they would be disdainfully ignored. In turn, Seidl let his own witnesses establish a portrait of a well-run clinic. Professor Franz Gerlach said the research facilities were excellent. Doctors testified to Issels' dedication and swore they had never heard him promise to cure anybody. The clinic's accountant revealed that the staff were paid handsome salaries, that Issels had a personal income, on paper, of DM 20,000 a month—but that most of his salary was ploughed back into new equipment and off-setting free treatment. Seidl deftly established the untruth of allegations about foreign bank accounts. He next mopped-up the charge of faking an X-ray plate in the case of Friedrich Dehm. He pointed to the testimony of the clinic's radiographer who admitted the mistake was hers entirely: she explained away the switch as 'a momentary lapse when sorting out many plates.'

The fraud charges relating to Karl Wiesinger and Richard Vogel had been dropped before the trial opened. Seidl moved that *all* the charges should be dropped for a similar lack of evidence. It was a cheeky ploy—largely directed towards the press box. The motion was swiftly denied. But next day newspapers all over Europe headlined Seidl's claim that the entire case was unfounded.

The defence had established a bridgehead far inside the prosecution lines. It soon emerged that Parsch's case was not faultless. The remaining fraud charges dangled from the slenderest of threads; whole segments needed to support, the manslaughter charges had been dangerously eroded under Seidl's probing.

In the press box, reporters polled each other. All agreed that so far Issels was *unschuldig*—not guilty.

No one suspected that there was a growing rift between Seidl and Fock. Fock felt his colleague was poaching on his province by mixing-up the fraud and manslaughter charges. Fock had been specifically retained to handle the latter cases; he felt Seidl's tactics weakened his chances. Seidl saw his role as undermining the carefully constructed prosecution case. He was a ruthless raider, attacking from a quarter Parsch did not always expect. The results were often devastating. Seidl had toppled more than one witness with a well-aimed thrust. Kurt Kirstein and Isa only partly succeeded in placating both counsel. At times the situation was tense and difficult.

The Public Prosecutor made valiant attempts to keep the case within a neat framework. He hammered away at a theme which increasingly revealed a strong medical influence behind the case. Issels was an exponent of 'fringe medicine', and the prosecution believed he was guilty on all counts because he flew in the face of accepted treatment. From time to time, expert witnesses lent support to that argument. They found themselves caught in devastating cross-examination by Seidl. He ridiculed them for failing to use words that were supportive of truth—such as 'fact', 'factual', 'genuine' and 'proven'. Instead, they preferred such substitute words as 'represented', 'designated', 'alleged' and 'opinion'. The defence called them words which fell into the category of 'that which remains to be proved'. Therefore, Seidl bitingly concluded, much of what they said deserved to be regarded with the same caution as they expressed in medical matters. It was dazzling stuff and the public benches lapped it all up.

Like all well-staged dramas the tension had steadily mounted. The supportive players firmly established themselves. The judges were a black-robed bloc occasionally questioning a witness. Parsch was the soft-spoken Bavarian gentleman, Seidl the nimble aristocrat, Fock the withdrawn ascetic, Kirstein the calm countryman who never mislaid a paper. Issels was the most natural of them all. He listened intently to everything. Reporters wrote he looked 'solemn', or 'serious faced'. But even those descriptions failed to explain away the words of the court President Seibert: 'The court will hear Dr. Teicher next. I hope when he appears the accused will not lose his poker face.'

It was, by any standard, an unusual observation for a judge to make. Seidl decided against challenging on the grounds that it would only make matters worse. But from that moment Issels became convinced he would not get a fair trial.

Teicher was an unprepossessing figure in the witness box. He was a balding, middle-aged man, with a habit of nervously darting his eyes around the court. One American newsman felt Teicher resembled 'a man who wished he was someplace else'.

Parsch, from his manner, made it clear that Teicher was as much a pariah to the prosecution as to the defence. Nevertheless, Teicher sketched a highly damaging picture of Issels and the methods practised at the clinic:

> The accused delayed surgery because of a misguided idea about the value of his treatment . . . nobody was treated free of charge . . . the diagnosis of cancer was incorrect in many patients . . . the Gerlach vaccine was useless . . . tonsilectomy and extraction of teeth was a death sentence on patients too ill to undergo such surgery . . . Issels was altogether too optimistic with relatives of patients . . . because of the bad conditions at the clinic I felt obliged in November, 1958 to start collecting evidence and to complain to the local medical association.

Parsch skilfully avoided any mention of Teicher's removal of case files and other confidential material from the Ringberg Klinik. It was all in vain. Seidl rose to his feet. For a long moment he sized-up Teicher. Then in a velvety voice the lawyer asked: 'Dr. Teicher, what gentleman of the Bavarian Medical Association asked you to collect material?'

'Objection!'

Red-faced, his cool ruffled, Parsch leapt to his feet protesting the question was irrelevant.

The judges deliberated. Then President Seibert pronounced: 'The question is disallowed because it is irrelevant to the matter of the witness's trustworthiness from which person employed by the Bavarian Medical Association he received the order or advice.'

Seidl was satisfied. That judgment linked the Bavarian Medical Association with Teicher's activities.

Parsch tried to retrieve the situation by guiding Teicher through the story of Richard Vogel, the janitor who died because he repeatedly refused surgery suggested first by other doctors and then by Issels. Teicher insisted Issels had never suggested an operation. That testimony brought him under attack from Judge Seibert:

Seibert: In a letter you wrote, 'up to now the patient has emphatically rejected operation'. In various other letters you have written you have expressed similar thoughts. How do you explain that?

Teicher: In this clinic one was allowed only to write positive things.

Seidl: So you intentionally deceived people?

Teicher: I was employed by the clinic.

Seidl: Besides you have constantly collected material against Dr. Issels. Why?

Teicher: I only collected material after I was dismissed from the clinic.

It was a foolish reply; he had stated to Parsch that he began gathering material in November, 1958, when he was still employed at the clinic. Tigerishly, Seidl moved in for the kill. He pinned Teicher down, forcing admissions about how the material had been taken. Teicher found himself in quicksand as he struggled to justify his behaviour. The more he threshed the more muddy a picture emerged:

Seidl: How did the files come into the hands of the Public Prosecutor?

Teicher: I was asked by the Public Prosecutor to submit the files.

Parsch: Objection!

Seibert: The court states that the statements of Dr. Teicher are of minimum importance.

Seidl: Dr. Teicher, did you submit your material to Professor Büngeler [secretary-general of the National Cancer Society] on your own free will?

Teicher: Is it enough if I say I did not do it on my own initiative?

It was enough. Seidl had shown that Teicher was not working alone. Büngeler, one of the most respected men in the German medical establishment, had been implicated in a very odd story.

Hitching his gown around his shoulder, Seidl pressed home the attack, determined to show what really lay behind Teicher's scrabbling in the clinic's archives through the winter nights of 1958. He pushed Teicher to the stage where the doctor revealed his 'orders to collect material came from a higher authority'.

Seidl: Is that 'higher authority' the Bavarian Medical Association?
Teicher: Yes!
Parsch: Objection!
Seibert: The question is not allowed because it does not shake the trustworthiness of the witness.

It was an unusual ruling for a trial judge to make. Seibert immediately made a further one. He produced a letter from the Bavarian Medical Association in which it was denied Teicher had ever been asked to gather material. Seibert said that ended the matter for the court. No member of the Association would be called to test the truth of that letter under cross-examination.

Dr. Rudolf Glaeser next swore to tell the truth. He had, one reporter noted, the air of a mouse approaching a trap—'eager to please and totally unaware of the danger.' His testimony swiftly became a fiasco for the prosecution. He had changed his story on many vital issues. For Glaeser the time had come to tell the real truth. He could not remember whether he had ever heard Issels promise a cure, or whether Issels had refused any patient surgery. He contradicted his own and Teicher's testimony.

Finally, Parsch lost patience. He began to hector Glaeser, reminding him he was under oath. Glaeser revealed the story of the wealthy old woman with land adjoining the Ringberg Klinik who believed cancer could be 'transmitted to her property'. She had given Teicher and Glaeser 'substantial sums of money' while both doctors plundered material from the clinic. Teicher, re-examined, denied the story. The full fury of the Public Prosecutor fell on Glaeser.

Parsch: You said you knew Dr. Teicher got money. You know you are on oath? I feel unwell when I see somebody committing perjury with open eyes.

Glaeser looked astonished; too late he sensed danger.

The rasping voice of President Seibert took up the questioning:

Seibert: Dr. Glaeser, you can't make jokes with us. Each word is important. Is it true that Dr. Teicher also told you he had got money from the old woman?
Glaeser: Yes. He told me he had received considerable amounts.

The court was silent. Seibert nodded his head, weighing something.

Seibert: Dr. Glaeser, I wish to ask about something else. Your visit to the Dehm house. Do you remember going there first *alone* without Dr. Teicher?

Glaeser could not remember. It had occurred nearly two years before. Judge Seibert looked at him frostily. Gunther Scheibeck, Friedrich Dehm's stepson, was called to the witness stand. He swore that Glaeser alone had paid a call on his mother and step-father. Scheibeck produced a diary to show he had recorded the visit.

Judges, prosecutor and assessors all looked at Glaeser. With a voice that one reporter likened as 'a trumpet of doom', President Seibert thundered: 'Dr. Glaeser, you ought to remember if you had been to the Dehm house alone or not.'

Glaeser shook his head.

It was his last public gesture. President Seibert ordered him committed to prison for 'suspected perjury'. A police officer escorted the doctor from the witness box and took him to jail. Glaeser spent several months in Stadelheim Prison before he was brought to trial—and found not guilty of perjury.

With both star witnesses discredited, the prosecution dealt with the specific cases. the fraud indictments were taken first. The ghost of Friedrich Dehm was resurrected by his wife, Emilie, as she repeated her story of a promised cure. Cross-examined, she amended her words: Issels had only talked of a chance.

'No more?' Seidl persisted.

'No. No more.'

The press box was agog as she paraded a long list of complaints about the clinic, its staff, and Issels himself. The testimony had a Brechtian quality all its own as Judge Seibert explored the reality of the situation:

Seibert: You have alleged that Dr. Issels drinks in the clinic.
Emilie Dehm: He came into my husband's room, sat on his bed, and I said to the doctor, 'the pulse of my husband is not in order'. Then Dr. Issels took my hand to feel my pulse. I said to my husband after the doctor had gone, 'either he drinks or takes morphine'.

The clinic's senior registrar, Dr. Georg Chyla, told the court that in his years at the clinic he never saw Issels touch alcohol on duty—'he has a carafe of apple juice on his desk. Frau Dehm has confused that with wine.' Seibert continued to question Mrs. Dehm:

Seibert: You have a further allegation?
Emilie Dehm: Yes, a nurse told us that patients who asked to leave the clinic got an injection to stay.
Seibert: An injection to stay?
Emilie Dehm: Yes.
Seibert: You mean a so-called staying injection . . .?

The judge shook his head wonderingly. Clinic doctors testified to the absurdity of Mrs. Dehm's statement. Seidl did not bother to question her. He directed his attention to building up the defence. A procession of doctors and nurses testified that Issels 'genuinely wanted to help'. . . 'Issels recommended surgery whenever it was still possible'. . . 'Issels never promised a cure, he only spoke of a chance.' No matter how hard Parsch tried, the witnesses refused to be swayed from those opinions.

The Dehm case had collapsed in a welter of laughter. Next came the case of Hermann Lang, the old architect, who had suddenly died on holiday in Switzerland. His widow, Magdalene Lang, was a colourful sight in a broad-brimmed hat and winter tweeds in the middle of June.

She stood in the witness box, glaring defiantly at Issels and repeated her story of being swindled. Seidl ignored her as he rose to his feet. Instead he addressed the court, a move allowed in German law, and revealed Magdalene Lang's background: she was a woman with a history of litigation—in one period she had sued, unsuccessfully, four lawyers who had handled other cases she had lost. She was a woman with a list of debtors, a woman to be pitied, but not a woman whose word could be relied upon. Scathingly, Seidl drew the Court's attention to the fact that the Ringberg Klinik's bill of DM 3,123 was still outstanding—and would remain so if Issels was convicted.

'We are not here to recover debts from Mrs. Lang or anybody else,' Seidl continued. 'We are here to hear the truth.'

He turned and looked at Mrs. Lang. 'When your husband died in a private clinic in Switzerland, an expensive place no doubt, did you pay the bill?'

'No! But I know what you mean. I am no fraud . . .!'

'Thank you. I have no further questions.'

He sat down. Thirteen days had passed since the trial started. The charge of fraud in the case of the American, Rudolf Schönek, collapsed without Seidl's probing. Magdalene Schönek, his widow, told the court that 'everything and everybody at the clinic did their best for my husband'.

Those words ended any hope the prosecution had of a conviction of fraud against Issels.

It was a hard-won victory—not made easier by the increasing conflict between Seidl and Fock. The chief defence counsel believed Fock: 'was one too many at our table. He came late to the case. Kurt Kirstein and I could well have managed. But Dr. Issels' other advisers felt he needed a specialist in medical manslaughter—so Fock was there.'

Fock had not endeared himself to Seidl, a staunch Bavarian, by one day drawing himself up after a squabble and coldly announcing: 'I am a Prussian.' The inference was clear: Fock was not going to take orders from a southern German. Wearily, Kurt Kirstein and Isa placated both men.

Only Issels showed no signs of strain. He had total concentration in court. At night, he sat with Isa in their hotel bedroom and pored over evidence still to be heard. Sometimes they read until the early hours. An exhausted Isa slept, but her husband continually played through his mind what the following day would reveal in court.

On July 1, the prosecution opened the second phase of the trial—the manslaughter charges. Parsch first dealt with the case of Karl Wiesinger, the fifty-nine-year-old commercial traveller with cancer of the penis. Parsch told the story of a man 'kept from surgery by the accused'.

Issels firmly denied the allegation. He outlined the clinical picture of Wiesinger's illness both before and after the two periods of treatment at the Ringberg Klinik. Issels told the court that on the day Wiesinger arrived in the clinic, July 7, 1954, he urged surgery, and had repeated the suggestion on numerous occasions.

Parsch called Wiesinger's family doctor, Dr. Friedrich Rink, who confirmed Wiesinger had a history of refusing surgery. It had been first suggested by one specialist at Würzburg University in 1952, by another in January, 1954, by a third in 1955. Only in June, 1955 did Wiesinger finally have his penis amputated at the University of Erlangen Hospital. He received follow-up radiotherapy, but died four months after the operation.

Two doctors from the Ringberg Klinik testified they recommended surgery to Wiesinger while he was in the clinic. A third clinic doctor stated he recommended radiotherapy, in January, 1955, to Wiesinger.

Parsch called Dr. Gunther Barth, director of the Radiotherapy Institute at Erlangen where Wiesinger received post-operative treatment. Barth felt it had not been successful because: 'The patient came too late into our care for surgery. If Issels had recommended surgery in time the patient would have lived.'

It was a bold prediction for any doctor to make. Seidl, for all his pressing, could not budge Barth from that view. Defence counsel switched the attack. He read the letter Barth wrote to Mrs. Wiesinger; Seidl underscored the words with telling effect. Barth was '*one of a dozen doctors*' interested in Wiesinger's illness and would like to '*use his case-*

notes for a scientific society interested in the cancer question'. Seidl turned to Barth:

Seidl: Why did you really write to Mrs. Wiesinger? Certainly not because you were interested in Wiesinger's life.
Barth: We were interested in the case.
Seidl: Why did you write that letter?
Barth: We were interested in the case.
Seidl: I ask again. Why did you write that letter?

Barth could not be drawn. Stolid and calm, he blocked Seidl's attempts to winkle out the story of how case-notes allegedly wanted for a serious medical purpose ended up in the prosecution's hands.

Professor Norbert Henning, rector of the University of Erlangen, and a professor of physical medicine, led the court deeper into the sad story of Karl Wiesinger. Henning's testimony was detailed and exact—a point Seidl seized upon:

Seidl: How do you remember so well the case of this single patient when you have seen so many others?
Henning: The case was so exciting for us because the patient would have been cured by surgery if it had been performed in time. There was a 'probability bordering on certainty' of this—and he would be alive now.
Seidl: How do you know?
Henning: Because the case-notes indicate it.
Seidl: How do you *know*?

But no amount of pressure shook Henning. Parsch, sensed a clear advantage, and called Professor Heinrich Gottron, the seventy-one-year-old director of the Dermatology Clinic at Tübingen University. Gottron read from a prepared statement that in his considered opinion Wiesinger would have lived if surgery had been carried out in time.

The defence did not cross-examine, believing Gottron could not be moved a single word from his stated position.

Seidl called Hans Kolb, a former patient who had been a close friend of Wiesinger during their stay at the Ringberg

Klinik. Kolb insisted Wiesinger had 'often said he would never have an operation'. Kolb was an engineer—and something of the precision of his profession came through in his manner. Parsch tried to unsettle him, casting doubts on Kolb's recollection, or that he had misunderstood Wiesinger.

Kolb : Impossible. I was quite clear what was said. Besides, I was cured by the Issels methods myself.

A rumble came from the bench. It signalled another intervention by Judge Seibert.

Seibert : We are not interested in the results of the treatment in general. We are only interested in this specific case. Do you remember details? What do you remember about an operation being recommended?
Kolb : One detail I do remember . . .
Seibert : What do you remember?
Kolb : He had just come back . . .
Seibert : Who?
Kolb : Wiesinger . . . he had just come back from the main building where he had a blood examination . . .
Seibert : I do not want to hear details! What do you remember about an operation?
Kolb : He told me one recommended operation.
Seibert : But at blood examination there are usually no doctors present.

The judge ordered the clerk of the court to note that the witness's 'answer' was that 'no doctors were generally present at blood examination'.

Seidl asked one question in his re-examination: was Kolb quite sure that Wiesinger had said he would refuse surgery? Kolb said he was.

Mrs. Christine Wiesinger, Karl Wiesinger's widow, brought a new sense of expectancy to courtroom number twenty-eight. The neatly costumed widow was reputed to have sensational testimony. It was not slow in emerging—though nobody could have suspected the contents. President Seibert opened the questioning:

Seibert: What was your husband's attitude towards an operation.

Christine Wiesinger: He was always against it. Only in the end, when the pain became too much, did he give way.

An audible gasp swept the court. Even Seidl was surprised. Parsch leapt to his feet, a stunned note in his voice.

Parsch: But Mrs. Wiesinger . . . what you have just said is just the opposite to your affidavit.

Christine Wiesinger: But it is true.

Seibert: What is true?

Christine Wiesinger: What I am saying now. That my husband did not want to be operated on.

Seibert: But in your affidavit you said that Dr. Issels kept your husband from operation.

Christine Wiesinger: No . . . no, that is not true. It was my husband's own fault he was not operated on.

Parsch moved that Mrs. Wiesinger be excused and Professor Henning recalled. He said that Mrs. Wiesinger once told him that Issels had refused her husband surgery. Christine Wiesinger was put back on the witness stand. She insisted she never said such a thing to Henning—or anybody else. Her husband died because he had steadfastedly refused to have an operation until it was too late.

Seidl did not cross-examine. In something close to uproar, President Seibert ordered the court recessed for twenty minutes.

Immediately the trial resumed there came a fresh sensation. The Public Prosecutor announced he had 'a surprise witness', Charlotte Hofmann, Karl Wiesinger's married daughter. Seidl lodged a heated objection. Mrs. Hofmann had been in the court room during all the testimony about her father and that barred her from testifying. President Seibert rejected the argument. Charlotte Hofmann, a pretty, demure young woman, made her way to the witness stand.

Parsch: Do you know if Dr. Issels was against operations or not?

Charlotte Hofmann : It was my father who was against surgery.

Parsch paled. Some reporters said he visibly trembled.

Parsch : But you have just said . . . in the corridor outside this court room that Dr. Issels had refused your father surgery.

Charlotte Hofmann : No. I never said that!

Seibert : Be careful. Only last week somebody was sent to prison from here because of perjury.

Parsch : But you must remember. It was just a short while ago.

Charlotte Hofmann : No . . . I did not say that.

Seidl rose to his feet, tugging his gown about him, a purring edge to his voice.

Seidl : It would be interesting to know to whom this witness is supposed to have said what the prosecution wants her to say.

Parsch : She said it to Professor Henning.

Henning was recalled. He said he just 'wanted to greet the witness and remind them of a conversation we had before Wiesinger died'.

Seibert : What conversation?

Henning : I had the impression the daughter could give evidence of Dr. Issels refusing to allow operation.

Red-faced the professor left the witness stand. His place was taken by Charlotte Hofmann: She stuck to her story—that her father had always refused surgery until the cancer finally forced him to change his mind.

Seibert : Are you sure?

Charlotte Hofmann : Yes.

Seibert : Are you quite sure?

The judge fixed her with his eyes. The room was totally silent.

Charlotte Hofmann: Yes, well . . .
Siebert: I see you are uncertain.
Charlotte Hofmann: I do not know anything any more.
Seibert: Very well. You can go. I want to avoid another case of perjury.

Present in court during this astounding episode was a German trial lawyer, G. A. Stolting, from Frankfurt. He wrote an 'open letter' to the influential *Welt am Sonntag* bitterly criticising Seibert's behaviour—'he is like a lion in the arena, he plays an additional role of prosecutor.'

That publicity expressed what many lawyers said in private about the judge's intervention in the trial. Seidl had made no objection to Seibert's behaviour. He later explained why: 'His remarks came well into the trial. To have objected would have meant possibly a new trial with a new judge. But that would also have meant the prosecution would have had a chance to plug the holes we made in their cases.'

Next came the case of Richard Vogel. Issels' version of the facts was that he had recommended surgery, even though the prognosis was dubious. Vogel refused the suggestion, grew worse, and was referred by Issels to the E.N.T. Clinic at Munich University. There, Professor Herrmann recommended radiotherapy. It was carried out in Vogel's home town clinic at Tübingen University Hospital under the supervision of Professor Schwarz. Irradiation only produced short-term relief and Vogel died in June, 1959. Afterwards Professor Walter Büngeler, then secretary-general of the National Cancer Society, wrote to Schwarz that Vogel's case might be used to end the 'peculiar' treatment at the Ringberg Klinik.

Schwarz testified that if Vogel had undergone surgery instead of going to the Ringberg Klinik he would 'have lived two to three years longer than he did'; he was sure enough to say it was 'a probability bordering on certainty'.

Seibert: How high is that probability?
Schwarz: Ninety-nine per cent.

Seidl swiftly saw an opening.

Seidl: Even with the dubious prognosis you had of the case, you still maintain that Vogel would have lived?
Schwarz: Yes.
Seidl: Yet your clinic wrote on his case file that the prognosis was dubious, that the patient was in an advanced state of metastases *before* Vogel went to the Ringberg Klinik?
Schwarz: Yes.
Seidl: Yet you still persist with your answer?
Schwarz: Yes.

Professor Herrmann of Munich University told a similar story. Seidl worried away at Herrmann, but failed to shake the professor from his belief that surgery would have saved Vogel.

The prosecution called as its next expert Professor Hans Leicher, director of the E.N.T. Clinic at the University of Mainz. Greying and distinguished-looking, Leicher was a clinician with an international reputation. His testimony shattered Parsch:

Leicher: No doctor in the world can say with 'probability bordering on certainty' how long a patient will survive surgery. There are statistics saying that 50 per cent of all larynx carcinoma patients, of which Vogel was one, survive surgery by three years, and 73 per cent by one year. Nobody can however say whether Vogel would have belonged to the 73 per cent survival group, or the 27 per cent who died. Nobody can say how quickly a malignant tumour grows.

Leicher turned towards the defence table, ready to answer questions. None came. Neither Seidl or Fock felt it necessary to improve on what the professor had said.

Schwarz was recalled by the prosecution. His confidence had gone. He insisted on revising his previous statement, changing 'probability bordering on certainty' to 'great probability'.

By the middle of July newspapers reported the trial entered a 'tense phase' with expert witnesses fencing with the defence. There was also a more pedestrian explanation. The court had sat for four weeks in stifling heat. Badly ventilated, the room grew increasingly warmer. President Seibert suggested to Issels that he exchanged his black jacket and striped pants for a lightweight suit. Issels politely declined the offer.

Seidl hammered away, with mixed success, at the medical experts whose language grew more clear-cut. They stoutly believed surgery would have saved the patients in the indictment. Fock joined the attack. He also discovered it was one thing debating strategy in camera, rising in court was something else. The experts remained largely unruffled when defending the finer points of their subject. Inevitably their measured answers slowed down the trial as the warm June days droned past.

On July 15, Seidl tangled yet again with Professor Herrmann—this time over the case of Albert Matzeit, the printer who had repeatedly refused surgery. Two doctors had already testified that Metzeit, with cancer of the left larynx, had shied away from operation. The court listened in silence as the clinical picture unfolded, of Matzeit's desperate hunt for an answer other than surgery. Dr. Herrmann Tross, a part-time consultant at the Ringberg Klinik, testified he had regularly urged surgery since Matzeit was admitted—and that Issels also strongly recommended operation. The patient's case-notes were read; they included a pointed reference that surgery had been suggested by Issels—and rejected. The magisterial Professor Herrmann brushed that aside. For him the case was simple.

Herrmann: The patient would have lived longer if he had been operated on in time.
Seidl: At what time should he have been operated on to have, as you say, lived longer?
Herrmann: In February, 1959, when he went to the Ringberg Klinik. If he had undergone surgery then, he would have had a chance of 75 per cent to 80 per cent.
Seidl: How can you be so positive?
Herrmann: It is my opinion.

Mrs. Anni Matzeit revealed under Fock's cross-examination that her husband feared surgery because two of his brothers had died after operations. Fock pursued the point, and found himself in unexpected difficulty. Anni Matzeit insisted that if Issels had persisted her husband would have undergone surgery.

Fock: How do you know?
Anni Matzeit: I know my husband. Dr. Issels told us that his tumour could be dealt with in two or three weeks. He said it was a little thing.
Fock: Then why did your husband not have surgery immediately he left the clinic?

Anni Matzeit did not answer. Fock waited, letting the significance of her silence settle over the court.

Fock: Why did another four weeks elapse before he went for operation?

Again the silence stretched between counsel and witness.

Fock: He left the Ringberg Klinik, saying he wanted an operation. Instead he went to yet another doctor to see if another way was possible. Then your husband had a choking fit. Only then, after Dr. Issels, after other doctors, had urged an operation did he finally have one. Had he delayed out of fear?

Anni Matzeit said she did not know. Fock had retreived some lost ground. But, in spite of her silences, Anni Matzeit had made a definite impression. Reporters began to have second thoughts over the outcome. The procession of experts, the sheer weight of their testimony, the evidence of relatives like Anni Matzeit, combined to leave the case wide open.

The tension increased still further as Issels addressed the court over the last charge, the case of the young Bremen housewife, Else Warnken, diagnosed with breast cancer, and urged to have both breasts amputated and ovarectomy. Facing the judges Issels stated:

For me the human being is important. If a woman says to me: 'I want to keep my breasts for the sake of my marriage, and to keep my husband,' then I respect her wishes—after first having warned her about the risk. That is what happened in this case. She was young and naturally anxious about the effects such surgery could have on her marriage. From the outset she said, before she came to my clinic—and that is important—before she came to me, that she did not wish to have such surgery. She honestly felt it could affect her marriage.

Issels understood her fears; he believed every doctor appreciated the psychological factors associated with such drastic surgery. Supporting evidence came from Else's family doctor, Dr. Irmgard Munchow-Schmerl, who said it took her over three years to convince Else to undergo surgery. In the meantime she had spent two periods in the Ringberg Klinik. Seidl's examination drew out the important fact that two full years had elapsed since Else left the clinic before she finally consented to operation.

His questioning of Dr. Franz Schroeder, the surgeon, who finally removed Else's breasts and ovaries in August 1957, drew another vital admission for the defence. Schroeder insisted that Else had never told him that Issels kept her from surgery: 'I would very well remember such a statement as it would insult the heart of a surgeon.'

Parsch called Else's husband, Artur. He told a different story.

Warnken: Dr. Issels told me on the telephone that he believed amputation was not necessary.
Parsch: If he had recommended surgery what would your attitude have been?
Warnken: I would have accepted.
Parsch: And your wife?
Warnken: She, too, would have accepted. But my wife's letters to me from the clinic show that Issels never recommended operation.

Fock began his cross-examination in a characteristic manner. He set out to show that the letters were open to interpretation—that even if they did not contain specific words showing surgery had been recommended, nor did they show that surgery had not been urged.

> *Fock:* Is it not understandable that a wife does not tell her husband about her fears over amputation of her breasts—and the possible consequences for her marriage?
> *Warnken:* That would never had been a reason for me to leave my wife.
> *Fock:* I never suggested it was. I am only stating the possibility that because she had not written to you about surgery, it does not mean it had not been considered.

Warnken finally conceded that was another interpretation.

But the prosecution had a further trump to deal. Professor Rudolf Zenker, director of surgery at Munich University Hospital, and a doctor with a world-wide reputation, took the witness stand. He said that if Else had been his patient he would have strongly urged amputation, which would have prolonged her life 'for ten or twenty years'. It had been 'irresponsible' of Issels to have not insisted on amputation. Calm and authoritative, Zenker remained unshaken under cross-examination.

Fock moved, and was granted, a defence request to call rebuttal evidence. Professor Fritz Demmer of Vienna University was heard on the thirty-fifth day of the trial.

Demmer had pioneered the 'restricted radical operation' for breast cancer. It had brought him international fame. A soft-spoken, quietly-dressed man he outlined his technique and believed it could have been used in Else's case as opposed to the amputation performed. If the reporters failed to immediately see the relevance of Demmer's words—after all he was still talking of surgery, albeit a different type—the medical experts in court clearly realised the full importance of Demmer's words. He had shown that Zenker had not been entirely correct in stating that amputation was the only surgical answer in Else's case. Demmer went further. He said he believed amputation often produced serious psychological upset, depression, even to the point where a marriage was endangered—

'it is good that Issels makes an effort to save the breasts'.

Parsch furiously attacked Demmer, and the Public Prosecutor found himself drawn deep into medical matters. Like a benign lecturer addressing a first-year medical student Demmer restated his methods:

> Local metastases occur more often, but can be more easily removed. But distant metastases, like brain tumours occur more seldom, because my method leaves the lymph glands in the armpits intact. In comparison to amputation what I do is a small operation, and so the patient has greater resistance . . .

He sat down.

On July 24, the trial entered its final phase. Parsch summed up for the prosecution in a speech lasting two-and-a-half hours. It was a cool restatement of the prosecution's view. Issels was not reproached for trying to find a new way of treating cancer. His crime had been to have claimed success with his methods—'just to lure patients to the clinic.' He had deceived and defrauded for money. The prosecution had clearly showed that money played a considerable role in the case. Turning to the manslaughter charges, Parsch said it was: 'Tragic that Issels, with his authority, did not insist on surgery . . . the trustworthiness of the accused has suffered an irreparable lesion by his manipulation of the case-notes.'

He called for three-months prison sentences, to run consecutively, in the cases of Dehm, Schönek and Lang. The Wiesinger and Warnken counts should be punished by six months apiece, and Issels should be sentenced to a further five months each on the Vogel and Matzeit counts.

The three defence lawyers vigorously called for an acquittal. Kurt Kirstein said that the 'prosecution has been misused by certain factions of the medical profession'. Seidl revealed the sort of oratory which had brought him headlines defending Rudolf Hess:

> Trials of this sort are of no use to anybody. On the contrary they disturb the whole doctor-patient relationship . . .

> the Public Prosecutor would prefer that instead of an atmosphere of optimism at the Ringberg Klinik, there be an atmosphere of despair and hopelessness . . . then there must be considered the whole background to this trial . . . there are those twelve doctors, and that so-called scientific committee, and all the others. They all had one thing in common: a desire to hunt Issels into the ground . . . the problem of medical trials is summed up in an old proverb, 'one crow does not pinch out the eye of another crow'. So it is with doctors. But the solidarity of doctors should not be at the expense of the truth.

Fock was briefer and less eloquent. He ended his plea by introducing an *Eventual-Beweisantrag*, literally a 'plea of eventuality'. The document ensured that if the court found Issels guilty then before passing sentence, it had to take account of the thirty cases of 'cures' that the defence had agreed to 'temporarily' remove at the outset of the trial.

The court adjourned on Friday, July 28, 1961 after one of the longest medical trials in post-war Germany. The case had been prosecuted with a harshness rarely seen in a German criminal court; there was something Kafkaesque in the zeal of the prosecution to see Issels banished to a prison cell.

At three o'clock in the afternoon of Monday, July 31, President Seibert began reading the verdict:

> The court had not to judge the effectiveness of the internal therapy of the accused . . . it had not been an expert's trial. The court does not wish to be a referee between orthodox medicine and outsiders. According to his own words, the accused is not an outsider, but only a representative of modified orthodox medicine . . .

Seibert read steadily through the seventy-page verdict. Fraud had not been proven.

> But in the manslaughter cases, the court is of the opinion that the patients only hesitated and did not wish to refuse surgery. They would have undergone surgery if the accused had insisted and not spoken so optimistically

about his methods. He has violated his duty by not foreseeing, as he should have as a cancer specialist, the dangers of such omission. In reaching a verdict the following question was decisive for the court: is it possible to predict with 'probability bordering on certainty' whether a patient would live considerably longer when surgery is performed in the early stage of the cancer disease?

All the experts said yes, except one, Professor Leicher. The court did not feel disposed to specially examine the differing opinion of Professor Leicher. In the cases of Matzeit, Wiesinger and Warnken, the court has recognised a casual connection between omitted surgery and the death of those patients. The court did not see this in the case of Vogel. The suggestion of the defence that Dr. Issels, through his cures, could rely on the effectiveness of his treatment, has also been taken into account. When the defence demonstrates out of 2,300 cases (almost all of the patients treated at the clinic in the years 1951–60) only thirty cures this means only one per cent. With this small percentage of cure he could not reject surgery or radiotherapy. Those thirty cases, some of which have no histological verification, deal with other sorts of cancer than we have dealt with here. Therefore the court has decided to reject the *Eventual-Beweisantrag*.

The court found Issels guilty on three of the manslaughter charges: Karl Wiesinger, Albert Matzeit and Else Warnken. He was sentenced to one year of imprisonment.

Issels showed no emotion at the sentence. Nor did Isa. They had planned it that way.

Kurt Kirstein lodged an immediate appeal on the grounds of mis-direction by the court. Issels was freed pending the outcome.

The sentence caused uproar in the press. Editorial writers castigated the court 'for hampering those doctors seeking new treatment methods'.

The prestigious *Die Welt* wrote on August 1, 1961:

Not only the accused and defence counsel will object to this verdict. It will also undergo a great deal of criticism elsewhere—and rightly. The consequences which this verdict will have for numerous cancer patients and their doctors must have extremely regrettable consequences.

The influential *Frankfurter Allgemeine* wrote:

It was unsatisfactory to have dealt out of context with seven single cases. The question, put without any emotion, is whether the accused received justice, or even more precise, could he have received justice? The answer is no.

The Bavarian Medical Association issued statements that they had in no way been implicated in the pre-trial investigations. Professor Hans Leicher, whose evidence had shattered the prosecution, wrote a paper commenting on the medical aspects of the trial and was attacked by the Association. Hundreds of letters swamped Rottach-Egern post office from all over Europe encouraging Issels to press ahead for an acquittal. Among those who wrote was Albert Schweitzer. He saw the verdict as: 'Peculiar. Manslaughter with three cases. Who ever will be able to judge manslaughter with a doctor. Yet those cases are what justice is based on. You are right to appeal.'

Both he and Isa were exhausted by months of strain and accepted a friend's offer to stay in her flat on the French Riviera in September. Three weeks later, sun-tanned and relaxed, Issels and Isa returned to Germany to prepare for the appeal.

Seidl was retained at a fee of DM 4,000 to argue the case before the Supreme Court of West Germany in Karlsruhe. The appeal was heard on May 3, 1962 before Supreme Judge Hans Geyer. After a day of legal argument, he directed there should be a second trial in the three manslaughter counts because the lower court made a 'formal mistake' in rejecting the *Eventual-Beweisantrag*. The thirty cures the defence submitted should have been heard.

Seidl, Isa and Issels left the court satisfied. But for all three it was also a sad moment. Seidl would no longer be defence counsel: he could not spare the months, and possibly years, needed to prepare for a second trial. It would be an 'expert's case', with the outcome turning on highly specialist testimony. It would need a lawyer who could devote all his time to the case.

Issels appointed Norbert Kückelmann as his new trial lawyer. Kückelmann was thirty-five years old, with curly black hair, and a relaxed, breezy manner. It masked an incisive mind, well able to grasp the intricities of complex medical arguments.

The hunt began in June, 1962 to find expert witnesses for the defence. The search widened to include former patients, their doctors, their relatives who could testify favourably. Doctors and nurses who had worked in the clinic were sought. It was a hunt, Kückelmann predicted accurately, that spread all over Europe.

For Isa, in spite of the pressures, life had never been happier because she had a feeling of being really needed. At weekends, Rolf and Uti Issels visited their father in Rottach-Egern; he made regular return trips to see his former wife, Irmengard, and the children in Munich. Both families were united by a common wish: that the man in their life should be free to practise again his first love—medicine.

13

Final Verdict

THROUGHOUT 1962, THE DEFENCE STEADILY ADVANCED towards a second trial. Kückelmann, retained for DM 10,000 was a tireless investigator, and ably supported by Kurt Kirstein. The continuing publicity over the first trial brought forth new defence witnesses. Kückelmann interviewed them all over Europe. Soon he had a formidable list of former patients and clinic staff eager to testify about Issels' methods.

Issels and Isa attended medical conferences, seeking experts. Many offered private support—but they simply refused to risk their own careers by stating publicly they approved of Issels' methods.

In August they travelled with a group of German doctors to Moscow to attend the International Cancer Conference. Issels found surprising, and for him satisfying, support publicly expressed for his theories. He was invited to tour cancer laboratories attached to Moscow University. The Russians were astonished how far down the immunological road Issels had already travelled.

Back in Rottach-Egern, Isa spent long days in the clinic archives compiling vital statistics about the types of cancer her husband had treated, his success ratio, specific treatments—anything which could be useful for an acquittal. It was tiring work—but highly rewarding. Isa established that in sixty cases patients had been referred for surgery by Issels *after* they had refused similar recommendations from other doctors. Fifty in the group heeded Issels' advice. Six refused, and were cured in the clinic—surviving more than the recognised five years without detectable cancer. The remaining four had been Richard Vogel, Karl Wiesinger, Albert Matzeit and Else Warnken. The last three formed the indictment for the second trial.

The prosecution was in no hurry. The State's case was in the hands of Prosecutor Karl Rüth, a moustached, stubby man with a reputation for toughness. By early 1963, Kückelmann was asking for a firm trial date. Vague excuses about a lengthy court list were tendered.

Issels devoted the winter months to reading when he was not travelling to medical meetings. He regularly received scientific journals from all over the world. In a back-number of *The Lancet*, a British weekly journal of high reputation, he found, in the issue of March 10, 1962, an article which considerably excited him. It was a long article, but Issels memorised lengthy passages of *Cancer: An Attack on Cytologism* by Professor David Smithers of the Royal Marsden Hospital, London. Smithers had a deserved reputation as a distinguished cancerologist as well as being a pillar of the English medical establishment. Yet he publicly expressed identical views to Issels:

> The impression given by much cancer research today, basic and clinical, is that it is still trying to find proof of ideas which formed part of an outmoded theory about the cause of the cure of a specific disease of the cells . . . the dilemma of cancer research is exemplified by the increasing obscurity of much of the writing, by the extraordinary remoteness, range and intricacy of the lists of papers presented at cancer meetings and by their failure to illuminate the scene. Information accumulates apace while understanding lags behind. We are in need of some simple bold statements once more.

Smithers attacked the popular concept of cancer, the conventional guiding beliefs, the standard wisdom, even the basic premises. All needed to be swept aside for 'more helpful ideas'. It was a clarion call echoing what Issels had urged for a decade. Smithers continued:

Progress comes from a readiness to be just as positive, if necessary in another direction, as soon as better evidence points clearly where to go. After treatment cancer patients may live or die, recover or be made worse, or pursue the course of their disease unaffected by our efforts. Too often the issue is beyond our control, but when controlled by us and not by chance it is controlled by taking action which must be based on reasonably simple understandable ideas. These ideas are seldom expressed in all their nakedness, perhaps for fear of exposing their inadequacy; but they are, none the less, the sources of action. It is important that we have them out from time to time, look them in the face and decide if they are worthy of our con-continued support. It is, I believe, high time that our present ideas were changed and that modified action flowed from principles more in keeping with the facts.

What then are the simplifications on which we act at present? Not much useful action seems possible on the diffuse thought reaching us from cancer research organisations and the empiricism of the new methods offered, especially the non-specific generally applied cell poisons of present day chemotherapy, which have little but hope to support them. To write down the ideas on which we act may well produce sharp reactions from those who have not performed this task for themselves for far too long. The test which each clinician must apply to himself if he does so react, is to give a frank answer to the question: 'If not these, then on what principles are my day-to-day actions based? What is my personal view of this process, for without one I am ill equipped to treat its manifestations in my patients?' Anyone who has a satisfactory answer, whose view of the neoplastic process has moved beyond the simple ideas here set out, should give them air. The time is ripe for controversy about our fundamental concepts in this matter. Sound basic ideas are lacking amidst a plethora of nostrums. The horrible position of having to adjust oneself to a new situation, giving up ideas which were hardly won, of altering practice convenient to one's skills and inclinations, and of having to think again, is only forced on the unwilling when the case against the conventional view at last becomes overwhelming. Until that

> moment, resistance usually hardens as the established position is attacked, arguments in favour of popular belief are paraded, authority quoted, and irrelevant complexities scattered profusely around. Once old ideas are seen to be no longer defensible in sanity, they are, however, quickly allowed to subside into obsolescence, and the new becomes, for the time being, the conventional wisdom. Practice may lag some way behind this change in ideas, being liable to last-ditch stands on the grounds that 'it has always worked very well in my hands', until younger men take over.

It perfectly expressed the essentials of Issels' defence to the charges his ideas were ill-founded. Smithers, at the hub of one of the major cancer research centres in the world went on:

> We need to restate conventional cancer theory in new terms more consistent with our history and with the observed facts and more in keeping with the logic of the situation. When we do this, much that has seemed to be obscure leaps into the light. We can then devise experiments to attack the new version of the theory at its weakest points and eventually see how to replace it by one which is more comprehensive and more fruitful of successful prediction.

Issels filed the article in a special folder he kept for material particularly relevant to his defence. He found its author refreshingly open-minded.

Throughout the summer of 1963 Kückelmann tracked down new witnesses whose testimony might demolish the manslaughter charges. They were patients and doctors who said Else Warnken, Albert Matzeit and Karl Wiesinger had consistently refused surgery until it was too late.

But the defence clearly needed its own experts. One finally emerged from behind the Iron Curtain. Dr. Leo Savnik was director of the Government Cancer Institute in Ljubljana, Yugoslavia. The seventy-year-old gynaecologist and oncologist was on a fact-finding tour of Germany when he met Issels and agreed to give expert testimony. Facing Savnik in court would be some of the most powerful medical men in Germany, including the legendary Professor Karl Bauer. Kückelmann had no intention of challenging the presence of such experts. He knew to achieve not only legal acquittal but also a wider exoneration Issels must overcome such formidable adversaries.

By early 1964 the prosecution still demurred over a trial date. Finally, late in the summer of that year, it was set: October 29. The venue: courtroom number twenty-eight. Only the bench was changed. President Göppner was joined by Judge Huber and Judge Pöll. One newspaper heralded the case as: 'never before in modern science have such formidable opponents faced each other over the fundamental questions of cancer.'

Isa and Issels moved back to the Munich hotel they occupied during the first trial. Apart from Isa being pregnant, everything was the same; the air of timelessness extended to the courtroom; all was exactly as it had been over three years earlier.

The mood of the trial came in an opening skirmish. The prosecution accepted that it was unnecessary to hear testimony from Teicher, Glaeser or other members of the medical cabal from the first trial. The indictment was brief. Issels had allegedly shortened the lives of Else Warnken, Albert Matzeit and Karl Wiesinger by not sending them for surgery in time.

In his familiar striped pants and black jacket Issels addressed the court. His speech was one David Smithers might well have written: nobody knew where the breakthrough in cancer would finally come. But certain things were clear. There was a poverty of ideas in the accepted attitude towards the disease, especially in the advanced state. There appeared to be no firm concept of attack; it was essential never to forget that *man* must be the constant object of all those seeking a solution to the disease. He went on to define the importance of basic treatment to reinforce resistance, of teeth and tonsil extractions in his concept that cancer was a chronic, degenerative disease where almost all essential organs were involved in the more advanced cases. Further:

With cancer there is often a permanent psychological strain. Psychological guidance of the patient is very important; therefore one has to be optimistic and give hope. If a patient has a special wish, such as placing a plaster of cabbage leaves on his body, as one patient in fact did, and providing it does no harm, then I fulfil the wish because I believe the psychological benefit is helpful.

His reference to the cabbage leaves was an open admission that bizarre things did happen in the clinic and that they only made sense when viewed from the psychological standpoint. Issels emphasised that his treatment began where other doctors stopped; that his patients were almost exclusively drawn from the *incurable* category—but that in the three cases before the court he had repeatedly urged surgery as a potential cure. It was a point President Göppner developed in the first case, that of Karl Wiesinger:

Göppner: Why did you not have a written release?
Issels: That was my fault.
Göppner: Why did you accept Wiesinger for treatment in the first place when he had refused surgery?
Issels: It is my duty as a doctor to treat him—otherwise I would be sending him into the hands of a herbal doctor.

Kückelmann securely stitched-up the Wiesinger case by calling three new witnesses, as well as others who had testified in the first trial, to show convincing proof of Wiesinger's opposition to surgery. Prosecutor Rüth failed to shake their stories.

The first sensation came when Kückelmann called Dr. Helmut Spohr, a former administrator of the National Cancer Society. Kückelmann wanted to show something of the under-currents of the trial. Spohr said he had been present at society meetings when Issels and his methods were discussed:

Spohr: Professor Büngeler said we should put a stop to his work.
Kückelmann: Was he alone in this attitude?
Spohr: No. For example, on November 28, 1958 there

> was a meeting at the Bavarian Medical Association between the Administrator of the Association, Professor Eder and myself. They had concrete ideas to undertake something against Issels because his principles did not fit the conventional concept. At the Cancer Congress in London, in 1958, the conversations were similar.

Kückelmann pressed no further: he had achieved his goal of implicating the medical establishment in the trial.

Spohr's evidence offered the reporters a welcome break from the tortuous daily unfolding of an extremely complex medical and legal situation. His testimony also set the seismographs of the German medical world fluctuating wildly and was a reminder this was still a *cause celebre*. The necessary ambiance and sense of high theatre was still there; prosecutor Rüth stalked the witnesses with the same skill as Leo Parsch; Kückelmann was as astute with every question as Seidl had been. But for all that the second trial was far different from the first one. The contrast lay in the way the second one was controlled. President Göppner maintained a proper distance with the rest of the proceedings. It made for a relaxed atmosphere, and left the reporters seeking colour for their stories elsewhere.

After a day of dry testimony the press played-up the presence of Irmengard, Uti, Rolf and Isa seated together in court. Irmengard had avoided the first trial, with its accusations of fraud, but testified in the second trial, with its newspaper-boosted glamour of being 'a medical trial of strength'. She was one of the character witnesses called by the defence.

Isa did not give evidence, but renewed her role as a court observer for the defence. In the recesses she provided Kurt Kirstein and Kückelmann with useful tips about a witness still to be called, or the reaction of the prosecution to a particular piece of defence questioning. Few in court suspected the true worth of Isa's contribution to her husband's defence. In maintaining minimal exposure of her help, Isa unwittingly presented an image of herself as an aloof, cold personality. Only Issels saw a warm and sensitive woman, one who was a cautious but decisive thinker working late into the night to help prepare him for the trial.

By the middle of November the court was preoccupied with the story of Albert Matzeit. Issels outlined the medical details of 'a man opposed to losing his voice'. He explained how he tried to lead Matzeit, step-by-step, to an operation by first persuading him to have some dead teeth and tonsils out. But Matzeit still shied away from having his malignant larynx excised. Dr. Hermann Tross, the E.N.T. consultant at the Ringberg Klinik, told a similar story. The deeply unhappy Matzeit had left the clinic searching elsewhere for a solution outside surgery to his case. He failed. Three new witnesses testified about Matzeit's fears of an operation. The prosecution failed to cast doubts on their statements. Professor Alfred Kressner, director of the E.N.T. Clinic at Munich's Rechts-der-Isar Hospital, called as a court expert, stated that even if surgery had been performed immediately Matzeit entered the Ringberg Klinik, 'the prognosis was already poor'. In the first trial, Professor Alexander Herrmann, a key witness, had stated virtually the opposite. Kressner's testimony, apart from revealing a real gulf between experts, also ended the Matzeit story.

The court recessed for the weekend. Issels and Isa returned home to Rottach-Egern to see their son, Hellmut, walk in the mountains, and read the lengthy newspaper accounts of the case. They felt the popular press were behind them; certainly several newspapers highlighted defence points. But most of the weekend was spent preparing for the case of Else Warnken. Kückelmann had predicted the final verdict largely depended on testimony over the young housewife.

Issels cleared the first hurdle by insisting he 'honestly cannot remember' the fateful conversation with Else's husband, Artur Warnken, in which the question of amputation was discussed. Issels went on:

> She threatened to go elsewhere unless I treated her. I tried to persuade her to have surgery. She refused because she feared the effects on her marriage of having both breasts amputated and an ovarectomy. I understood her fears. But I still tried to persuade her to think about an operation.

Artur Warnken took the stand. He was quieter and not so

dogmatic as he had been in the first trial. Gently, but firmly, Kückelmann drew out valuable admissions. Else had been 'strongly opposed' to amputation from the outset—'her mother and a girl friend had died during similar surgery'. Even after leaving the Ringberg Klinik she still sought non-surgical solutions. Warnken agreed his wife's fears were so deep-seated that it had taken years of intensive persuasion long after she had left the clinic to consider surgery—and then the operation was far too late.

'Fear,' said Kückelmann. 'That is what this case is about. Fear, not manslaughter, but fear. The understandable fear of a woman who does not wish to be disfigured.'

A succession of doctors expanded on that fear. They had treated Else over the years of her illness and all swore she firmly rejected amputation. A clinic doctor testified: 'The patient told me: "Doctor, you are a man. I am a woman. You will never understand me."'

A clinic nurse said that Else had rejected surgery 'because she did not wish to be mutilated'.

> *Rüth :* Who talked of mutilation?
> *Nurse :* The patient did. It was she who said she did not wish to be mutilated.

The prosecutor sat down, well aware that further questions might further sap his case.

The court heard expert testimony from Professor Karl Blumensaat, surgical director of the Knappschaft Hospital at Bottrop. He had inspected the clinic some years before, and had reported favourably on its methods. Nevertheless Blumensaat felt that amputation was the only answer in Else's case. Kückelmann questioned the professor as to why he could be so certain in this specific case, but Blumensaat clung to his opinion. Kückelmann then called Professor Georg Salzer, professor of surgery, at the Lainzer Hospital, Vienna, who offered another surgical solution—the 'restricted radical operation', pioneered by Professor Fritz Demmer. Salzer added that biological follow-up treatment would be recommended in such a case.

Again, the defence had scored an important point. A respected surgeon had shown that even with surgery, there was no need for the emotionally crippling amputation that had been urged on Else. Her fears of surgery had stemmed from that very first day when a Bremen surgeon had told her that both her breasts and her ovaries would be removed. When Issels later pressed her to consider surgery that would not be so drastic her fears had overridden all other considerations.

The prosecution sought, and was granted, leave to call yet a third expert to rebut Salzer's testimony. Rüth said he needed time to introduce a suitable expert—and the court put back Else's case until he could appear.

That ruling marked a new phase in the trial; the hearing from both sides of expert testimony over cancer and its treatment.

The defence was heard first. Its answer that cancer was not a local disease was rooted in the words of Professor David Smithers, who wrote of the need for a revised cancer image. Smithers, who had yet to meet Issels, expressed a view that conventional cancer theories contained too many incompatibilities, that it was so hedged about by compromises and obscurity that it could not be seen for what it was—outmoded. Smithers had not referred specifically to Issels' views on cancer, but much of what he wrote came remarkably close to the defence's attack on conventional attitudes.

The first blow came from Dr. Primarius Kretz editor of *Krebsarzt*, the journal of the Austrian Cancer Society. Like Smithers, he believed there was a need for a new concept in cancer—but went further in his belief in the need for a general recognition that it was a 'whole body disease with psychological side-effects'. Kretz developed his argument with a rare lucidity: medical science had eliminated the totality of the natural biological rules of the human body, mostly by dividing up research into so many specialities: medicine had forgotten that every part was only a piece of the entire body: '*Ganzheitstherapie* is not new but it is different. It looks on the patient as a whole. It affords no risks, no mortality. It only offers a chance, an improved chance of a cure.'

It was a theme other defence witnesses expounded on.

Many were practitioners of *ganzheit* methods. In spite of fierce attacks on their credentials they maintained their composure. The prosecution did not attack Professor Werner Zabel's standing: as the promoter of modern *ganzheitstherapie,* he was still a powerful figure in German medical circles. He insisted that 'before a growth starts, the function of the organism must have been abnormal. That is a real blow to the concept that the tumour is a locally limited disease.'

Slowly but steadily a defence picture emerged of cancer being a chronic disease where it was not enough to only recommend surgery or radiotherapy; the primary tumour was a local manifestation of a general disposition to cancer. Some of the defence experts were not well known, and did not have the status of university posts. The prosecution pounced on them. Cross-examination revealed that the doctors held a sophisticated view of cancer, even if only by appreciating some of the many discrepancies in conventional dogma about the disease. By the end of November the defence presentation ended.

On November 30, the prosecution experts were heard. Courtroom number twenty-eight was not big enough to hold the press and television crews who wished to record that part of the trial, so the hearing was transferred to the enormous main court of the Palace of Justice.

There was an immediate sensation when Kückelmann objected to the presence of Professor Karl Bauer, professor of surgery at Heidelberg University, and the most powerful single voice among European cancerologists; Professor Herwig Hamperl, professor of pathology at Bonn University; Professor Julius Ries, director of the Gynaecological-Radiotherapy Institute at Munich University. Kückelmann asked they be barred from speaking on the grounds that:

> Bauer belongs to a small, but powerful, group of university professors who have persecuted Issels. He has discredited Issels' work without knowing anything of it because of personal reasons, not only scientific reasons. He has attacked the accused before this trial with subjective acrimony, using all his authority and power to do so.

> Hamperl has shown a clear attitude of bias and prejudice. Ries has shown a very negative attitude towards Issels when he was a prosecution adviser at the time the accused was originally imprisoned pending investigation. His philosophy towards the accused can be summed up as 'it is easy to cure cancer when there is no cancer'.

The court rejected the petition. Kückelmann promptly produced another. He wanted leave to call Dr. Mark Sauthem, a cancerologist at the Sloan-Kettering Institute in New York and Professor I. Kosaki, from Tokyo University. Counsel told the court that both men had shown cancer was not a local disease. The motion was denied on the grounds it was irrelevant.

Professor Karl Bauer took the stand. Small, slightly built and precisely-manner, he revealed a surprisingly clear voice as he addressed the court.

> It is impossible for this court, for any court, to judge about the genesis of cancer. That is a matter for experts who can prove they are experts . . . nobody will deny that the cancer problem is not yet solved. But I will not have it suggested that I am against outsiders. All I say is that they have to prove scientifically their claims. The thesis of cancer as a general disease cannot be proved scientifically. Cancer starts on one spot of the organism, and the whole organism is then involved later. The cancer cell is the primary, and the general disease is the consequence.

Bauer turned to Issels' methods. He dismissed them as little more than 'putting cabbage poultices on patients'.

President Göppner intervened. He sternly reminded Bauer: 'I want to draw your attention to the fact that such allegations have already been settled.'

Bauer shrugged off the rebuke: 'In my whole career I have not met a single patient who has refused surgery. If Dr. Issels had insisted on surgery as strongly as he did on tonsilectomy he would not be here . . .'

It was heady stuff for the press. Surrounded by photographers and film cameramen Bauer tilted away:

> To be able to judge the efficiency of Issels' treatment would need a committee of experts. But in this trial it is not a question of whether Issels has another weapon against cancer, but whether it was his duty to apply or recommend the only successful treatment in the early stages—surgery.

He came to a stop, looking around the court. Kückelmann waived cross-examination. The lawyer saw it as the most effective way to express the defence's contempt for Bauer's views.

Professor Julius Ries was next on the stand. He was tall and portly with the manner of a born lecturer:

> We cannot believe that the accused has cured cancer, even one genuine case of cancer. He should have remained running a sanatorium for follow-up treatment; with his claim to have cured cancer his misfortune started. He overreached his capability and this led to the situation where operable patients became patients refusing operations.

Ries was in full stride about the difficulties even he had in recognising cancer symptoms at various stages of conventional treatment when Issels rose to his feet. Like his defence lawyers he was entitled to cross-examine expert witnesses on points of medical interest.

> *Issels :* You have stated that in general gynaecologists, not having your standing and experience, often cannot discern tumour recurrence from the after-effects of radiotherapy?
> *Ries :* That is correct.
> *Issels :* Then how many women in ordinary clinics are mutilated without it being sure they definitely have cancer?
> *Ries :* Mutilated? They are not crippled. The patients still have their legs and can walk.

Professor Hans Erhard Bock, then President of the German Cancer Society, testified that there was no known cure for cancer outside surgery and radiotherapy.

Bock: Issels uses too many drugs and measures to the point where they cannot be critically evaluated by anybody.
Kückelmann: He has had cures.
Bock: I do not deny that he has had results. But I am of the opinion that the drug 'doctor and hope' plays an important role. Issels fails to examine the effectiveness of single measures. If you shoot shrapnel you will certainly not know which piece hit the target. But you must look.
Issels: I do look. I look at every piece. Every measure of my system of treatment has its part to play.

There was an audible rustle of expectancy as Kückelmann rose to present the next stage of the hearing: the examination of thirty-four cases of cures performed at the Ringberg Klinik. Among them were the cases of Thea Döhm and Käthe Gerlach. Both patients and their doctors testified that Issels had cured them. It was a dramatic moment, made more so by the prosecution's medical experts doubting how the women had been cured. It set a pattern: one case after another was challenged on that ground. Soon the courtroom became bogged down with highly technical medical arguments. Issels followed attentively; he had briefed himself thoroughly by reading the latest medical literature. The defence table was piled with books and journals. But the press and public were often bewildered by the exchanges. Only momentarily did the fog lift and the spectators sense the drama behind the questions and answers in such cases as that of Helene Koch.

The fifty-three-year-old housewife's case was enlivened by the appearance of Professor Peter Stoll for the prosecution. Mrs. Koch had been diagnosed as having inoperable cancer of the uterus. She received radium treatment and later radiotherapy. Two specialists, Dr. Klaus Klöppner and Professor Hans Busse saw her separately and decided no further treatment was possible. But after two periods at the Ringberg Klinik she had shown, according to Klöppner, 'a complete remission'. Professor Stoll disagreed that Issels' methods had played any specific part in her cure. Issels took issue:

Issels: Professor Busse diagnosed the patient, and with his experience and standing, how can you dispute his conclusion?
Stoll: In general, an ordinary clinical gynaecologist cannot judge whether it was a recurrence or the after-effects of radiotherapy.
Issels: On that basis you doubt the qualifications of literally hundreds of ordinary, clinical gynaecologists who every day irradiate their patients without being sure whether they are actually treating cancer or not?
Stoll: It is difficult even for me, with my experience, to always know if it is cancer.
Kückelmann: Can you exclude that this case was cured by Dr. Issels?
Stoll: No. But for me it is not proof.

Stoll, Professor of gynaecology at Heidelberg University, was still more revealing in the case of Renate Werner, a twenty-eight-year-old bride who had been diagnosed as having cancer of the uterus. She had received a preliminary curetting of the womb, but refused a hysterectomy. After two spells at the Ringberg Klinik she was discharged as 'free of detectable cancer'.

Stoll: She was cured by the curetting. It was not an invasive cancer. I even doubt if it was cancer at all.
Issels: You say that in spite of three independent diagnosis of cancer by pathologists at reputable institutes, including the Histo-Pathological Institute of the University of Zurich, whose director, Professor von Albertini diagnosed invasive carcinoma?
Stoll: Yes. In my opinion it was not cancer.
Kückelmann: I must conclude that the expert is shaking the very foundation of surgery and radiotherapy in cancer treatment in order not to admit that Issels cured this patient.
Stoll: We must never accept a diagnosis.
Kückelmann: Especially one in favour of the accused . . .

The lawyer sat down. Stoll left the witness box looking every bit as confident as he had appeared at the outset.

The case of Elisabeth Dreyer caused an unexpected sensation.

The thirty-four-year-old widow, mother of two children, was one of many patients Issels had treated free of charge. Her medical story began in early 1952 when she was diagnosed with progressive, 'stage three' cancer of the uterus. A hysterectomy had been performed, but it had not been possible to remove all the growth. Elisabeth received follow-up radiotherapy. But, in June, 1952 she experienced a relapse. She received further irradiation 'to the limit of endurance'. In July, 1953 she suffered a second relapse, and was said to be beyond further conventional aid. She received four months' treatment at the Ringberg Klinik: on the day she was admitted, one of the clinic's outside consultants found: 'her whole abdomen filled with tumorous mass'. After leaving the clinic she continued follow-up treatment at home, returned for a further six weeks as an in-patient, and by 1958 the gynaecologist who performed the original hysterectomy verified she had undergone a complete remission.

It was, said the defence, a classic case of Issels succeeding where all else failed. The prosecution contended that Elisabeth had survived because of surgery and follow-up radiotherapy.

Professor Bodo Manstein was called as an expert witness. The exchanges between him and Kückelmann electrified the court:

Kückelmann : The patient is alive?
Manstein : Yes she is alive.
Kückelmann : Why?
Manstein : I am sure the patient would have died without the systematic treatment of Dr. Issels.

It was the breakthrough the defence sought. It hammered home its advantage by calling its own expert. Dr. Leo Savnik, one of Yugoslavia's leading cancerologists. He was 'positive' that Issels had effected a cure, and had done so with a specific cancer treatment.

Prosecutor Rüth and his aides were invested with a proper crusading spirit. But they must have felt their confidence ebbing as the defence presented the case of Gerta Kaiser, a sixty-four-year-old housewife with a tumour of the thyroid gland. The diagnosis that it was malignant had been made by the Pathological Institute of Berlin University. Professor Heinz Oeser, director of the world-famous Radiotherapy Institute at the university urged surgery and radiotherapy. Mrs. Kaiser had rejected the advice. Without receiving any previous form of conventional treatment she spent twelve weeks in the Ringberg Klinik and, after follow-up treatment at home, doctors diagnosed a complete remission. She sat in court as the prosecution sought to prove that she had never suffered from cancer.

Oeser took the stand. The distinguished doctor, immaculately dressed, exuded quiet confidence as he faced a tense courtroom. He created an immediate sensation:

Oeser : In retrospect I believe it was a case of a non-specific inflammation.
Rüth : Why do you say that?
Oeser : The whole course of her disease indicates it cannot have been cancer. Retrospectively, it cannot have been cancer.

No defence grilling matched the ferocity of Kückelmann's attack on Oeser. In biting language he fired a volley of questions:

Kückelmann : We have three independent pathological diagnoses from reputable clinics. All three state the same. It was cancer. How do you explain that?
Oeser : I can only say that I doubt the pathological interpretations.
Kückelmann : You doubt all three?
Oeser : Yes.
Kückelmann : Even though you do not doubt the reputations of the Institutes concerned?
Oeser : Yes, in this case, yes.

Kückelmann shook his head wonderingly. Issels rose to ask a question.

Issels : Had the patient been operated, and then irradiated following the diagnosis, then this diagnosis would have been right?

Gerta Kaiser leapt to her feet shouting:

Kaiser : Then I would be dead now!
Oeser : You would be here exactly as you are now!
Kaiser : No I would not!

Uproar filled the court. Spectators shouted at Oeser, standing flushed with anger in the witness stand. It took minutes for the judge to restore order. Issels lunged into the attack:

Issels : You have admitted recommending both surgery and radiotherapy after you first saw the patient. Why?

Oeser remained silent.

Issels : Now you have a different opinion? Have you decided it was not cancer because the patient is still alive?
Oeser : Yes.

Issels sat down, leaving Kückelmann to deliver the final questions:

Kückelmann : Can you exclude it was not cancer?
Oeser : No.
Kückelmann : Can you exclude it was cancer cured by the accused?
Oeser : No . . .

That clash marked the virtual end of the prosecution's attempts to seriously discredit the cures. In all the defence presented eight cases of cancer of the cervix, six uterus cancers, five breast cancers, two brain tumours, two lung cancers, two cases of cancer of the ovaries, and single cases of cancer of the colon, rectum, testes, stomach, thyroid, sarcoma of the spine, sarcoma of the leg, a case of lymph-sarcoma in a child and a case of Hodgkin's Disease. Five defence experts testified the cases illustrated the effectiveness of Issels' treatment. Among others the prosecution countered with Professor Stoll and Professor Manstein. In the end both experts made remarkable concessions. Stoll said Issels had dealt 'with progressive cancer in a remarkable way'. Manstein admitted:

> It is important to have such clinics, and we are receptive to the efforts of Issels. When he has performed cures then we should recognise them, examine how they were achieved and follow the principles of *ganzheit* medicine. I recognise the exactness of the case-notes and the responsible work carried on at the clinic.

On December 3, the presentation of cured cases was followed by the evidence of Dr. Heinz Laprell, medical director of the Tegernsee Hospital, near the Ringberg Klinik. He said that in a four-year period Issels referred forty-nine patients to him for surgery. Another nail had been driven into the prosecution coffin.

Rüth made one last attempt to retrieve the situation by returning to the case of Else Warnken. He had found his expert, Professor Werner Wachsmuth, director of surgery at Würzburg University. He 'heavily reproached' Issels for having kept Else from surgery. Once more the spectre of Issels' 'lack of sense of proper duty' was before the court. Issels was 'irresponsible' in not insisting that Else had a full amputation of both her breasts: 'if she had been so operated she had an 85 per cent chance of a cure.' The defence poured scorn on such an exact prognosis. Finally, Kückelmann produced his trump: new witnesses who testified that Else Warnken had always emphatically spoken out against surgery before, during and long after her stay in the Ringberg Klinik.

On December 8, 1964, Prosecutor Rüth called upon the court to sentence Issels to four months' imprisonment for causing the death of Else Warnken, to be followed by three years probation and to be fined DM 3,000.

Kückelmann, visibly tired at the end of the six-week trial, spoke quietly and firmly. He began with a quotation from Emile Zola:

'The truth is coming and nothing can stop it.' The very essence of this trial were the prosecution witnesses whose attitude can be summarised by the motto, 'as it must not be—it cannot be' . . . one phrase in Professor Bauer's textbook is that not one case of cancer has been cured by *ganzheitstherapie*. But that has now been shaken by the evidence heard here. If this trial shows nothing else, then it shows a need for the concepts of the accused to be examined thoroughly.

Kückelmann, like Kurt Kirstein, the other defence lawyer, called for an acquittal. All eyes then turned on Issels. He rose slowly to his feet to speak for the last time in the trial. It was a concise resumé of his whole treatment philosophy, his beliefs as a doctor, his abiding concern for the welfare of his patients:

I have always taken my profession seriously, perhaps more so than some other doctors. I went on where other doctors gave up. I never acted against my duty. I always acted in the best interests of my patients. I can honestly feel no guilt over the deaths of the three patients because they repeatedly refused my pleas that they had surgery. I always acted to the best of my conscience and knowledge. But I had to respect their decision—they alone had the right to decide what was to be done with their bodies. In Roman law it is clearly stated that the will of the patient is the highest law. In spite of their refusal of surgery, I tried to give them maximum help.

He paused to sip some water. It was the only sound in the stilled courtroom.

I saw my task as developing a treatment for the so-called incurables—but not ever to keep curable patients from conventional treatment. Science should not be an end to itself. It should serve doctors to give our patients the best chance of success with the minimum amount of damage to their bodies. A doctor has always to act to best meet the individual circumstances of a patient. Statistics alone should not determine his actions. I have often asked my-

> self what is the real purpose of this trial. I think I have at last found it. It has been a fight to gain freedom for a new way of treating and research for cancer patients beyond conventional help.

His statement lasted for almost an hour. He was visibly affected when he sat down in the middle of the afternoon of December 9, to thunderous applause.

The verdict came two days later. A packed court heard President Göppner find Josef Issels not guilty. The judge's words were lost in tumultuous applause.

Isa had a corner seat in the courtroom. Few saw her crying behind sun-glasses. Issels bowed his head and wept into his hands. Irmengard, Uti and Rolf also blinked tears. Composed again, Issels and Isa were ushered by friends from the courtroom, jammed with press and television cameramen.

In all Issels had spent DM 250,000 of his own money to clear his name. The court ordered the State to repay his costs. During the four-year legal battle he had practised no medicine. As he left the Palace of Justice, a reporter asked him what he wanted to do. Issels replied: 'I just want to get back to my patients.'

14

Renewed Struggles

THE BAVARIAN MEDICAL ASSOCIATION WAS ANGERED WITH the verdict and said so publicly in its monthly journal. It was an unprecedented attack on the proceedings, the trial judges, defence lawyers, and Issels—a polemic that belonged to a byegone age of denunciation. Nor did the Association stop there. The editor of its journal penned a further article libellous enough for Issels to obtain an injunction. The revised text was finally published in a Munich newspaper. National press interest in the case remained high. Former patients found magazines eager to buy their stories of alleged cures. Irmengard was paid for a series rehashing her working life and times with Issels.

From the day he and Isa returned to Rottach-Egern, Issels was bombarded by the press for the rights to his story; publishers made approaches for a full-length book. He rejected them all. Some magazines then adopted a new tactic. They told Issels that unless he co-operated with them they would run their own version of his life story. Perturbed, Issels sought legal advice. He was told the only way to kerb the excesses of the Continental press was to make a contract with one magazine for an 'authorised first person' story. Issels was not wildly enthusiastic, but accepted the advice. Late in December, 1964, the mass-circulation *Quick* began serialising his life. They paid DM 40,000 for the rights. Every mark went to reopening the clinic. It was the opening the Bavarian Medical Association needed. Issels was hauled before its Disciplinary Committee charged with unprofessional conduct. He was fined DM 5,000 and cautioned over further contact with the lay press. The verdict angered him: other doctors regularly wrote for newspapers and escaped censure.

Isa foresaw, correctly, that the articles caused raised eyebrows even among doctors sympathetic to Issels. *Quick* was a brash weekly—and not an accepted forum for serious medical views. It was one more burden for her to cope with. Isa was exhausted by years of strain. Her second son, Christian, was born in February, 1965. A combination of sleepless nights with the baby and long days planning with her husband the re-opening of the clinic took its toll.

Issels found a necessary relaxation by going to Munich where he wined and dined a succession of pretty girls. He did so with Isa's blessing. She trusted her husband completely and believed their marriage strong enough to survive such moments. Issels also called regularly on Irmengard, Rolf and Uti. Isa also encouraged that contact; she was that rare woman, one without jealousy. Her motives were misunderstood. Uti and Rolf looked on their father's regular visits to Munich as a sign of unhappiness in his second marriage. Uti recalled:

> There was a sadness about him. He would have preferred it if Isa had gone out with him. For years he had told us how good she was at everything—including speaking fluent French. That was the big point with him. She could speak fluent French and we couldn't. I remember my mother once said that you didn't choose a wife because of a linguistic fact. Of course Isa could do more. She showed that at the trial. But when that was over she seemed to fade away. So Father had to go out alone. It was such a shame for him that his beautiful wife often seemed too unwell to be with him.

It was an unjust picture of Isa. It took no account of the sheer hard work she put in for years, or the patience and buoyancy she showed in nearly seven years of marriage largely overshadowed by outside conflict. Isa had sacrificed her health and strength for her husband, and he appreciated it. He also recognised her genuine attemps to establish a meaningful relationship with Uti and Rolf. Both were grown-up and found it hard to reciprocate her friendship. There was little more than an outward show of politeness. Rolf summed up his relationship with his step-mother as: 'Respect. Just respect. No more, no less.' Uti: 'I have no real relationship with her, though my father has asked me to try.' It saddened her father immeasurably when he learnt that his dream of a united family would not be possible.

Uti, in particular, found the situation intolerable. She claimed that her father had told her:

> When he married Isa he had told her that his work came first, then his family from the first marriage, then Isa. Now when I met him he seemed so sad. Isa had become ill, or weak, or having to go to bed early. It all added up and he was tired of it. That's why he went to Munich alone just to talk to some young girl . . . nothing more, just talk.

Uti found it easier to stay away from Rottach-Egern.

Issels felt that was a distorted picture. Isa had only been ill twice in her marriage. Uti's view failed to express totally what only her father knew; that his second marriage was secure; that the sadness came from a totally different source. On more than one occasion he had even wept at the thought of the five years he had lost as a doctor.

Yet, if Issels wanted a life of pleasure the temptation was there. The *Arbeitsgemeinschaft*, the welfare agency leasing the clinic, offered a ten-year extension contract with the guarantee of a generous monthly stipend for Issels. He received further offers to act as a handsomely salaried medical director of various clinics. He refused. His only ambition was re-opening the Ringberg Klinik and treating those he regarded as 'incurable' cancer patients.

By the summer of 1965 his plans were well advanced. The welfare agency agreed to hand back the clinic as soon as Issels was ready. He recruited nurses and doctors. Professor Franz Gerlach and his wife returned to work in the research laboratories. Gerlach said he needed two years to develop fresh batches of immunological vaccines. Issels set about finding a stop-gap drug.

On September 15, exactly five years since being arrested in his offices, he sat there again briefing his doctors on how to help those seemingly beyond hope. The ghosts of Huneke and Rühmkorff were clearly present.

There were fifteen patients in the clinic the day it re-opened with one ward. Within a month there were eighty 'incurables'. Several of them died soon after admission because they were virtually moribund on arrival.

Issels keenly felt the old and familiar strains of coping with the dying, and afterwards the bereaved relatives. He was fifty-eight years old, an age when he was beginning to consider the approaching imminence of his own end. He was convinced dying need not be a time of fear for anybody. He observed that many close to death were influenced by entrenched attitudes and fears of dying, but still that did not mean that during the act of dying unpleasant thoughts of death dominated. Quite the contrary was often true: dying patients displayed a humbling serenity rarely seen in healthy people.

Issels' religious beliefs also widened in late middle-age, and that also influenced his outlook on death. He rejected religious dogma where death was used to encourage spiritual laggards. Though still a believer in Catholicism, he increasingly turned to the teachings of Buddhism and Hinduism. He was attracted by Eastern thought with its view that man must renounce the world to accept life. He grew increasingly concerned with such questions as relating his own thoughts to the life he lived and those same thoughts to the universe in which he lived. He concluded it was impossible attempting to explain the universe. Once more he was guided by the words of Albert Schweitzer who wrote that the glories of the universe were matched with equal horror; that the very spirit of the universe was both creative and destructive: it created what it destroyed and destroyed what it created and because of that would always be a riddle. Schweitzer had died a few days before the clinic re-opened. But of all the influences on the philosophical side of Issels' character, Schweitzer's remained constant. Issels came to the same conclusion that Schweitzer had: the universe was morally, objectively and rationally neutral. It was unbiased—it was simply there. Man was biased—it made life meaningful. It was essential to take sides, to make a consistent commitment. Issels believed he had done so by his treatment of terminal cancer cases. But he was still hurt and bewildered that his acquittal had not brought recognition; he had a strong feeling of isolation. Yet he also saw the logic of his life as strikingly clear: there were new dreams to be fulfilled. He refused to accept that leisure was the principal benefit of longevity. On his fifty-ninth birthday he demonstrated the same application which he revealed thirty years earlier—putting in a fourteen-hour day at the clinic and then hosting a lively party in his splendid new home.

Few other homes have attracted so much speculation and rumour as the house Josef Issels built beside the Tegernsee. It stands in a park of 5,000 square metres of trees and lawns. Outside, it has been photographed from every conceivable angle. Once, a helicopter was hired to see if it was possible to trace from the air the course of a secret passage leading from Issels' bedroom suite to an exit point near a clump of trees. The underground tunnel was never found because it did not exist. But the story persisted to this day.

That particular yarn was the creation of an Englishman, a former patient, whom Issels showed around the house one evening after dinner. In Issels' bedroom, the patient noticed a seemingly solid glass wall. It contained a concealed door. Behind the door was a dark recess. Issels, ever fond of a joke, winked at the patient, and said: 'my bolt hole'. It was enough. The Englishman returned to London, and soon newspapermen were offered another juicy tit-bit to the Issels story: he had a secret passage through which he brought in girls—a route unknown to Isa who had a separate bedroom suite. It was pure fantasy. The recess was no more than a landing which led onto the main staircase. There are other tales:

Vision:
Beneath his six-bedroomed house there is a dance hall about fifty metres long, and there with his private orchestra the doctor likes to throw his parties, to which anybody may be invited. The district around the Issels clinic is

peppered with retired generals who may find themselves rubbing shoulders with their own gardeners or with an international film star. Two or three hundred guests is a fairly cosy evening at one of Dr. Issels' parties. His wife has only just persuaded him to install ash trays on the basis that it was costing them too much in scorched furnishings.

Sunday Express:
It is a quietly rich house with massive beams in the Bavarian tradition. It is full of antiquities. One of the things for which Issels' enemies cannot forgive him is that he has made money out of cancer, and he is sensitive about this accusation. Some of his pieces were sold to him cheaply by grateful patients. 'I am a baroque man. I love the baroque,' he says, 'and antiquities are my hobby.'

Yoga and Health:
He sleeps alone. It is a strange awakening at 6.30 a.m. About one metre above Dr. Issels' pillow is set a calisthenic bar. As soon as the doctor awakes he starts doing pull-ups and exercises on this bar. Then, at the foot of the bed, there is another bar higher up, on which he swings and stretches himself until it is time for him to move to the bar bells, the weights and the rowing machine, and so until he is dripping with perspiration at the end of forty-five minutes of gymnastics. Do not forget this is the routine of a man who nearly starved to death in a Russian prison camp. Then there will be a quick shower, a shave and into one of his well-cut suits, always with a white shirt and white silk tie—he has dozens of them.

B.B.C. Television:
While he was still on trial for fraud and manslaughter, Dr. Issels began building his home. The cost was considerable. It was put up at one end of Rottach-Egern's Millionaire's Row. His nearby neighbours include a member of the Krupp family and wealthy retired German generals. Dr. Issels' home is carefully furnished with *objects d'art* from all over Europe. He has a taste for Dutch masterpieces, tapestries, sculptures. It's a big house, a luxurious home that needs a staff of three to run

it. But it's a style of living that attracts speculation from orthodox doctors who believe that it provides a clear indication of his motives for running the clinic. Dr. Issels and his wife are aware of this. If he minds those charges he doesn't show it. The man who has been twice imprisoned in his life, once by the Russians, once by the Germans, looks upon this house as a necessary place of comfortable refuge.

The author has always been particularly fascinated by the paintings, tapestries and wood-cuts that adorned the walls of Issels' house. Some reporters have estimated that they cost around DM 2,000,000.

That figure approximated the market value of the entire property in 1972. Issels had bought the plot for DM 100,000 in 1964, plus a monthly rent of DM 1,200. He raised the payment through a bank loan. Another DM 500,000 was borrowed from a building society on a twelve-year mortgage. The loan was effected by Isa's father and brother handing over their building society securities to Issels. The house was entirely in his name.

It was, as the reporters and television men said, a splendid house. But there was no secret passage, no bedroom gymnasium, no underground dance hall, no private orchestra, no Dutch masterpieces, no antiques hocked-off by grateful patients. There was a party room in the basement. It contained a small bar, some hand-hewn tables and chairs, and a record player. It held forty people in comfort—not three hundred. There were excellent paintings, some costing DM 12,000 each. But they had not been gleaned from all over Europe. Issels picked most of them up in Munich art shops. Isa had two maids and the clinic's gardener mowed the grass. Unlike his neighbours Issels had no swimming pool, and ran a four-year-old car. Nevertheless, the house gave rise to speculation. One English professor said after visiting it: 'The place is every bit as big a drawback for Issels as his insistence on tonsilectomy.'

Rolf found it difficult just being the son of Josef Issels—though in 1967 he took the first move to follow his father's footsteps by becoming a medical student. He found his professors held widely differing views to those of his father. But he steadily came to the conclusion he: 'Believed in my father's methods. I want to follow his ideas. But I want to make them even more scientifically understood to all doctors.'

With all his enthusiasm for pure science it is doubtful if Rolf could have offered an acceptable explanation for Prodan Christoff and his substance, CH23.

Prodan Christoff was a Bulgarian, forty-seven years old, handsome enough, with a flair of showmanship not normally associated with a cancer researcher. He came to the clinic with an extraordinary story: on New Year's Eve, 1959, as he peered down a microscope in his private laboratory in Vienna, he saw what the world needed: a non-toxic antidote to cancer made from alpine plant extracts. He promptly called it CH23, after the first letters of his surname, and the twenty-third combination of particular plant alkaloids.

He and his brother, Christo, who described himself as an independent financier, patented CH23 and offered it to one cancer institute after another for evaluation. Finally Graz University Klinik, in Austria, injected CH23 into cancer patients under the direction of Professor Franz Spath. After six months all the patients were dead from the normal progress of the disease. But Spath wrote to Prodan Christoff: 'With highly effective doses of CH23 it is possible to observe tumour reductions or tumour dissolutions hitherto unknown.'

It was a handsome testimonial, even if it did not come from one of the world centres for cancer research. Christoff picked up a couple of more useful reports from Dr. Erich Berger in Klagenfurt—he wrote of an 'unprecedented inhibition of tumour growth'. Professor Hans Fleischhacker at Vienna University Hospital also reported favourably on the substance. Six institutes reported it was 'non-toxic'.

Christoff was anxious for wider recognition. Issels, eager to provide effective substances for his cancer patients, arranged to meet Prodan Christoff. The two men met with Christo hovering in the background to tie-up the business loose ends. Issels, having verified CH23 was non-toxic, found he had acquired Prodan Christoff for the duration of a full-scale clinical trial of the substance at the Ringberg Klinik.

Christoff's arrival soon brought problems. His colourful personality was tailor-made for the popular German Press. They expanded considerable efforts hoping to discover his formula, even trying to bribe clinic staff to pass on data about patients treated with CH23. One magazine went so far as to hire a private detective to filch Christoff's secret.

To all intents and purposes the Bulgarian revelled in being centre-stage. He swept through the clinic like a one-man Cossack charge; he insisted on mixing his substance behind locked doors; he was every bit the Bulgarian Merlin. Gerlach, a distinguished cancerologist, felt Christoff was, as he delicately put it: 'Not quite the sort of person you normally expect to have found the answer to cancer.'

Tension between the two men reached a point where Christoff delivered an ultimatum: either Gerlach was banned from the clinic or Christoff withdrew from the clinical trial. Issels found himself in a dilemma. The trial was well under way: early indications suggested it might indeed have a part to play in the combined treatment. Issels persuaded Gerlach to confine himself to his own laboratory. In November, 1966, Issels noted that Christoff's insistence on stepping-up the dosage of CH23 was producing 'a bad reaction' in patients. He reduced the injected measures of the substance. In 1968 he published a clinical paper concluding:

> CH23 is a maligno-static preparation of *Verbascum* and *Paeonia* (two alpine plants). Applying CH23 in the terminal phase of a malignant disease can significantly extend the short life-expectancy of patients due to its immediate tumour selective effect. It allows these patients to benefit from the slower acting immunotherapy with its long term effects. Thus, CH23 improves the chances for a further extension of life or even a cure.

In all 1,056 patients received CH23, in addition to Issels' basic treatment, and the case-notes indicated some remarkable remissions. Issels reported:

> By means of the dosages tested up to now, visible success could be achieved in about 60 per cent of our patients within the observation period, namely: (*a*) a standstill of the tumour process, (*b*) a decrease of the tumour or the metastasis (partial remission), (*c*) in some cases a complete remission.

But personal relationships between Christoff and Issels became disturbed. Issels was particularly angry at Christoff constantly seeking publicity for CH23. Popular magazines called it *wundermittel*, a miracle drug. Issels realised the professional dangers of being associated with such wild claims. But the publicity continued, further harming the clinic's standing in serious medical circles. Finally Christoff and Issels parted company, though CH23 continued to be prescribed at the clinic until May 16, 1967 when the Bavarian Medical Association condemned the substance as 'toxic and injurious to patients'. Issels immediately stopped prescribing it, although his experience showed it to be non-toxic.

In November 1967 Christoff's resident's permit was not renewed. He left Germany and dropped out of the headlines.

But the Ringberg Klinik continued to make news, largely through some magazine or newspaper. Issels disliked such publicity, but was powerless to stop it. Since re-opening the clinic he took every precaution to avoid medical criticism. All patients signed a form accepting there was no promise of a cure. Yet the word appeared in countless headlines around the world. In the first three years since restarting, 1,545 patients from thirty-six countries were treated, several of them free of charge: in that period Issels prescribed over DM 250,000 of free treatment. Yet the profits from treating cancer patients aroused increasing curiosity. Issels guarded such details carefully, being well aware of the implications behind questions about money. But by 1968 a B.B.C. investigator scanned book-keeping records to provide a picture of the clinic's income and expenditure:

	£ per annum
Income:	
Patients' fees	720,000
Legacies (average)	60,000
Total:	780,000
Expenditure:	
Drugs	350,000
Nurses' salaries	110,000
Doctors' salaries	75,000
Administration salaries	30,000
Research laboratory	15,000
Food	38,000
Equipment replacement	15,000
Heat, lighting	9,000
Telephone	40,000
Insurance/mortgage	10,000
Misc. (post/stationery etc.)	5,000
Total:	£697,000

This means that the clinic makes a profit of £83,000 per annum. Out of that comes Dr. Issels' personal salary, believed to be in the region of £20,000 per annum.

It was by no means a complete budget: no mention was made of the DM 40,000 worth of free treatment given that year; the profit returns were far lower than a comparable private clinic elsewhere in Europe—and almost miserly compared with American private clinics. Nevertheless the B.B.C. decided that on those figures, the Ringberg Klinik's profits were not excessive and began its in-depth investigation. Urging them on was one of the most remarkable patients Issels ever treated. Peter Newton Fenbow, whose very presence at the clinic had been innocently engineered by the production team.

Fenbow, a sociologist and his wife, Wendy, a schoolteacher, had founded in 1965 in Britain an organisation called the Association for Cancer Education and Prevention. In spite of its imposing title it had little standing in medical circles. Fenbow, an intense, volatile man, had been diagnosed in April, 1957 with an osteoclastoma of the sacrum, or a sacral tumour. The diagnosis was made by Sir Stanford Cade at the Westminster Hospital, London. Cade recommended surgery. Physically Fenbow was in poor shape; the tumour had paralysed both legs and medical opinion was doubtful if he would walk again. He underwent a thirty-six day course of radiotherapy at the Westminster Hospital. It gave him partial relief, including being able to walk once more. But by October, 1960, his condition deteriorated. He was seen by Mr. Standley Lee, consultant surgeon at the Westminster Hospital, who ruled out further deep-ray treatment. He was given a course of chemotherapy but showed 'negative response'. In June, 1961 he received cobalt treatment. His case-notes revealed:

> Now has a large tumour massing out of the pelvis and out of the glands of the right groin. Tumour is tender and there are small tender tumours left iliac fossa. X-ray examination reveals there is destruction of the bone of the body of the first piece of the sacrum and of the alae of the sacrum possibly due to metastases of the vertebrae. To combat this he received cobal treatment 20.CO: 60. He did not respond. Patient happier by going home, being aware of the prognosis.

Fenbow later claimed the prognosis indicated a fatal cancer and that was why he began to devote a great deal of time furthering lay interest in the disease. When researchers from the *Man Alive* team approached him in May, 1966, he accepted a part in a television documentary called *Living With Death*. He was filmed with his wife discussing intimate details of their lives, including a wish for a baby before Fenbow died. It was highly-charged programme material, filled with tragic and romantic undertones. It caused a brief sensation when it was screened. A journalist obtained a transcript of the programme and sold it to various continental magazines. By sheer chance Issels read on account of Fenbow's part in the tele-cast and was moved by his courage. He wrote to the programme producers offering to treat Fenbow for nothing. They conveyed the offer to Fenbow's English doctor.

Meanwhile the German magazine, *Neue Revue,* sensing a useful circulation booster, persuaded Fenbow and his wife to let the magazine fly them to Germany in return for the exclusive rights to their story at the clinic. On February 3, 1967, the Fenbows arrived in Rottach-Egern. They were given a small private suite free of charge.

Clinically Fenbow was in a low condition with a growing tumour, failing kidneys, a rising blood urea, considerable pain and frequent nausea. After three months' treatment, he showed considerable improvement. He decided the time had also come to tell the world about his remission. He and Wendy were filmed by German television. But when the programme was screened, Fenbow claimed it had been edited out of context. More important for Issels, the programme contained an interview with Dr. Willy Reichstein of the Bavarian Medical Association. Reichstein condemned Issels' methods. The interviewer asked him:

> 'Then how do you account for Mr. Fenbow's apparent improvement since he arrived in Germany?'
>
> 'That is quite simple', Reichstein replied. 'If he has improved since arriving in Germany then he has never *had* cancer.'

It produced a new crop of headlines attacking the clinic's methods. Fenbow caused further embarrassment to Issels by issuing a lengthy press statement violently attacking the Bavarian Medical Association. Finally, while still a patient, Fenbow and his wife founded a small 'Committee Against Tyranny In Medicine' whose only stated aim seemed to be 'more militant actions should the blatant abuse of power continue'.

Issels was unaware of Fenbow's tub-thumping. He was content to confine his writing to Fenbow's clinical notes. By June 4, 1967, the day the Fenbows returned to England, his clinical picture had improved considerably. In the next year Fenbow returned four times for further short spells of back-up treatment—all free of charge. In August, 1968, his clinical picture showed: 'The tumour in the abdomen no longer exists as a tumour, but is only passive scar tissue. The original tumour of the sacrum appears clinically dormant. The sacrum has recalcified.'

Fenbow was still anxious the whole world should know about the Ringberg Klinik. He became an unpaid, and unauthorised, standard-bearer for the clinic.

On a warm autumn evening of 1968 Fenbow arrived in the B.B.C. Science and Features Department. He was questioned for several hours by the co-producers investigating Issels. Both were considerably shaken by Fenbow's remarkable good health and his insistence that it was all due to Issels. Fenbow left the producers with the impression he would work with them on any proposed documentary for a suitable fee. The television men had no intention of employing Fenbow in such a capacity. They believed to do so would create an impression they were Issels' protagonists—an issue that had already been raised, and vigorously denied.

After consultation with senior executives the co-producers were told to press ahead with research. Again they were cautioned to show extreme care in their attitude towards the investigation, and it was made clear to them that under no circumstances were they—and therefore ultimately the B.B.C.—to appear to be championing the claims Issels was making. The fear was understandable enough: cancer, and especially the suggestion of any cure for the disease, was highly emotive. But the production team after months of investigating, believed it could maintain a proper perspective.

Some clues as to how the B.B.C. team probed around the world are available in Issels' own notes of various telephone conversations with Corporation employees over this period.

> —— —— telephoned. Says Wilmans (Dr. Hilman Wilmans, medical director of the German firm which developed Endoxana) had no idea we use the drug 'in such a clinic'. —— agrees with me this is very odd as I have given him a complete file of correspondence between Wilmans and myself over using Endoxana in the clinic.

Or:

> Long walk with —— today. Says they have a big file now of doctors who deny sending patients here; or patients

who refuse to admit they have been here and drug houses who deny supplying us with drugs.

In December 1968 Issels minuted:

> B.B.C. very confident. I agree that they can bring specialists from England and America to carry out a full clinical investigation here of my methods. B.B.C. plan to bring Shimkin and Haddow for at least a week, and maybe longer. I am very impressed at the power of television.

Professor Michael Shimkin of the University of California, San Diego, was one of the world's leading authorities on the clinical chemotherapy of cancer, cancer statistics, and international aspects of medicine.

Professor Sir Alexander Haddow, Director of the Chester Beatty Research Institute in London and Past President of the International Union Against Cancer was a scientist intimately in touch with the entire field of cancer research. Both men were known to Issels as usually open-minded and his confidence of being medically accepted soared.

Weeks passed before Issels learned that Shimkin and Haddow had declined to visit the Ringberg Klinik. Haddow subsequently said the 'whole idea was a foolish one'. Shimkin said it would have been 'inappropriate' for him to have flown to Germany.

Issels' keen disappointment at this outcome was quickly softened by the news that one scientist had agreed to come. He was Professor John Anderson, professor of physical medicine at King's College Hospital, London.

Anderson had a brilliant academic background. As well as impressive medical qualifications he was a Rockefeller Research Fellow. His written work on aspects of cancer had firmly established him as one of the liveliest minds in British medicine. At the age of forty he held a key post in a great teaching hospital and was a consultant to the World Health Organisation. He had considerable experience in managing cancer patients and was an international authority on computerising medical statistics. The production team found him refreshingly frank: Issels, with his homoeopathic

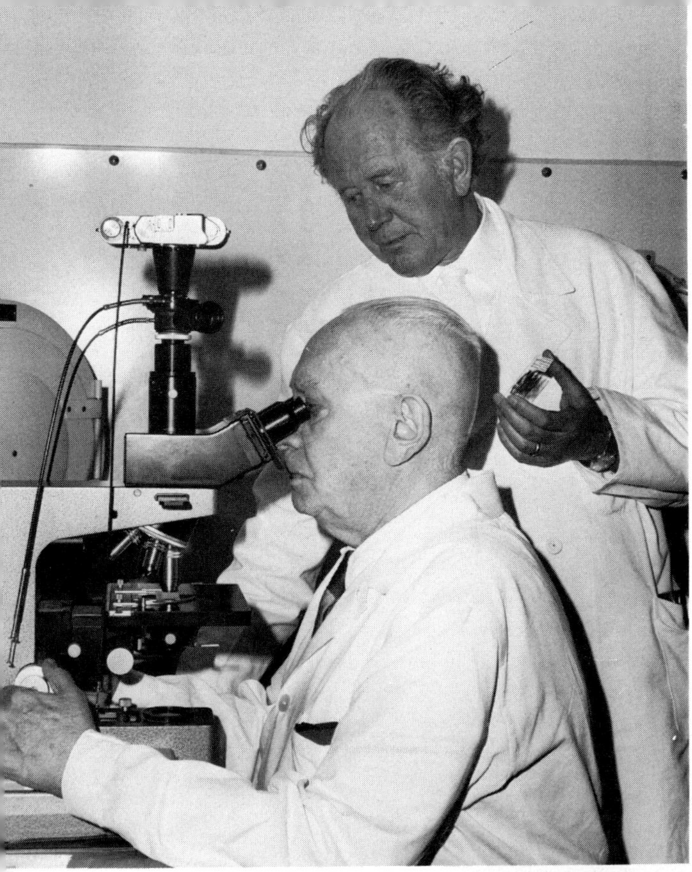

Dr. Issels and Professor Gerlach examining blood slides from a patient

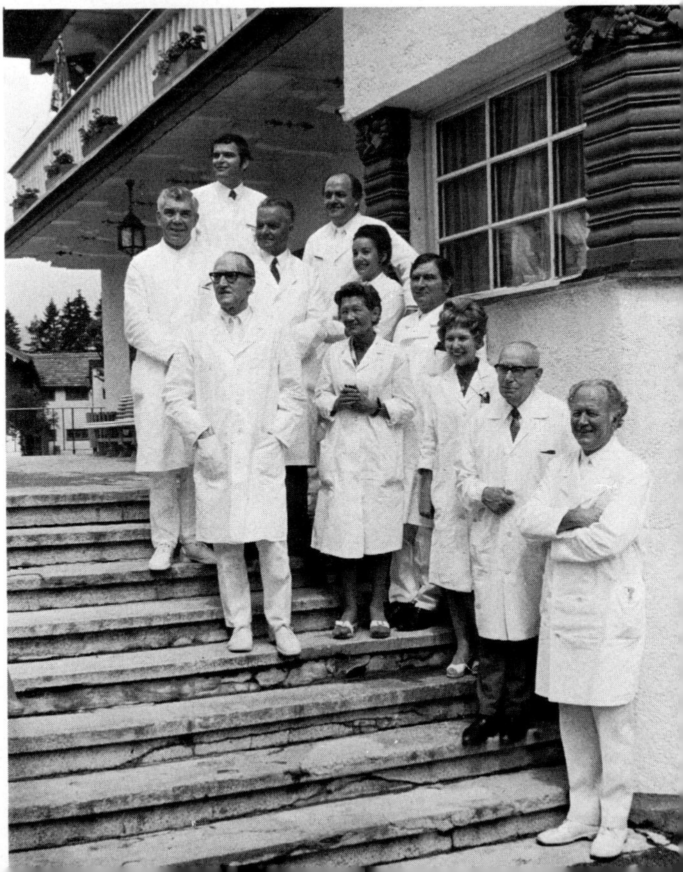

Issels and the Ringberg Klinik medical 'team'

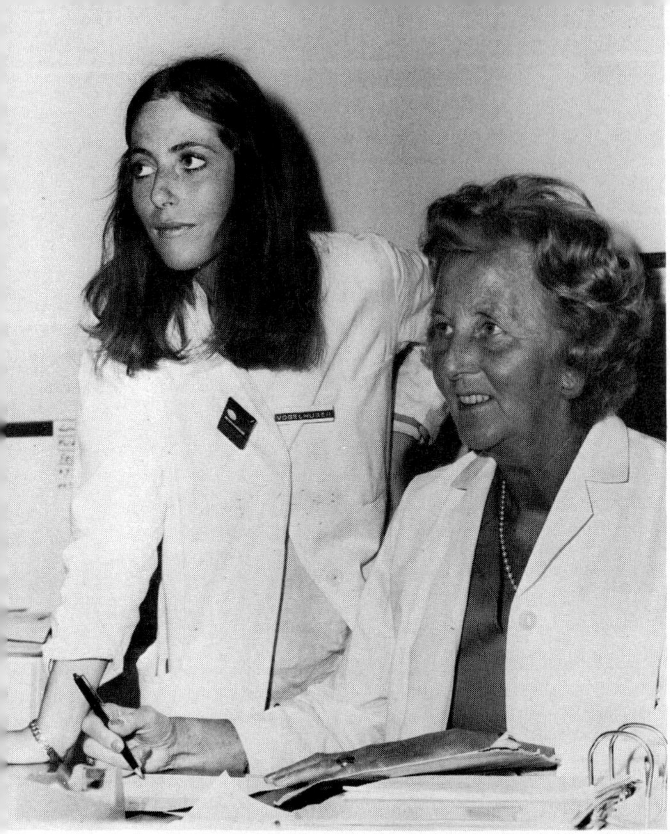

Mrs. Margot Findheisen (*right*), Issels' favourite sister, who is the chief administrator of the Ringberg Klinik, with one of her staff

Dr. Issels and two members of his team making a ward round

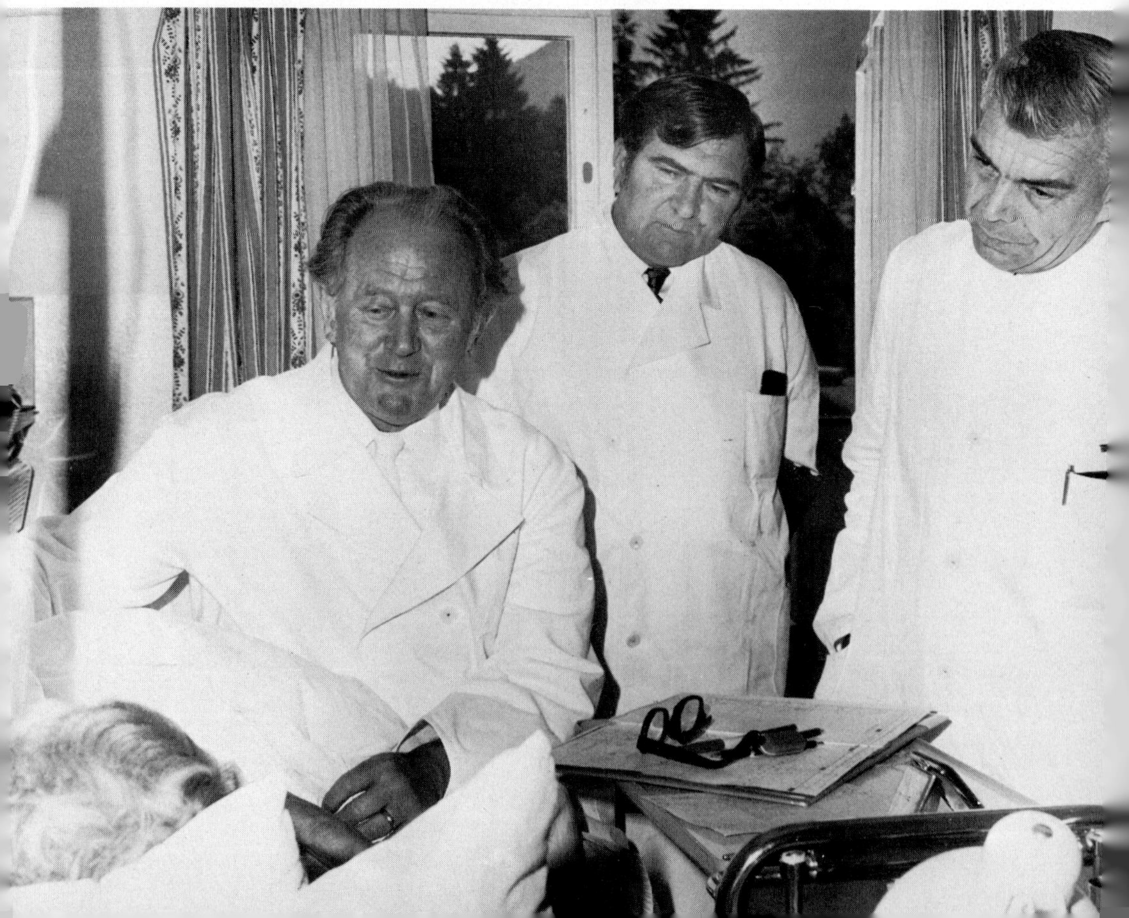

treatments, neural therapy, infusions of ozone, insistence on teeth and tonsilectomy was outside Anderson's ken, but that did not mean he had nothing to offer. Anderson had been immediately struck by the statistical proof prepared by Dr. Arie Audier of Leiden University, Holland, nearly ten years earlier. Anderson agreed to fly to Germany.

He was preceded by a B.B.C. team gathering evidence throughout Europe. Among them was Bob Symes, a former Intelligence officer, charged with establishing the truth about Issels' Nazi background. Symes investigated with the same zeal he once ran down suspected collaborators. The B.B.C. men finally translated nearly two million words from foreign medical reports and papers. They had taken a 'crash course' in the fundamentals of cancer and medical statistics. They interviewed patients like Thea Döhm and Käthe Gerlach; eventually inquiries spread to America, South Africa, India as well as all over Europe: in all two hundred patients were located, interviewed and their medical stories verified by independent doctors. Audier was traced to a small village in the northern Belgian Congo where he was conducting field trials. He explained the background to his statistical evaluation. The American Cancer Society Incorporated was reluctant to explain in detail its black-listing of Issels. In Vienna, Professor Hans Wrba, Director of the Institute for Cancer Research and a member of the Executive Committee of the Austrian Cancer Society said that Issels undoubtedly produced results but they 'needed proper scientific evaluation'.

On Thursday, February 27, 1969 Professor John Anderson arrived at the clinic to carry out such an assessment. His journey had been arranged by Symes, who treated it, with the same seriousness as if he still worked for British Intelligence. Anderson was given a cover name—John Smith—whisked in and out of airports by fast cars and installed in an adjoining suite to the watchful Symes. Symes was concerned that some newspapermen might spot Anderson and reveal the whole story.

Anderson had a plan allowing him to have the maximum amount of relevant information in the short time available. The afternoon he arrived he toured the clinic, met the staff, studied the methods of note-keeping and the response-charting and made requests for the information he wanted available: statistical evidence of all kinds. He visited the dispensary to see what drugs were used and checked-out the clinical laboratories and Gerlach's research unit. Then he moved into the archives. He selected 550 cases by random sampling that represented 10 per cent of all those the clinic had treated. With the help of translators he assessed them over several days. At night Anderson arranged his notes in tabular form, analysing the data and drafting a report to the B.B.C. On March 3, 1969 he submitted his findings:

> There are three general conclusions to be drawn from the short visit to Dr. Issels.
>
> 1. The first is that the therapy routine for primary and secondary cancer carried out at the Ringberg Klinik under Dr. Issels is unique. To my knowledge it is not used elsewhere in the form Dr. Issels prescribes at any other clinic. Based on a survey of the clinic and its patients and on statistical evidence about the survival of these patients, I am of the considered opinion that this is a new approach to cancer treatment and appears to be a considerable improvement on what is usually offered.
>
> 2. In essence the treatment is to encourage the normal mechanism of the body which already deals with a large number of cancer cells to be so strengthened that they bring about a natural remission of the disease. Some of the cases I saw at the clinic would have been regarded as hopeless by physicians in the United Kingdom. My overall opinion is that the Issels' approach to the treatment of cancer is a unique and pioneering solution to a very difficult problem.
>
> Dr. Issels is an able physician, a shrewd and penetrating clinician, whose principles and practice of medicine I admire. He is a shrewd observer of clinical conditions and has probably had more practical experience with his six thousand patients at medically treating cancer than anyone else. There can be no doubt that he is genuine in what he does and the results he gets. He has a good competent supporting medical and nursing staff and the staff/patient ratio is higher than that generally seen in the United Kingdom.

My overall impression is that the clinic is well ordered and fulfils the best clinical traditions of medicine.

3. I am prepared to set up a double blind clinical trial in the Department of Medicine at King's to reproduce and test the Issels therapy regime as far as possible under the conditions under which I have observed it. Given certain prerequisites it should be possible to start such a trial by the summer of 1969.

An indication of how it is progressing may be available towards the end of this year, but this would only be an impression and I doubt if we could expect to have any really worthwhile information until well into 1970 or later, depending on the survival times of the control groups of patients treated by standard methods.

The prerequisites are as follows:

The Ethical Committee at King's College Hospital will have to give their consent to this trial and in view of its expense and the allocation of nursing and medical resources, will have to review it carefully.

I shall have to talk to the Dunlop Committee and let them know of my intention and the problems in relation to a treatment not well understood at present.

I shall also have to arrange with a drug firm to supply the treatment used by Dr. Issels.

I do not anticipate undue difficulties but there is going to be a considerable amount to be done but I think that we can consider that this is worthwhile. It will have to be remembered that at present much that is being done by Dr. Issels is not standard treatment and so far no other clinic has produced his results which is essential if we are to bring the benefits he claims to patients.

While Dr. Issels is a sound and able clinician who has kept to the traditional medical procedures, he has kept no adequate records of his work and his experience in organising scientific clinical trials and the problems raised in relation to carrying out such a trial and carefully measuring the results of such investigations is limited. Recently he has taken a medical statistician on to his staff to help with the great problem of analysing his existing records. However, the difficulties in relation to retrospective research are quite great. Nevertheless, looking at the data which is available I accept his findings of a long remission rate of nearly 17 per cent in 'terminal' cases. The difficulty with his statistics as a whole is that there are no other satisfactory results elsewhere to compare them with.

I understand very well why Dr. Issels has never really attempted to undertake the type of trial I have proposed for he feels that his therapy is an answer and that he would be wrong not to treat all patients with it. He confides in his patients a great deal and they are very well aware of their condition and he allows them to actively participate in the treatment. He has, however, compared different treatment regimes in different wards and incorporated the results into this therapeutic regime. From a clinical scientific point of view, an independent trial is essential if his treatment ideas are to be accepted more widely and further research must be undertaken to evaluate what he has studied.

We had some difficulty in communicating with Dr. Issels as he relies on medical terminology which has either been forgotten in the course of clinical progress or is basically only applicable to his treatment. It will be essential for me to produce a glossary of his terms so that we can get agreement between us, and also with present-day medical people, about what he really does mean. This is a difficult semantic problem and will take some time. I shall have to look at some of the past homoeopathic work in which I have had little interest and will try to evaluate the work of Spengler as some of Issels' treatment is prepared according to his formulae and treatment. As you will imagine, all this is written in German and I feel it is essential to have someone of the calibre of Bob Symes to translate and make clear the problems of communication in medical terminology. I wonder if it would be possible at this stage to have his intermittent help. I am quite certain that without his assistance we shall be a considerable time in arrears with our clinical programme in trying to evaluate all this material.

There are also two other major problems in relation to the clinical side of Issels' treatment:

The first is the psychological approach, in which the patient is told all about his disorder, including a great deal of medical detail and is encouraged to help to try and fight his cancer. The patient actively participates in all phases of investigation and treatment. This I think I certainly can do, but I doubt if all of my staff will have the same views and this may not be so easy to do in a double blind trial.

The other problem is that of equating the ecology of Rottach-Egern, a small idyllic village in the Bavarian mountains with those of Denmark Hill, London, S.E.5. It is impossible for us to recreate the clean atmosphere or the walks that the patients take outside the clinic. It was interesting to see what I would have considered quite seriously ill patients climbing mountains with grossly enlarged livers and secondary cancer in their chests and elsewhere. Part of the treatment is to keep the patient solidly on the move from sunrise to sunset and they are encouraged to take as much time as possible to get out and about into the surrounding countryside. It is going to be impossible to reproduce these exact conditions even if we transport our patients to Crystal Palace, but we must try.

A more intensive medical and nursing service would be necessary if we are to carry out such a trial and this is not available at the present time, which is one of the reasons for not beginning the clinical trial until the summer as we will have a gross nursing shortage until June. While I can overcome many of the problems of staffing and surroundings, these will not be exactly the same.

Overall, I advise that Dr. Issels has a new approach of interest to doctors and patients in the United Kingdom. The Issels story has a great deal of human interest. Without doubt he is a remarkable man doing something which is much needed. He is undoubtedly producing clinical remissions in patients who have been regarded as hopeless and left to fall back on their own resources. I also accept that even when he cannot produce a long remission he aims to allow the patient to live out his life in a worthwhile manner with more quality than would be possible. This project deserves recognition as does the work of Cicely Saunders who cares for terminal cases in the United Kingdom.

> Before I undertake such a venture, I would like to point out that a premature explosion of information about the work of Issels could jeopardise the clinical trial, for if public opinion felt that it was right this would result in patients besieging their own doctors with a request to be sent to Bavaria under the aegis of the National Health Service. This would not benefit Dr. Issels in any way and would only make it more difficult for us to set up a double blind trial. Neither would I wish my colleagues or King's College Hospital to be besieged by the world's press and television networks. Could we therefore treat this matter with discretion until we make up our minds whether it is worthwhile and until you decide at which point you think it would be appropriate to inform the public about it.

The Anderson report caused a sensation within the B.B.C. Science Department.

Anderson approached the Ethical Committee at his hospital to permit a double blind trial in which forty fatally ill patients, all suffering from various kinds of cancer, would be divided into two groups. One group would receive the Issels treatment, the other group would not, acting as 'control'. No patient would know who received *ganzeitstherapie*, and who did not. The Ethical Committee authorised the trial. Anderson approached the Dunlop Committee, a Government-appointed watchdog on all drugs used in Britain. They flatly rejected his proposals. On April 14, 1969, Anderson wrote to Issels:

> They are not prepared to authorise such a treatment, largely because of its multiple nature and the fact that the drugs, are not, according to them, acceptable in the United Kingdom. However this does not prevent me carrying on the trial on my own initiative but I would obviously need a drug company to co-operate with me.

Anderson hoped the company would not only provide the necessary drugs, but also the £100,000 to stage the trial. The drug house could by-pass the Dunlop Committee's strictures by importing Issels' medicaments for 'clinical analysis'.

Nevertheless, the Dunlop Committee's attitude was an odd one. All the drugs Anderson had submitted to them for clearance were German ethical preparations, appearing on the *Rote Liste,* the equivalent to the British Pharmacopea. He felt he was: 'In for a hell of a ride. The block was being put on before I even started.'

Yet it seemed in that hot summer of 1969 that his fears were groundless. The production team fed him regular bulletins about former Issels patients and much else. Hoechst Pharmaceuticals offered to back the clinical trial. It was a major step: Hoechst was one of the world's largest ethical drug firms. They told Anderson they 'were sure' they could get him all the 'raw materials' he wanted. Anderson wrote to Issels: 'We all believe you have something important to give the world.'

He asked permission to bring a three-man team from Hoechst to look over the clinic. Issels agreed and in September, 1969, they arrived in Rottach-Egern. The Hoechst men inspected the clinic—and urged Issels to beware of the B.B.C. production team. Issels was surprised—it was the team which after all had introduced Anderson to him. Issels was told that television was not the best medium 'to present such an important thing as your method'. He readily saw the sense of that; he had complained on more than one occasion to the production team that they were behaving with a harshness more in keeping with 'police prosecutors than television researchers'.

Yet in spite of it all, Issels believed his life-time of struggling for recognition was ending. Anderson agreed to co-operate on an English-language paper about the *ganzheit-therapie* and Hoechst were 'seriously interested in promoting the treatment in England'. The company's divisional director, Dr. G. T. Basil wrote to Issels on September 16, 1969:

> We are all deeply impressed by your clinic and the work you are doing. From what we saw it is obvious that there are many extremely interesting ideas to be followed up in depth in addition to the proposal to repeat the general therapy in London. From our side we are willing and eager to help Professor Anderson. In the meantime we

shall look forward to your publication in a British journal.

Letters like that ensured further healing of the wounds Issels had received in a life-time of battling. The words of Anderson and the drug-house men were balm for the scars of thirty years.

The co-producers pursued its inquiries in a number of countries. They were satisfied on a number of points: Issels had nothing to reproach himself over during his days in the Nazi Party or in World War II; he had, according to other doctors, achieved cures; he was the victim of constant rumours about his professional and private life.

Then, in October, 1969, the inconceivable became fact. Powerful factions within the medical world moved to pincer-out the B.B.C. and Anderson. Exactly what happened is not clear; to this day B.B.C. executives maintain silence; nor will Anderson discuss the pressures he faced. But certain facts are beyond dispute: the already costly B.B.C. investigation ground to a halt; Anderson postponed his clinical trial indefinitely; Hoechst faded from the scene.

Confused, and not a little angered, Issels tried to find out what had happened. He became convinced that at least one B.B.C. employee was involved in some sort of conspiracy against him. It renewed his belief that he was forever the victim of the Fates and underscored his conviction that the Fates had powerful allies in England.

Against this background the irrepressible Peter Fenbow launched himself on the media. Physically, he was in good shape and wanted the world to know why.

Fenbow was a man of astonishing energy and directness, and he used both to attract the attention of reporters. But those who listened noticed he had periods of great inner turmoil, frequently suffering from nervous prostration. Nevertheless, there was something moving, and sad, in his conviction he was still alive solely due to Josef Issels. Set against this was Fenbow's own personality, so structured that some situations he could anticipate with blinding clarity, while others he only saw dimly.

He failed totally to realise that the claims he made in his capacity as a patient was hardly the way for Issels to be taken seriously. Fenbow frequently spoiled his argument by overstating the opposition of the medical establishment towards Issels. Soon, like Shigalov in Dostoyevsky's *The Possessed*, he became perplexed by his own data and the outcome of his crusade became a direct contradiction to the original idea with which he had started. His demands for Issels' acceptance was like a lever attempting to turn the medical world on to an orbit more to Fenbow's liking. Because he pressed too hard on the lever, his claims about Issels were not taken seriously by, among others the B.B.C.'s production team.

Finally, rejected by them, but far from dejected, Peter Fenbow called upon Professor Anderson. By all accounts Anderson gave him a sympathetic hearing, but bridled at the suggestion that he joined forces with Fenbow to get Issels accepted. Thereafter, the relationship between Fenbow and Anderson markedly cooled.

But Fenbow was still determined to ensure that Issels received coverage in Britain; he contacted Granada's *World in Action*. Its programme-makers listened carefully, and decided here was an excellent chance to pip the B.B.C., always an incentive in the world of television.

Granada approached John Anderson. Worried at the possibility that the commercial company's approach 'might not be quite right', Anderson contacted the B.B.C. production team 'for advice'. The upshot was the B.B.C. resumed its investigations and Anderson once more began to plan a clinical trial.

The first Issels heard of all this was when a member of the production team arrived at the clinic with a world-exclusive contract. Clinic staff recall the Corporation man waving a piece of paper about 'as if he was a cross between Chamberlain returning from Munich and an insurance salesman offering a particularly good life policy'.

The B.B.C. man tried to smooth out all the weeks of frustration Issels had experienced with the Corporation. Then, having got Issels signature on the contract —— the £25 fee gave the B.B.C total rights in a proposed film— the executive astonished Issels by revealing that the production team in Issels' later aide-memoire of their conversation, had:

Without my authority passed on data of case histories obtained months before with my consent from the clinic's archives, to Dr. Robert J. C. Harris, (Head of the Department of Environmental Carcinogenesis at the Imperial Cancer Research Fund). They had been passed over to Harris in a form I would never have allowed. I would have been perfectly willing to have sent Harris any information he would require on a doctor-doctor basis. My immediate reaction was to abandon the whole idea of doing this film. There had been all that funny business with the B.B.C. earlier in the year. But —— —— insisted to me that from now on things would be different. Only the continued presence of Professor Anderson in the project convinced me, in the end, to go on. Anderson was a powerful force in medical circles.

Issels made one stipulation: The £25 fee from the B.B.C. should be promptly paid over to the Imperial Cancer Research Fund in London.

In London John Anderson undertook to co-operate only with the B.B.C. Granada's *World In Action*, on hearing of this, abandoned their plans to make a programme. Peter Fenbow, the man who had restarted it all, dropped out of sight. Only his death, in the autum of 1972, brought him back into the headlines.

Throughout the first weeks of 1970 the production team maintained the closest contact with Josef Issels as the final stages of its investigation gained momentum; some days he took up to a dozen telephone calls from Corporation researchers checking on and seeking further information.

The B.B.C. later opposed publication of any details of the production team's enquiries. In 1973/4 when this book was being prepared, the B.B.C. exerted considerable legal pressure in this matter. It is therefore impossible to fully evaluate the truth of stories, which have already appeared in the European and American Press, to the effect that in the early weeks of 1970 the B.B.C. were 'warned off' by powerful cancerologists from going ahead with their film. If there is no evidence that the B.B.C. will now allow to be published which points directly to such pressures, there is such an abundance of clues that it is impossible to deny such attempts were made to influence the co-producers of the investigation.

In the end small clues amount to a large clue; some of the evidence is unsupported and by itself would scarcely amount to a bill of accusation that doctors tried to interfere with the co-producers' traditional freedom. But when supported by transcripts of various telephone conversations between the production team and Josef Issels, the accusation must be taken seriously. These aide-memoires Issels kept of his endless dialogue with the production team, are fragmentary, and in no way offer a complete view of what was happening in London and elsewhere: their importance lies in the fact that the B.B.C. men, innocently or ingeniously, add their share of circumstantial evidence that there was pressure from certain medical men to stop the film. That the film survived was due to the courage of Dr. Robert Reid, then Head of the Science Department, who fought a brilliant tactical battle to keep the production afloat.

Issels viewed the struggles calmly: there was nothing he could do to influence the outcome. Further, he believed that if the film-makers triumphed, they would have a better appreciation of the many years of battling he had endured.

He put events in London out of his mind, turning his thoughts to the wider aspects of patients' welfare. For many years he had been concerned with the issues of whether a doctor should tell his patients they had cancer. Issels believed implicitely they must be told—with the rider that they should be informed there was positive treatment open to them after conventional methods had failed: *ganzheitstherapie*.

His interest in the matter was renewed early in 1970 by details of a survey carried out in a large hospital in the north of England, on patients who were told *after* treatment they had cancer. Some found the knowledge made them uncomfortable. But seventy-five percent welcomed confirmation from their doctors of what they had suspected all along. They experienced real relief that the 'white lies' were over, that they could return to the 'two way partnership' which is the essence of all good doctor/patient relationships, and one which Issels had always laid store upon as an additional recuperative aid. In his mind the survey prompted the question: how would those patients have reacted if they had been told *before* treatment that they suffered from cancer? The thought formed the basis for another medical paper. In a few hundred words Josef Issels encompassed the essentials of the problem, offering at the end a sound and human solution to every doctor's dilemma:

> Much of the superstition and fear in people's mind towards cancer can be largely laid at the door of that body of powerful medical opinion which argues that the present state of conventional treatment rarely allows open honesty. In advancing this argument those doctors are also implicitely admitting the limitations, and even failures, of standard methods for controlling cancer. Knowledge alone, does not, of course, conquer real, exaggerated, or imagined fears about cancer. Nor indeed does it play a direct part in the active treatment of the disease. But suspicion is a breeding ground for psychological stress—and that can affect the course of the illness. The important thing is to convince these patients, by word and deed, that medical science can offer more than only the surgeon's knife, or the radiotherapist's cobalt gun; that, important though they are, these weapons can only be much more effective when they are incorporated into the whole-body concept of treating cancer.
>
> The question then, in whole-body therapy, is not *when* to tell, but *how* to tell the truth. Firstly, there is a need for a careful psychological assessment of the adult patient. Fear is a very necessary part of man's defence mechanism; after all it is fear that makes a person become a patient in the first place. It is important to understand that fear, and assess it in each patient before revealing the truth to him. Having done this, the next step is to present the clinical symptoms as succintly as possible. This is the time for plain speaking where cancer is called by its name, and in doing so, where the fear is taken out of the word. It should be presented as one more chronic illness which can be effectively treated by approaching it on the lines of whole-body treatment, while at the same time recognising the value of standard surgery, radiotherapy and chemotherapy. It is this combination, presented properly to the

patient, which can help remove his fear, make his cancer an acceptable word, and open the door to awareness that whole-body treatment is the best possible approach to the disease.

None of this is possible without the right attitude from medical and nursing staff. Apart from proven professional skills, other attributes are essential. Pessimism must never be allowed to take root. The aim must always be to shape in the patient's mind a positive attitude towards cancer. Having established such a framework of honesty, realism and mutual co-operation, it is only then that cancer can be viewed as no longer an 'incurable' disease. When all this is achieved only then can we progress; only then can we expect to see surgery and radiotherapy and the other aids, play a more curative role, as opposed to a more palliative one. And perhaps only then will the 'white lies' cease to be the stock-in-trade of so many doctors.

On the day he completed this paper, January 24, 1970, the B.B.C. film team arrived at the clinic.

The arrival of the film crew turned the clinic upside down. For two days helicopters swooped over the grounds filming establishing shots. They were grounded when Arndt Friedrich Alfried von Bohlen und Halbach, the last of the Krupps who lived in Rottach-Egern, complained his afternoon nap was being disturbed. Reporter Raymond Baxter said his statements to camera and departed in a snow storm, leaving some of the clinic staff with a lasting impression that an oracle had been briefly among them. Members of the film crew struck the Germans as being somewhat eccentric. The director spent long periods walking around with one eye closed, declaiming, 'I have it visual'; an associate producer collected small pots of jam, hoarding them in his room. After a week, the sound recordist believed he had contracted cancer: it needed a series of tests by the clinic's pretty laboratory technicians to reassure him. Nevertheless, the film progressed swiftly. Cameraman Fred Hamilton captured several poignant exchanges between Issels and his patients. After two weeks, and several parties, the final sequence was shot: a dozen patients doing physical exercises on top of the 6,000 feet Wallberg Alp in a blizzard. It provided a title for the film: *Go And Climb A Mountain.*

The team returned to London and edited the film—unaware of another gathering storm.

15

Further Complications

THEY HAD ALL LEFT BEHIND 'CONTACTS' IN THE CLINIC; doctors and nurses with whom they had become involved with during their stay, either professionally, or, in most cases, socially. In the weeks following their return to London a regular two-way communication was maintained between the film-makers and clinic staff. Amidst all the ardent promises to return to Germany, the crew slipped in details of what was happening to the film. In turn these snippets were passed on to Josef Issels. What he heard made him increasingly uneasy as to whether the film would ever be shown. His attempts to discover whether his doubts were justified were, he recalled, met with official rebuffs. His understandable frustration was summed up in the belief that:

> The B.B.C. have spent a small fortune investigating me and making this film. I have opened every door to them. But in the end, from all I hear, pressures will stop the film coming out. As such, I do not mind if the film is shown or not. It's only importance, indeed, the only reason I ever agreed to co-operate with the B.B.C., is that the film could turn out to be the trigger-factor that could create further, and more serious interest, in my whole-body approach to treating cancer. That is all I am concerned about: getting across the message.

His feeling of perplexity deepened when the co-producers finally invited him to London to view the show-print of the film, and to be present when the question of whether it could be transmitted would be debated by other English oncologists. Issels' feelings over this were encompassed in a diary note in March, 1970:

> This is not at all what I expect from the B.B.C. with its image of standing aloof from pressures. From what I understand, the B.B.C. are so much under pressure that two camps exist, each with their team of experts. This is by any account an extraordinary situation. None of these experts have ever been to my clinic; none of them, I am told, have any first-hand knowledge of my methods; some, I understand, have never even heard of *ganzheitstherapie*. Worse, they are expected to pass a value judgement on a serious way of treating cancer, and all on the basis of a television programme that I have now been told must have a strong entertainment quality as well as being full of what the B.B.C. may decide is their idea of science.

When Issels arrived in London with Isa, their anxiety was somewhat allayed by being met at the airport by that eminent oncologist, Mr. Denis Burkitt.

Burkitt explained to Issels that, having already viewed the film, his appetite had been aroused to discuss matters with Issels more fully. The two doctors subsequently remained closeted alone in a London hotel for hours discussing the full implications of Issels' methods. Afterwards, Issels wrote up the customary detailed summary of that meeting; once more it caught his thoughts on the wing:

> Mr. Burkitt made a profound impression of me. He was totally open-minded. What especially interested him was my views on enhancing immunological competence. He said this was still relatively new in standard thinking about cancer, and he was openly astonished when I explained to him that I had long regarded immunological competence as being of paramount importance. Later, when the conversation turned to more general things, Mr. Burkitt said there appeared to be a great deal of opposition within and outside the B.B.C. to showing the film.

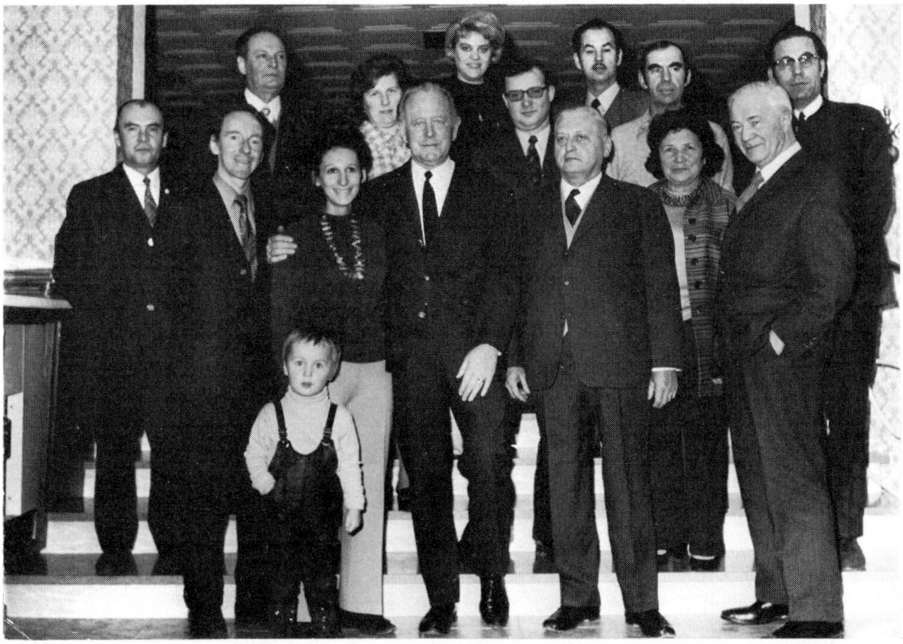

Issels with several of his cured patients

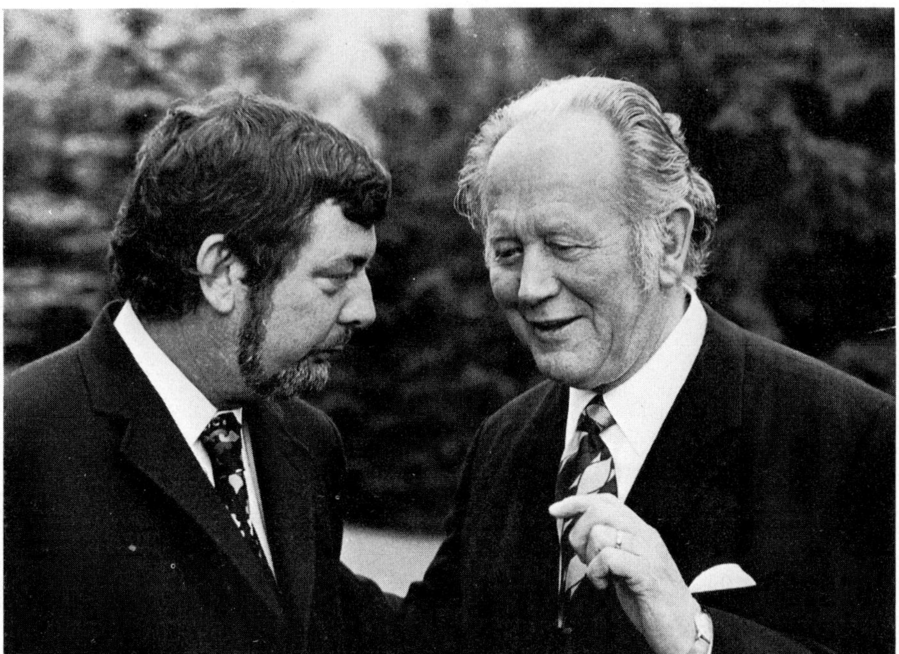

Dr. Issels with the author

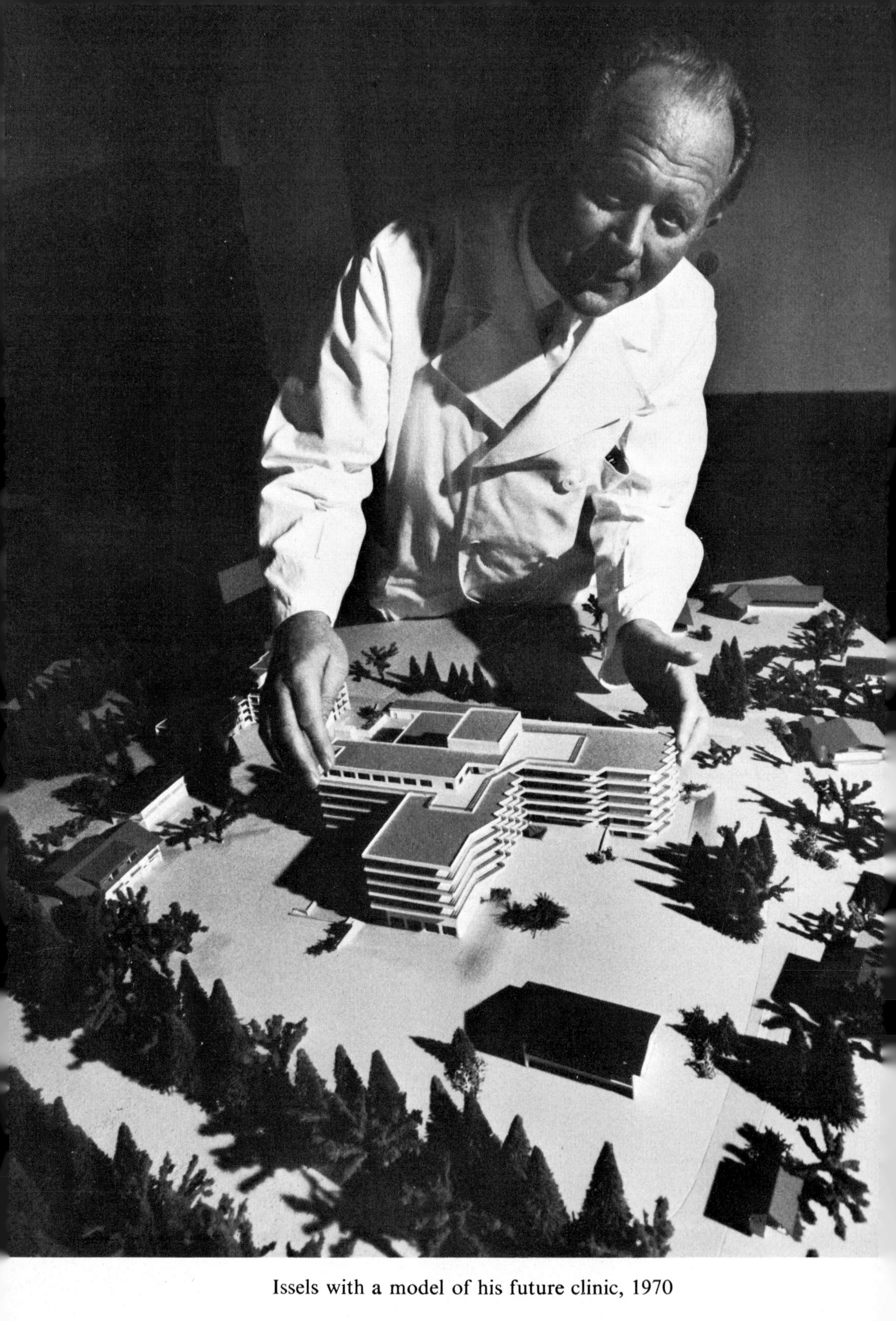

Issels with a model of his future clinic, 1970

A further hint that the Corporation was not united was later made to Issels at a private dinner party. A cancerologist, renowned for his bluntness, told Issels it was 'High time the B.B.C. stopped fooling around with the film'. When Josef Issels visited the B.B.C. studios the full realisation dawned on him that, in some way, this was not to be the film he had expected to see:

> The pictures were excellent—as pictures. Fred Hamilton [the cameraman] could be proud of his work. So could Ted Reid [the sound man]. But the film had been so constructed that no adequate space was given to my treatment methods. Everything had been edited for a dramatic effect. Worse, the proposed commentary was hostile in places. There were references to people accusing me of being a charlatan, a quack, a peddler of false hopes. There was also an emphasis on my personal life which I did not think was warranted.
>
> After a few minutes my instinct was to walk out. Isa stopped me, suggesting I made my objections and see what happened. A B.B.C. executive, obviously embarrassed by my attitude, quickly explained that things would be changed. With that promise I sat back and watched it through. After the showing, I was told that some fifteen English cancerologists had already seen the film. Among them had been Sir David Smithers and Dr. Gordon Hamilton Fairley. Smithers I knew from his published work. In *The Lancet* years before he had pointed out that cancer was no more a disease of cells than a traffic jam was a disease of cars—or that a life-time's study of the internal combustion engine would not help anybody to understand traffic congestion. A man who could talk like that about the cancer problem was worth meeting. But when I suggested this to the B.B.C. men they quickly changed the subject. So I suggested they might arrange for me to see Dr. Hamilton Fairley. After all they had told me he was a man who thought along the same lines as Smithers. But once more the idea seemed to create a very real embarrassment among the B.B.C. team. I put it all down to the fact that it was a clash between 'orthodox' and 'unorthodox'. It really was very understandable, but sad.

Issels attended a further viewing with the B.B.C. experts. Introductions, he recalled, were perfunctory. But he was pleased to see that the commentary had been changed; it had lost some of its hostility, and the more pointed references to his private life had been subdued. When the showing was over there was, Issels recalled, a brief discussion and everybody then made their way to the B.B.C.'s Kensington House Club:

> Somebody told me this was where all the real decisions were made [recalled Issels]. A more senior B.B.C. man overheard the remark and clearly did not think it amusing. But then the whole atmosphere was hardly funny. The B.B.C.'s experts would come over to me, ask a question and then go into a huddle again. God knows what they were deciding. Certainly they could not hope to have made any serious assessment of my work, especially as we had all become familiar with the B.B.C. attitude that the film had to be entertaining as well as instructive. I could see the need for that in terms of getting a large audience. But in that case I could not understand why all those experts were there. Nobody told me what they said. But I could guess by some of the questions that they didn't understand the basic principles of my ideas. I invited them to come to the clinic and see for themselves, and they behaved as if they had been asked to commit professional suicide. I recognised the attitude too well. I had seen it too often in other doctors over the years. The whole attitude of some of the experts was summed up for me by a B.B.C. man saying 'you see if they went to look at your clinic they would feel themselves guilty by association. . .'

Josef Issels was glad when he finally left the B.B.C. and an atmosphere which he regarded as being oppressive. He had flown to London willing to believe that the rumours he had heard in Rottach-Egern were largely baseless. Instead, his doubts had been all too clearly confirmed. He had detected a clear undercurrent of hostility whose mainspring could be traced to sources he now believed were both inside and outside the Corporation.

Not unnaturally he became depressed that an organisation as influential as the B.B.C., the world's largest film organisation, could, on what he had been told, be put under pressure. He wondered what hope could he, a private individual, with no powerful lobby behind him, with only limited funds, have of ever achieving the breakthrough for his ideas?

The only crumb of comfort was a message from the co-producers that 'all being well' the film would be screened on March 17, 1970.

He had his doubts. But he kept them to himself.

The visit to London had been worthwhile in one respect. Both Denis Burkitt and John Anderson had carefully explained to Josef Issels the need for him to produce a clear exposition of his work in an English language clinical paper. Both scientists argued only in this way could Issels hope to counter the growing opposition for his ideas in certain medical quarters.

It was not enough, Burkitt told Issels, to be utterly sincere in a belief that *ganzheitstherapie* worked; such a conviction needed to be rationalised in scientific terms. Burkitt also told Issels he had urged upon his fellow cancerologists to reserve any judgment on *ganzheitstherapie* they may have formed from the film. Instead, a small team of specialists should be co-opted to visit the clinic and carry out a thorough study of the treatment.

> Mr. Burkitt summarised for me the terms of reference such a team should have [Issels recalled]. Its members should be competent to evaluate all the evidence before making any judgment. At the same time it must retain an open-mindness which would not assume an unscientific attitude; that, in Mr. Burkitt's words to me 'a result had not been achieved because it could not have been achieved'. It was the most heartening thing I had heard in London.

Professor Anderson also urged that Issels should regard the film as no more that a 'latch-key to open the door' for a team of recognised authorities going to the clinic. He was confident, he told Issels, that such an investigation would be impartial, even if it contained members who had seen the film. But nothing could be done until Issels produced an acceptable scientific paper.

Both Anderson and Burkitt, highly experienced in the art of writing clinical papers, offered Issels useful guidance. They said an important thing was to overcome the impression that the treatment could only be carried out at the Ringberg Klinik that it somehow depended on Issels' own personality for its success.

This was a view Issels had discovered was already circulating in London. He dismissed it as a not very subtle move to discredit him. What did upset him was to learn, on the eve of his return to Germany, that John Anderson had also become the target of a smear campaign.

Anderson explained to Issels that he (Anderson) had transgressed one of the unwritten commandments of the medical establishment by continuing to support a medical heretic. Anderson shrugged aside the matter as a clumsy attempt to 'get him'. He was still confident that publication of Issels' paper would end such a campaign.

Issels greatly admired the courageous stand Anderson continued to take. With the strong hint that writing a successful paper would see the collapse of medical resistance and pave the way for a serious investigation, Josef Issels returned to Rottach-Egern. He now genuinely believed that whatever the B.B.C. decided to do with their film it could have little effect on the future of *ganzheitstherapie*.

Hardly had he settled back into his clinical routine before Josef Issels received a telephone call from a member of the production team. Issels kept a careful note of what was said:

> —— —— said the film was cancelled. He said the opposition was too hot. He was personally very upset about it all, but he said there was nothing he could do because two of the B.B.C. experts had written a letter to the Corporation saying the film should not be shown. Because of that the B.B.C. had decided not to go ahead. Worse, in the opinion of some of the B.B.C. experts my treatment was worthless. I could not believe it. How could anybody have made a serious judgment on my work on

the basis of a film? —— —— said that as far as he knew some of the experts had never read any of my work, never seen any of my patients, and, until a short time before they had never even heard of me! But they were politically powerful, and in medicine that is as important as treating people. What a thought said —— ——, and I agree. He said the only hope of getting the film screened was for me to publish an English language paper which the B.B.C. could use as an excuse to justify the film. Such a paper would also end all the fighting in the B.B.C. Finally —— —— said that another expert argued that even though I got a 17% cure rate with incurable patients, a fact he accepted, my work should still not be looked at. The expert had told —— —— that to come to my clinic would need three months proper investigation.

In the next weeks Issels worked on a draft of the paper, interrupted from time to time by anxious calls from the production team checking on his progress. They told him that publication would lift the ban on the film. Anderson offered continual encouragement and the promise to place it in a reputable journal. By the end of March Issels had completed *Immunotherapy in Progressive Metastatic Cancer: A Fifteen Year Survival Follow-up*. He paid proper tribute to the work of scientists like David Smithers, and went on to claim:

Combined general and immunological treatment based on the concept of cancer as a chronic systematic disease of the body can offer a chance of a fifteen-year remission in about 10–15 percent of patients with rapidly progressive tumour growths not responding to existing treatment.

John Anderson sent the paper to *The Lancet* on April 30, 1970. He believed 'there will be no difficulties over publication'. He was wrong. It was rejected. He sent the paper to the *British Medical Journal* in June, 1970. It was swiftly rejected. Finally, late in September, 1970, *Clincial Trials Journal* accepted it for publication.

Meanwhile there were other stories circulating about Issels and his clinic. A Dutch journalist had somehow obtained highly confidential memos between Anderson, Issels and the B.B.C. He interpreted what he read as 'indicating a conspiracy' to keep the film off the air. More important, the correspondence revealed that Anderson had been discreetly trying-out *ganzheitstherapie* at King's College Hospital, London, one of the bastions of the medical establishment. Anderson did not wish for any publicity stating he was working with a new 'cure' for cancer; he also was trying to negotiate for more funds for his trial—and publicity would hamper that hope. But the journalist offered the story to *The Sunday Times* and *The Observer*. They tackled Anderson—who strongly denied using Issels' methods. The newspapers approached the B.B.C.—who denied the film existed. *The Sunday Times* dropped the story; *The Observer* pursued its enquiries.

Meanwhile another story began to circulate. It had been fashioned out of the imagination of a German freelance writer with a contact inside the clinic. His source revealed the B.B.C. appeared to have abandoned screening the film. The freelance believed a more sinister reason than mere medical politics lay behind the Corporation's decision: The B.B.C. had been told by British Intelligence that the clinic was under surveillance by German secret servicemen because it was, 'unknown to Issels, being used as a meeting place by Soviet spies'. The yarn had all the ingredients of an episode in a James Bond film: patients from behind the Iron Curtain were said to leave the clinic carrying microfilm in their blankets—being so ill they were never searched by German border guards. The film was then handed over to Soviet Intelligence.

Like all good fantasies, this one contained a grain of truth. The clinic did take patients from the Communist countries; there were no border searches of the acutely ill. It was enough to send journalists scurrying around Europe. Issels flatly denied the story. But it took weeks for the story to die—finally killed by the military attaché at the German Embassy in London insisting it was totally untrue.

On October 18, 1970, *The Observer* published a long exclusive article on the front page: 'CANCER FILM BANNED BY B.B.C.'

It revealed much of the background to the filming and

a fair summary of Issels' methods. Aubrey Singer was quoted as saying, 'the film is in the final stages of editing'. The team who made it were surprised at that statement: they knew the film had not been touched since final editing and dubbing of a commentary occurred eight months earlier.

The story caused a new outcry within the B.B.C. The *Daily Sketch* caught a whiff of the grapeshot flying around Television Centre with a story the following day headlined:

> B.B.C. CHIEF STEPS INTO T.V. STORM.
>
> The Head of B.B.C.–1, Mr. Paul Fox, will today step into the backstage row over the scrapping of a £100,000 documentary about cancer.
>
> The hour-long programme spotlights German expert Dr. Josef Issels who claims to have found new treatment methods to save cancer patients.
>
> Mr. Aubrey Singer, head of B.B.C. Features Group is refusing to submit the programme for screening because some officials fear it could give unfounded hope to British cancer sufferers. The B.B.C. screened the programme at secret previews for 15 leading medical experts. Nine of the experts backed the programme, but the other six opposed it.
>
> Mr. Fox, who is senior to Mr. Singer, will call for a screening today to make his own decision.

Precisely what happened between the two executives is not known. But Fox issued one order: *Go And Climb A Mountain* was to be aired at the earliest possible moment—at peak viewing time on November 3, 1970. Extra time was allocated for a medical discussion after the programme. Singer issued his own verbal order-of-the-day to the elated production team: 'Boys, nothing will stand between us and showing the film. I'm with you all the way.'

Issels heard the news during an evening ward round. He was telephoned and told the film would be shown in the main lecture-theatre of the prestigious Royal Institution. It would be followed by a discussion to be transmitted live throughout Britain.

—— —— added that though the film was going to be

shown, the opposition was still trying to do everything possible to stop it. But he was quite sure that with the B.B.C. having made the decision nothing could stop the film. I asked if I could see the film before it was transmitted, reminding ——— ——— that in my contract with the B.B.C. it was implicit I could have this right. He sounded embarrassed, and just kept on saying 'it will be all right on the night'. When I asked if the film had been changed because of the pressures he finally admitted it had been altered after arguments inside the B.B.C., and the outside influence of certain doctors. I pointed out this was an extraordinary situation in so much that for eight months after visiting London I had been given no chance to discuss any changes or approve them.

——— ——— agreed it was not a happy situation, but kept on saying the matter was out of his hand. He gave me the impression that the film had become a political tool in the hands of certain people and that really the production team had little or no say in the matter.

One thing was very clear to me from the entire conversation and it was that extensive pressures had been exerted to not just stop the film, but also to halt the progress of *ganzheitstherapie*.

Knowing some of the B.B.C. men involved I knew how hard they had fought. But it was clear that their work had been seriously interferred with by doctors who simply could not see that my methods of treating cancer are not a threat to them.

In the days leading up to the screening Issels was constantly telephoned by the production team on the need to avoid the Press. 'I had the feeling the B.B.C. wanted to stage manage every move I made. It did not make me very happy.' What worried him was the plan to reveal during the live debate following the film screening that *Clinical Trials Journal* would publish his long-awaited paper. He thought it smacked too much of 'entertainment and not science'. But here, too, the B.B.C. men soothed his fears.

With the B.B.C. finally committed to showing the film the medical opposition decided to make no further move until after the screening. They were thunderstruck by John Anderson's revelation he had treated patients with *ganzheitstherapie* at King's College Hospital. The news made headlines around the world—and assured the B.B.C. of a massive audience for *Go And Climb A Mountain*. Anderson had called a press conference to reveal his news simply because he feared 'some sensational paper would get hold of the story and blow it sky-high'.

Late in the afternoon of November 3, 1970, a distinguished panel of medical men and women gathered in the Royal Institution to view the film and discuss its implications. They were surprised, and gratified, to find Lord Snowdon in the audience. He had heard of Issels and his struggle and felt that public recognition by a Royal presence might be beneficial; later, in private medical circles, he was condemned for involving the Royal Family in such a manner.

The Netherlands Cancer Foundation sent an official delegation; there were doctors from all over Europe. Raymond Baxter controlled the debate in a manner which ensured it remained calm and moderate. Dr. Stuart Phillips, Editor of *Clinical Trials Journal* revealed the Issels paper was soon to be published; Anderson elaborated his now familiar views that the Ringberg Klinik demanded serious recognition. Baxter deftly moved from one speaker to another; many agreed there was a need to have 'an open-minded look' at Issels' work.

Issels flew to London to see the film and discussion. He was impressed.

The film had been edited and rescripted from the one he recalled seeing the previous March. The follow-up discussion gave it a validity he had not expected. That night, the B.B.C. production team took Issels for a champagne supper. In the early hours of the morning the mood of conviviality evaporated when the talk turned to the future of *ganzheitstherapie*. The B.B.C. men, who had been in close contact with the Corporation throughout the night, were now convinced there was trouble ahead from the medical profession; the B.B.C. had received many hostile calls from doctors.

In subsequent telephone calls with B.B.C. executives

during the following days, Issels learned with a sense of shock, that the film had unleashed a vitriolic campaign against him. What especially stunned him was that Sir David Smithers had joined in the attack:

> —— —— telephoned to say Smithers had written a furious letter over the film. He said it had been totally unscientific. He said it was quite wrong to say that the channels for changing attitudes to cancer were not open to everybody. —— —— said that Smithers had insisted he was willing to go 'anywhere to see anything', but that this sort of film was just trouble-making.

The B.B.C. objected in 1973 when details of Smithers' letter were about to be published in this book.

But Smithers could not have seriously argued that for Issels 'the channels' for a new attitude towards cancer treatment were open to everybody. There was the evidence of rejection by two British medical journals after Issels' paper had been sent out for refereeing. If Smithers did 'willingly go anywhere to see anything'—why did he not go to the Ringberg Klinik to examine for himself the evidence? The B.B.C. would pay his expenses if he wished to go. But Smithers refused to entertain the idea. After one of the film's producers talked to him he was left with a clear impression that Smithers was totally and utterly opposed to Issels and his methods. Smithers had joined that group of powerful medical men Denis Burkitt castigated in a note to the B.B.C. on November 22, 1970: 'I would like to congratulate you on your courage in showing the Issels film. I am sure you did right. Claims like this deserve investigation. It is quite unscientific to say "it can't happen: therefore it didn't happen".'

The B.B.C. received hundreds of telephone calls and letters following the programme. One of the callers was a young journalist, David Emery. His fiancée, Lillian Board, was dying of cancer, and the B.B.C. gave him the address of the Ringberg Klinik. For Josef Issels, a new, and in some ways, frightening chapter in his life was about to begin.

Lillian Board was one of the world's great athletes. She was an Olympic medallist, a sprinter with the world at her feet. For two years the sports pages around the world called her Britain's 'golden girl' for the 1972 Olympic Games in Munich. She was, in the words of one newspaper 'beautiful, brilliant, brave'. For months she had been dying of cancer. Early in September, 1970, her surgeon, Mr. Peter Hawley, at St. Mark's Hospital, Islington, London told David Emery that Lillian's life expectancy could be 'two months, maybe three'. A colostomy had been performed, but it had little effect on a rapidly growing cancer of the rectum. After the operation Hawley told Emery: 'we can only pray for a miracle now.'

Issels, as portrayed in *Go And Climb A Mountain,* seemed to Emery and the Board family as being that miracle. Emery telephoned Sir Francis Avery-Jones, the consultant who originally diagnosed Lillian's condition. He was discouraging. He felt Lillian was better off dying at home. Emery refused to accept the idea. He telephoned the Ringberg Klinik, discussed her condition, and was told a bed would be available for Lillian. Emery said he would bring her on the next possible plane. His newspaper, the *Daily Mail,* gave him leave of absence, and a cheque to help pay for Lillian's treatment. The Board family were willing to sell everything to help save Lillian's life. Emery's worst moment was breaking the news to his fiancée that she had cancer; Lillian took it well. On Saturday, November 7, the *Daily Mail* ran an exclusive front page story that the 'golden girl' was flying to Germany that morning. Within an hour every national newspaper in Britain remade its front page to carry the story. A fund, the first of many, was opened by the mayor of Ealing to meet the costs of treatment. Eventually, a considerable sum was raised by public subscription as a result of Lillian's cancer becoming public knowledge; her illness was a remarkable exercise in British public sentiment.

Issels was totally unaware on that first Saturday in November that his methods, indeed his very life was about to be subjected to intense international scrutiny. He had flown from London after the film to address a medical conference in Baden-Baden, Germany, where he presented data about sixty patients he claimed to have cured.

Meanwhile in Britain opponents to such a claim were mounting their attacks. One group of doctors chose to also involve the B.B.C. Fearing publicity they took great care to ensure they remained anonymous. They drafted a resolution which they wanted the Central Ethical Committee of the British Medical Association to act upon:

> The B.M.A. Council is concerned that a documentary programme appeared on B.B.C. at 9.20 p.m. on Tuesday, November 3. This described and showed a private nursing home on the continent where patients with advanced cancer are treated by a special regime. The address of the nursing home and the name of the doctor were given. Such an advertisement by doctors working in Britain has been unacceptable because it was considered that it was not in the best interest of the patient. The B.M.A. would like to discuss the propriety of this type of programme with the General Medical Council, other professional bodies, and the B.B.C.

The resolution sounded mild enough—but a clue as to what lay behind it was in a covering letter to Dr. Peter Wilson, assistant secretary of the British Medical Association from one of the resolution's draftees:

> I was present at the original showing and discussion and saw the subsequent television programme. If advertising is not in the patient's interest when undertaken by doctors working in Britain is it desirable to allow doctors from overseas to advertise in this country?

It was the first move to use official channels to bring pressure on Issels.

John Anderson also felt the whiplash of hostile criticism. Pressure from various quarters forced him to 'rethink' about continuing using Issels' methods at King's College Hospital; finally, with his research grants threatened he virtually abandoned using *ganzheitstherapie*.

The B.B.C. drew considerable fire from the medical profession and the press for screening the film. The production team found itself bogged down for days replying to letters.

Over a hundred had been answered by the time Lillian Board and David Emery flew out of England. Late that Saturday afternoon, Issels received a telephone call from the Ringberg Klinik. The young couple had arrived. For them all an ordeal was about to begin.

David Emery claimed Issels' first words to Lillian were:

> You know I can make you better? You believe me? Good. Together we will fight. You and me. Together we will beat the cancer. Tomorrow he will know we are coming to fight him when we start the treatment. He will always feel the strength of our forces. We will have no secrets. Always I will tell you what I am doing and why. Do you trust me? Will you fight with me?

Issels cannot recall literally making such a speech, but he had always believed it vital to encourage all patients. After he completed a full clinical examination, Issels talked frankly to Emery: he feared Lillian had come too late to be saved—but nevertheless he would try to help. Issels emphatically remembered making such a statement; equally Emery believed Issels said there was 'a chance'. Both agreed on one thing: Issels had immediately insisted on treating Lillian for nothing.

By Sunday, November 8, 1970, the world's Press and television networks had settled around the clinic. In one day the switchboard took over five hundred calls from the media in all parts of the world. Telegrams poured in for Lillian. Emery became the official spokesman about her condition. Issels did not relish the publicity, and forcibly said so on more than one occasion: equally there was no way of stopping it. The media pandered to the morbid curiosity of millions by highlighting 'the golden girl's latest race', or as the London *Sun* called it, 'a race against Big C'. Lillian was a month short of her twenty-second birthday and Emery was a handsome enough young man: *Love Story* was the romantic novel of the year—a tale of a young girl who died of cancer after finding true love. Lillian and Emery became living symbols of that best-selling fiction.

Clinically, Lillian was an acute case. X-rays showed her

big intestine impacted with barium; it was a left-over from her treatment in England. Issels regarded that as:

> Very serious. This blockage of an important organ made it more difficult for the combined treatment to have an effect. She was remarkably brave, and I warmed to her courage. Her whole outlook was summed up in a telegram somebody sent her. It just said 'Win'.

In London Jack Ashley, Labour M.P. for Stoke-on-Trent, tabled a series of Parliamentary questions asking whether Issels' claims were valid. Sir Keith Joseph, Secretary for Health and Social Services, replied:

> Treatment at the Ringberg Klinik uses conventional as well as unorthodox methods, of which the former are available in National Health Service Hospitals to all cancer patients. It will be open to the medical profession to study the information when published on all aspects of this treatment and to adopt those methods that are supported by medical evidence. The fact about the methods used and the results obtained in the Ringberg Klinik have not yet been published in a form which will enable a judgment to be given. Publication is said to be imminent and inquiries are being made from the West German Federal Health Department.

The conventional treatment prescribed at the clinic was not often available in the manner given by Issels; for example his high, single doses of Endoxana was not generally given in English hospitals. Issels' work had been published in Germany. It would have been a simple matter for the British Government to find a competent translator. Further, proof copies of the English-language paper were available at the offices of *Clinical Trials Journal*. No Government approach was made to get hold of an advance copy—or to translate his other papers.

Precisely what those inquiries produced from the West German Government only became clear later. A confidential file was sent from Bonn to the Department of Health in London. It had been compiled, by members of the German Cancer Society. Its exact contents remained a secret, but one eminent cancerologist said it damned Issels.

On November 2, 1970, Ashley, a former television producer, made a discreet approach to the B.B.C. to see whether they could find out whether Issels would accept another famous patient. That day, in *The Times*, Leslie Cannon, one of Britain's most powerful trade union leaders, revealed he was dying of cancer. He added:

> For myself I have conditioned my mind to the prospect of death and I am not afraid of the disease. The course of treatment which I am now undergoing will never cure me and no one knows that better than I do. But it will, I hope, provide me with the extension of life I need. During that time someone may come up with a permanent cure and that is what I and thousands like me are banking on. For all I know Issels may be the man.

Cannon was one of a number of powerful lay voices beginning to demand that the British Government acted—and send a medical team to study the Ringberg-Klinik. All the same it must have taken great courage on Cannon's part for him to publicly declare that his own life was virtually forfeited.

The B.B.C. production team arranged for a telephone link to be established from their offices to the Ringberg Klinik and on November 16, Cannon's doctor telephoned Issels.

He explained Cannon's wish to come to the clinic, but felt the prognosis was hopeless. Issels questioned him carefully. Finally, after a lengthy discussion, Issels agreed that Cannon was beyond his help, adding that in any case the clinic was already full.

Cannon died soon afterwards.

By then a new and even more extraordinary development had begun—aimed at discrediting Issels. An anonymous 'top cancer expert' told the Newcastle *Journal* that Lillian Board might not be suffering from cancer. In other parts of Britain similar unnamed specialists were telling newspapermen an almost identical story.

16

Renewed Opposition

LILLIAN BOARD HAD A RAPIDLY WORSENING CANCER.

Yet Issels saw the story as part of a concentrated campaign by British doctors opposed to him. They remained for the most part anonymous. One 'expert' told the London *Evening News* that 'honestly' he thought the sad journey of Lillian Board was unnecessary because she could have received adequate treatment in Britain. Another 'physician' told the same newspaper there was no hard evidence that Issels' treatment was effective, that 'in probably four years' time' he would be a forgotten man, and it was therefore pointless to even examine his methods. The *Morning Star* 'expert' said: 'There is something very distasteful at the thought of doctors and their financial supporters doing very well at the expense of seriously ill and dying patients.'

A 'leading medical expert' told the *News of the World* that his colleagues were: 'Shocked because Issels opened the door to TV before independent doctors could check his records . . . the fact is that most cancer patients DO NOT need the spartan, almost inhuman regime of the Ringberg Klinik.'

A 'specialist' told the *Daily Telegraph*: 'British specialists do not abandon patients however grim the outlook. The patients are supported to the end.'

Some medical opponents allowed their names to be used. Professor Theodore Crawford, chairman of the British Empire Cancer Campaign Scientific Committee announced it would be 'tragic' if people spent money they could not afford on seeking an unproven treatment. Crawford told the *Guardian*: 'There is no acceptable evidence that he [Issels] gets better results than you might call the orthodox profession.'

Crawford told the *Daily Sketch*: 'I'm afraid that the statistical evidence on remission rates doesn't stand up to critical examination.'

He told the London *Evening Standard* that if Issels was: 'In fact getting better results than other forms of treatment, you are faced with the problem of which of the many forms of [Issels] treatment is responsible.'

Dr. Graham Bennette, secretary of the British Cancer Council told the London *Evening Standard* that: 'We simply do not know how he [Issels] defines a patient as "terminal" or the particulars of previous treatment, the methods used in confirming the diagnosis and the stage of the illness.'

He told the *Guardian*: 'If Dr. Issels' work has been in progress for many years and really has merit, then it is likely that the German medical authorities would have launched some evaluation of its work.'

The *British Medical Journal* questioned whether British experts, busy with treatment and research, should even consider looking at Issels' methods: 'Ought the inquiry not to be left to German experts . . . was it worthwhile for Miss Board to be flown to Bavaria to undergo the rigorous measures Dr. Issels' treatment entails?'

Professor Henry Miller, Vice-Chancellor of the University of Newcastle, launched a long attack on those methods in *The Listener*: Miller swiped at everything in sight, including the B.B.C. who owned the magazine. But he reserved the full majesty of his fury for Issels, 'the Herr Doktor' and his methods:

> A package tediously familiar to those who have investigated treatments for chronic disease. Such routines comprise orthodox drugs together with mumbo-jumbo of widely variable types, and they are almost invariably so complex as to defy rational assessment. They are not unknown in Britain but flourish especially in the private sector of medicine in continental Europe. I have in mind

a compatriot of Dr. Issels who obtained excellent results in Parkinson's disease with massive doses of the usual drugs combined with an elaborate routine during which the patient was pursued up hill and down dale by a posse of physio-therapeutic Valkyrie. Unfortunately improvements did not long survive the calling-off of the Valkyrie and the patient's return home. A much publicised Franco-Belgium treatment for multiple sclerosis combines the not entirely irrational employment of live wide-spectrum antibiotics and hot baths impregnated with an extract of seaweed obtainably only from a Bordeaux pharmacist—and injections of camphor, a nineteenth-century elixir.

Miller undoubtedly believed what he wrote. It is more difficult to accept the sincerity of some of Issels' other detractors. By the end of November, 1970, a fresh rumour circulated freely. It was simple—and potentially deadly. It said that Issels' English-language paper had come under suspicion—'the figures have been cooked' was how one doctor heard it. It was an almost identical allegation to that made years before when Dr. Arie Audier published in a German medical journal statistical proof showing Issels obtained a 16·6 per cent cure rate. Issels claimed a similar result in his own paper. Dr. Stuart Phillips, Editor of *Clinical Trials Journal* stoutly denied there was anything wrong with Issels' paper. But the rumour succeeded. Before publication, the claims Issels advanced were suspected. Newspapers became cautious. The paper was played down. Issels suffered another reverse.

The opponents had still not finished. With the Lillian Board drama filling the front pages, the anonymous experts returned to advise editors that if Issels saved Lillian then possibly his treatment might be taken more seriously. In the public mind the issue became a simple one: if Issels 'cured' Lillian he was a medical hero; if she died he was a charlatan.

In every way it was the most effective, and cruel of all the propaganda.

While deeply admiring her courage and determination to live, Issels was not blinded to the clinical picture of Lillian

Board's illness. He knew it was virtually hopeless, but apart from telling David Emery, Issels kept his views largely to himself. He had no desire to alarm anybody—or find his medical opinions quoted in the world's press.

In the middle of November, 1970, Lillian's parents and her twin sister, Irene, flew to be at her bedside. They had comfortable suites in a local hotel and a car paid for by public subscriptions in Britain. They were entranced by the towering mountains, the glassy, calm Tegernsee, the picture-pretty inns, alpine shrubs in window boxes, waitresses in *Dirndls*, folk music and the general *Gemütlichkeit* of Rottach-Egern.

The town had a sizeable English colony by December: press and television crews covering the Lillian story; English patients and their families. The media filled in the time by filling out the stories of numerous cancer victims. There was Patricia Parsons, a forty-year-old Londoner, a mother of four children, whose husband died of cancer of the brain in 1968. Doctors at Guy's Hospital, London diagnosed her with cancer of the liver. Mrs. Parsons 'gladly' spent her £1,500 to come to the clinic. Another widow, Sylvia Harvey, brought her seven-year-old son, Jonathan, seeking a cure for his leg cancer. A Manchester surgeon had advised amputation; funds had been found to bring him to Rottach-Egern. He joined another English child, David Towse, aged five years, from Luton, Bedfordshire. David had lymphosarcoma and doctors at Great Ormond Street Hospital, London, said his prognosis was bleak, Britain's largest private medical insurance company, British United Provident Association, announced it would consider claims from members wishing to be treated at the clinic; the first claim came from theatrical agent Robin Fox. Those English patients joined others from all over the world. They were photographed and interviewed in a score of languages. The clinic received unparallel attention, including notice from the editorial columns of *The Times*.

Some of what was written was critical, but for Issels nothing provided strength so readily as did opposition. He set down in his private diary on the eve of his sixty-third birthday on November 21, 1970, his own attitude: 'In spite of the hostility, the recurring results give me the strength to go on and do my best. I can only wonder at the real motives of those opponents who have never read my work or been here.'

He was hurt and genuinely astonished at the venom of some of the attacks on him and the clinic. He had never hoped that everyone would ever agree completely with him over his ideas, but he was dismayed at the bitterness of some of his opponents: they challenged his very existence as a doctor. Yet Issels remained steadfast in his beliefs that public opinion must be awakened over the need to remove the *fear* of cancer. The tragic case of Lillian Board had brought the word into the headlines as never before. Issels deliberately used the opportunity to express the fundamentals of his theories to newspapers all over the world. Inevitably, he suffered a certain amount of personal publicity, and he accepted it as a reasonable price to pay in exchange for an unprecedented platform for *ganzheitstherapie*. The motives of all the visitors to the clinic varied, but Issels welcomed them all.

Many callers felt that Issels displayed loneliness, and in a way that was true. Issels was a man on a summit, one he had created to climb himself. Few understood the reasons behind that climb; perhaps because of that he showed undue compassion towards his detractors. He forgave them while at the same time holding fast to his own integrity. It was yet another facet of a highly complex personality, a man of great depth, ever ready to face censure and controversy by rejecting esteemed medical truths. Millions came to realise what those close to him had known for years: Josef Issels was a dissenter, and proud of it; a non-conformist living a life with a highly individualistic perspective—something never easy in a profession steeped in organisations, institutions, colleges and power blocs.

Unknown to him the first moves by one of those groups had begun to select a team of British cancer scientists to investigate the clinic. The Co-ordinating Committee for Cancer Research in Britain met in London to consider suitable names. One expert was ruled out. Professor John Anderson's views were already known. Not generally known was the fact that since he continued supporting Issels, Anderson suffered serious difficulties with research grants;

at one stage he feared he would lose everything for his beliefs. But, in his later words: 'I would not have backed away from Issels.'

At the end of the Co-ordinating Committee's meeting, Brigadier David Gribbin, secretary-general of the Cancer Research Campaign said there was a growing body in favour of an investigation into Issels:

> It would mean sending a team of busy high-grade experts to spend several weeks in Bavaria . . . it would be impartial and not be influenced by any other consideration than to evaluate the truth of this man's work and to report on it in a proper scientific manner where nothing would be prejudged.

Issels was delighted by those terms of reference. They confirmed what he still largely believed—that in spite of all the attacks he would get a fair hearing from a British medical team.

It brought extra joy to his birthday party which was held that evening. Among those present were his children, Uti and Rolf. They brought warmest greetings for Issels from his first wife, Irmengard. Outwardly, family discord was put aside for a planned night of fine foods and wines and the kind of music Issels enjoyed most of all, soft and sentimental.

Shortly after nine o'clock, Issels received a telephone call to return to the clinic. Lillian Board had taken a turn for the worse. He arrived to find her surrounded by nurses, a duty doctor, Lillian's twin, Irene and fiancé, David Emery, who recalled:

> Issels looked grave as he examined Lillian and then nodded for Irene and me to talk to him outside. Lillian was busy with one of the nurses, so we slipped out quietly. 'The tumour in her stomach has swollen,' Dr. Issels said. 'If it does not go down her condition is very critical. Her parents should be told.' I looked at Irene and the expression on her face told me she was feeling the same as me. 'I know it sounds bad,' I told her. 'But I'm sure it will be O.K. I've just got that sort of feeling.'

Issels said little more because he did not wish to cause further alarm. He authorised injections to help her over the crisis and suggested Emery camped-out in Lillian's room for the night.

He left, not to return immediately to the party, but to ponder over the case and its implications. In the hundreds of telephone calls from the mass media, several journalists told him that if Lillian died he faced a professional holocaust from doctors who mistook his initial certainty in his treatment of Lillian to be conceit. Issels knew it was essential to sustain proper hope in both Lillian and her family—as he knew their greatest wish was that he extended the length of an enjoyable and useful life for her. He believed that no longer possible. Though death might perhaps be deferred the signs of fatal illness were increasingly evident.

He returned to the birthday celebration, his mind still filled with the problem of the young woman on the second floor of Ward Five. Since coming to the clinic Lillian had never admitted to herself, or anyone else, that she was dying. Her conversations had contained such assertions that all 'would be well' or 'I'll be fine' or 'I'll win through'. Undoubtedly Lillian felt little reason to think otherwise, and her family and Emery fostered the illusion. It was clear to Issels they never wanted to think of death. He understood well their outlook: it was a protective function of their own minds subconsciously rejecting any thought over Lillian's end. He respected and sympathised with their attitude—with its bland cheerfulness, firm beliefs, a point of view perfectly captured in David Emery's words: 'It will be O.K. I've just got that sort of feeling.'

Issels did not share that optimism.

In the last week of November Lillian rallied. She grew excited about her approaching birthday, December 13. In London, newspapers planned to fly out reporters and photographers with sacks of gifts from their readers. In return they hoped for interviews. On December 1, Lillian underwent surgery at Tegernsee Hospital to try and remove the blockage in her lower abdomen. Issels attended, and saw her abdomen was filled with a mass of tumour. He knew that he could do little more, and told Emery.

On Friday, December 11, back in the clinic, Lillian collapsed and was moved to Ward One. The emotional undercurrents remained in Emery's later recollection that it was a move to 'the death house'. Ward One frightened him: 'Its sparse business-like furniture and the huge statue of Christ which overhung the main staircase brought home so forcibly the reason we were there.'

His undoubted and understandable shock over Lillian's move clouded his recollections. He later remembered Ward One as carpetless, without ornaments, nothing that afforded a hint of welcome:

> There was no illusion of glamour here. Even the nurses, handpicked for their attractiveness in the other wards, were highly competent, but ordinary. This was the nerve centre of Issels' clinic, a grim area of life and death struggle, that had no place for the squeamish and the sensitive.

Ward One was not that cheerless. There were landscape prints on the walls, flowers on side tables, and judging by the attention they received from the reporters, the nurses were every bit as pretty as anywhere else in the clinic.

Nevertheless, Emery had been right over one thing:—Ward One was for the acutely ill—and Lillian was certainly that.

A new crisis came on December 12 when her abdomen had to be drained. On December 13, her twenty-second birthday, she showed further deterioration. Issels spent a sleepless night knowing there was little hope of her even surviving a few more weeks. On Monday, December 21, Lillian had a further collapse. Issels feared peritonitis. He called the Board family and Emery to his office and explained death was only a matter of days, possibly even hours, away unless she underwent surgery.

At nine o'clock that night Lillian was driven by ambulance to Munich University Surgical Clinic where Professor Rudolph Zenker hoped to operate. From Munich Emery conveyed the full drama of the occasion in an exclusive interview with his newspaper, the *Daily Mail*.

An operation was performed on the Wednesday, December 23.

Issels was on hand before and after surgery. He remembered that she smiled at him and whispered after the operation: 'The last hurdle . . . marvellous.'

They were the last words she spoke to him. Issels drove back to Rottach-Egern immeasurably saddened, tears on his cheeks, by the sure knowledge that she would be dead by the end of the week. The end came at two minutes past four on Saturday, December 26, the second day of Christmas.

That evening television stations throughout the world carried the news. The Queen sent a telegram of sympathy, so did Britain's Prime Minister, Edward Heath. Opposition Leader Harold Wilson penned a glowing tribute. The media linked her death with the fact that Britain's Co-ordinating Committee on Cancer Research was sending a team to investigate the clinic. The news bulletins gave no details. Issels found the further details in a letter written on December 18 by Dr. R. C. Norton, secretary of the Committee:

> As I am sure you know, the methods of treatment of advanced cancer used in your clinic have recently aroused great public interest in this country. The available information about these methods has recently been considered by an officially sponsored scientific advisory committee known as the Co-ordinating Committee on Cancer Research of which I am the Secretary. This Committee has been set up jointly by the Cancer Research Campaign, the Imperial Cancer Research Fund and the Medical Research Council, which are the three main bodies responsible for supporting all kinds of Cancer Research in this country.
>
> The Committee did not feel that the information which they had received so far was sufficient to enable them to form a valid opinion, and they agreed that, subject to your being willing, a visit to the clinic by a small party of experts in the treatment of cancer might provide more information. These experts could then advise whether a further longer-term study should be recommended.
>
> I am accordingly writing on behalf of the Cancer Research Campaign, the Imperial Cancer Research Fund

and the Medical Research Council to ask whether you would be willing to receive such a visiting party and to give them whatever facilities might be necessary to enable them to make a preliminary report, which might in due course be published in this country.

In the event of your being agreeable to receiving such a party the experts who are listed on the attached sheet have been nominated by the sponsoring bodies and have agreed to be members of it.

The three sponsoring bodies would be glad to know whether you would be agreeable to receiving this visiting party and they would be most grateful if you would do so. If you are willing, it appears that the most convenient dates for the party to make their visit would be either the week beginning January 4th or that beginning January 25th. Could you please let me know whether one of these times would be convenient to you? May I also ask whether it would be possible for the visiting party to be accommodated in the vicinity of the clinic?

The letter proposed five members for the visiting party. They were:

Professor Sir David Smithers, Director of Radiotherapy Department, Royal Marsden Hospital and Institute for Cancer Research; Dame Albertine Winner, Deputy Medical Director, St. Christopher's Hospice, London; Dr. Gordon Hamilton Fairley, consultant physician, St. Bartholomew's Hospital, London; Dr. R. J. C. Harris, Department of Environmental Carcinogenesis, Imperial Cancer Fund Laboratories, Mill Hill, London; Dr. V. C. Medvei, formerly Principal Medical Officer to Her Majesty's Treasury.

They were distinguished names. Issels was particularly pleased to see the name of Dame Albertine Winner on the list. Her reputation was known to him as somebody passionately concerned with the problems of managing the dying. Professor Anderson had spoken warmly to Issels about Dame Albertine's compassion and understanding for her patients. Issels believed he would have much in common with her.

Smithers' name prompted him to turn again to Sir David's well-thumbed *Lancet* paper. What he read there reassured him. Smithers, too, had a similar attitude in that paper towards cancer as Issels. Issels believed the team would be objective and without pre-conceived ideas. He wrote in his diary for New Year's Eve, 1970: 'They are British. The British are always fair in everything they do. They may be hard. But they will be fair, as they cannot overlook the facts. Unlike the Germans they won't have made their mind up before coming.'

He drank a toast to 1971, believing that international acceptance was only a matter of a short time away.

Mr. W. Dempster, Reader in Experimental Surgery at the Royal Post-Graduate Medical School, Hammersmith, spoke for a section of the medical establishment when he wrote to *World Medicine*:

> The medical profession has set a spineless precedent, bowing to uninformed, highly emotional public pressure. Instead, our profession should have issued a confidential and reassuring statement indicating that nothing new had emerged in cancer therapy in years. The public should have been told that assessment of cancer therapy takes years and involves clinical trials, observation and debate and cannot be based on a visit to one clinic 'by public demand'.

Dempster voiced a fear many scientists felt uneasy about: the visiting team planned to spend only five days in Germany. Yet Brigadier Gribbin, secretary-general of the Cancer Research Campaign had publicly stated a month before that scientists needed to spend 'several weeks' at the clinic. Gribbin had not been the only one to say that.

For months cancerologists had maintained that the statistical evidence was a key factor in any proper inquiry into the Ringberg Klinik. Dr. Arie Audier had conclusively shown a 16·6 per cent cure rate. Professor John Anderson had verified that figure. Issels' own clinical paper showed a similar rate of remission. Yet the percentage had been doubted simply because it was so staggeringly high. Anderson calculated that Issels obtained eight times better results than almost anywhere else in the world in managing properly verified terminal cases of cancer. The World Health Organisation comparative figures showed a 2 per cent remission rate. Anderson had given evidence to the Co-ordinating Committee for Cancer Research describing his own investigation at the clinic; he urged that the inquiry team must have a competent medical statistician able to process the case-notes into a form whereby they could be analysed by computer.

Yet the team contained no recognised medical statistician. It was the most curious omission of all.

Issels prepared to meet the team calmly, an attitude fostered by Isa, who immersed herself completely in what she called 'The Task', her shorthand for doing everything possible to help her husband. In the years of marriage Isa had repeatedly demonstrated her complete imperturbability, remaining sensible, completely interested in Issels' work. Painstaking in her efforts to get things right, she was never dull. Nor did she suffer fools gladly, sending them politely about their business. Never were those qualities more needed, or appreciated, in the weeks before the English team arrived.

There was excitement and tension in the clinic in spite of Issels' effort to dampen down things; some of the staff had invested the English scientists with power of life and death over their future.

There was also continuing tension between Issels' older children and Isa. She understood only too well the problems Rolf and Uti had in making adjustments, and she made all the allowances possible for their attitude, even though at times she was deeply privately hurt. She subjugated her personal feelings, and often her pride, for the sake of their father. Because of this, harmony of a kind was finally established. Rolf and Uti said they recognised their behaviour had been hurtful towards their step-mother, and promised at least to accept her as having a full role in their father's life.

The weekend before the English team arrived Issels flew in, at his own expense, thirty-one former patients from all over Europe to be presented to the scientists as so called 'incurables' who had shown tumour remissions after the clinic's treatment. Among them were Peter Newton Fenbow, Käthe Gerlach and Thea Döhm.

On Monday, January 25, 1971, Issels and his senior doctor met Smithers and his party at Munich Airport. Issels was impressed by Dame Albertine Winner's friendliness, but found the others distantly polite. Smithers informed him that they planned to stay about a week.

Later, Issels expressed to Smithers how much he had enjoyed his paper in *The Lancet*, adding: 'My philosophy about cancer is nearly the same as yours.'

Smithers made no reply.

The team began work immediately, following an almost identical pattern to that devised by Professor Anderson when he had investigated the clinic for the B.B.C. Issels was impressed by the team's hard work, even though they showed little reaction to what they saw. A change came with the presentation of cured patients. Fairley and Smithers showed signs of awakening interest; Dame Albertine Winner was often openly incredulous.

Harris, the party's microbiologist, spent three days with Gerlach, who explained, among much else, that his original vaccine had not been used in the clinic for four years, and that his current work was isolating mycoplasma from human and animal tumours, culturing in broth, or agar, and testing them for tumour production in mice. By the end of their meeting, Gerlach had formed the opinion that Harris was impressed by what he learnt.

It was a view Issels also held over the attitude of the other members of the team in the three days they toured the clinic. On the fifth day, they compared notes and left, having spent a combined 220 hours scrutinising the treatment methods.

From Munich Smithers wrote on Friday, January 29:

Dear Dr. Issels!

All the team which came with me and I myself would like to thank you for your hospitality. You made us welcome, when we came on a difficult mission, you allowed us freedom to see everything we wished and you saw to our transport and our comfort.

We found ourselves in agreement with many things in

your clinic particularly your approach to patients who were desperately ill. We could not agree with all your conclusions I fear. This letter is to convey our thanks to you for your frankness and your welcome. From us all.

Yours most sincerely,
David Smithers.

During the whole of February, 1971, the visiting team drafted versions of the report. How many is not clear, but informed observers like John Stevenson, then medical correspondent of the *Daily Sketch*, believed there was a genuine conflict between members of the visiting team over what to say. A number of stories circulated in the lobbies of the House of Commons, the Department of Health and the B.B.C. that the differences were so deep that the report was being vetted by Treasury Counsel because it was so vitriolic. Government spokesmen denied the story—but it persisted.

Meanwhile Issels accepted an invitation to address the Royal Medical Society in Edinburgh, and drew one of the largest audiences in its history when he addressed them on February 24, 1971.

He returned home to find a letter from the British Medical Research Council advising him that the Government-sponsored report would be flown out by special messenger immediately prior to its publication on March 3, 1971.

When he read it, Issels was dumb-founded. *A Report on the Treatment of Cancer at the Ringberg Clinic, Rottach-Egern, Bavaria* was worse than he had ever expected.

17

Tomorrow is Another World

The Report had been approved by the Cancer Research Campaign, the Imperial Cancer Research Fund and the Medical Research Council and published by the Stationery Office on the authority of the Department of Health and Social Security. It bore all the marks of a document worried over by many hands. Yet much remained not ordinarily found in a Government-sponsored paper. There were references to Issels and his staff which they regarded as casting personal scorn, doubt and ridicule on their work:

'Gerlach's mice are well cared for by his wife. He does not do any histology but sends all his material to Vienna for "independent" examination.'

Or: 'The selection of patients is done by correspondence. Dr. Issels says he really has no means of choosing, since how can he refuse someone if he has room, and the letters often give no clear idea of how ill the patient is.'

Issels regarded those statements as well short of the truth and a deliberate attempt to discredit the Ringberg Klinik. No mention was made of Gerlach's distinguished background or of his contribution to cancer research. Gerlach had provided Harris with the fullest details of his life-time's work, and the English scientist apparently expressed considerable excitement and interest at what he had seen and been told.

It was true that the Ringberg Klinik had no method of selecting its patients—any more than other cancer hospitals picked and choosed whom to treat. But the Report implied that the clinic operated something akin to a medical mail order service, where patients were taken on the strength of a letter containing little information. No reference was made that cancer specialists all over the world sent patients to the clinic with proper medical documentation.

The Report particularly stunned Issels because he believed he had proved his theories to the visiting team; he had been encouraged by Smithers' note from Munich. He had even hoped that the Report might endorse many of his ideas and urge a further investigation into them. All his dreams and trust were synthesised in the words: 'The British are fair.' The twenty-two-page Report sent his optimism crashing.

One elegantly damning phrase followed another:

> We searched for every possible indication of tumour regression not due to cytotoxic drugs and found none that was convincing . . . a few patients seemed to us to suffer from lack of investigation and of treatment which they might have been given elsewhere. A diagnosis cannot be confirmed or rejected here . . . every reaction is explained in terms of action taken the day before. In the early stages bad signs are said to be good reactions, but if the same signs persist they become bad reactions and then the patient either has cytotoxic drugs or failure is admitted . . . the main cause of confusion about the successes claimed in this clinic has arisen in our opinion from the acceptance of misdiagnosis made elsewhere . . . the fact that so many patients go to the clinic to find something they fail to receive at home is really more a reflection on the medical service they leave than a credit to Dr. Issels' particular treatment.

The Report dealt with two of Issels' earliest patients, Lydia Bacher and Käthe Gerlach, conceded they were 'dramatic cases' but doubted if they had been helped by Issels, or even whether Lydia Bacher had cancer at all when she had been admitted to the clinic blind, deaf and paralysed with a brain tumour. Then came a surprising admission: 'We were not there, we cannot know precisely what happened, but in both these patients the records provide a picture of a slow recovery from gross over-irradiation.'

Issels was baffled. The case-notes showed in his mind a steady recovery from cancer brought about by *ganzheitstherapie*. Professor Anderson, medical expert at the trials, and later doctors from all over the world, had checked out the two cases and come to a similar conclusion. In Issels' later words:

> The documents of both those cases were prepared by physicians who were *there* during treatment—who knew *precisely* what happened. They had the clinical picture before them, with a clearly fatal prognosis. They followed the progression and regression of the tumours during the months and years of treatment and recorded their findings. Such findings serve in the medical world as the basis for acknowledgment of cures achieved.

The Report contained faint praise for the psychological support and nursing care—and Issels detected the hand of Dame Albertine Winner behind those remarks. But there was little else of comfort to be drawn from the conclusions. The harshest words were reserved for an accusation Issels had lived with for twenty-one-years: his diagnostic facilities were 'sparse' so he could not tell if a patient actually had cancer on admission. Therefore, in the Report's opinion, a large proportion of his 'successes' were no more than patients suffering from over-irradiation. They had been 'cured' before coming to him and he had mistaken cancer for the after-effects of radiotherapy. He had faced, and overcome, similar stories at his trials. He was staggered to find them repeated years later, more so in view of his clear recall of painstakingly pointing out to the visiting team that, while the Ringberg Klinik did not diagnose cancer in the first instance, 99 per cent of all patients were admitted with a properly verified diagnosis of cancer: of those, about 90 per cent had been pronounced 'incurable'. Nor was a diagnosis ever accepted 'without criticism'. Outside consultants with regular sessions at the clinic checked out every diagnosis. If further histological verification was possible without endangering the lives of already critically ill patients, it was done in pathological institutes in Munich.

The Report caused an international outcry in the mass media and medical circles. Issels issued a brief statement rejecting the findings. It was lost in a welter of headlines attacking him. More than one newspaper reminded its readers that he had failed to save Lillian Board.

The verdict left Issels with a strong feeling that it had been penned by complacent hands; that all was well in the world of conventional cancer research and there was no place for his theories. It hurt him deeply, not because he had ever wanted to be hailed as the man who changed medical history, but simply because he believed a magnificent opportunity had been lost to help more lives. His disappointment was the more so because he believed Smithers, of all cancerologists, had given every impression of sharing similar views to his own. On March 9, 1971, Issels wrote to him:

Dear Sir David,

Now that the smoke has cleared a little, I feel I must write a few words to you personally as the leader of the visiting party.

It was really a valuable experience for me and for my colleagues to receive your visit to our clinic and to follow your efforts to assess our work. Our discussions were indeed very rewarding for me.

I very much appreciate your largely positive comments on our medical and nursing work, and I should like to thank you also on behalf of my staff.

It is true, of course, that your conclusions have resulted in conflicting impressions. It is very difficult to accept that scientifically-based histological or clinical diagnoses, often provided from several completely independent sources, have been later doubted, subsequently leading to a strict conclusion, i.e. the rejection of the therapy.

There is no difference of opinion as to the fact that my therapy seems to be largely unspecific. By consistent retuning of the organism, it aims to support the rehabilitation of the body's defence mechanism, providing a better pre-condition for any specific measures. Our experience speaks for this assumption.

The therapy practised at the Ringberg Klinik should only be judged from this point of view.

I believe that in the cancer therapy of the future, besides the removal of the tumour, great importance should be placed on the field of improvement in the natural resistance, also significantly to ameliorate the results which today are achieved by the classic weapons. We all know that these methods, in spite of the high standards achieved appear to have reached a certain point of stagnation.

It is a complete misinterpretation of my intentions to presume that with my therapy I wish to give the impression of offering competition for the classic weapons.

That this is *not* the case (which would not only be presumptuous, but also completely unrealistic) can be seen very clearly from all my papers and statements—also from the fact that my therapy is almost exclusively put into action where conventional therapy can no longer be applied.

Smithers replied from the Royal Marsden Hospital, London, on March 29:

Dear Dr. Issels,

Thank you for your letter.

There are really two matters at issue, only one of which is my direct concern. This resulted from a programme put on by the B.B.C. here about your clinic, this made grossly misleading statements, caused a great deal of publicity and anxiety in this country and your clinic was represented as having a method of curing cancer, regarded as incurable by other people, in some 16 per cent of cases. This we were asked to investigate, this claim we found to be without foundation on the evidence presented to us and we so reported. We found much to admire in the way you handle difficult patients and did not think that our duty extended beyond reporting to Britain on this first question.

The second question is not a matter of public discussion as far as I am concerned but since you raise the matter in private correspondence let me reply in the same vein.

Of course patients with cancer should be put in the best position to combat their own disease, there is, and has been for some time, a move in this direction in cancer departments all over the world, particularly in relation to immunological research. For any department or clinic to state that this is one of their objects makes no progress, it is merely recording a pious hope. If you are to convince the world that you have made any advance in this direction whatever you have to produce scientific evidence, so far you have not done so. Your only publication in Britain was inaccurate, misleading and really not a scientific publication at all in the strictly accepted sense of the word, it will carry no weight. I am sure your intentions are excellent, I am sorry that you have not produced any evidence of their efficacy but that is the fact of the matter as it stands at present.

You say that it is difficult to accept that scientifically based histology or clinical diagnoses provided from independent sources should be doubted; I am afraid that this is what we do every day, all diagnoses are doubted until they are confirmed, but your case is I think rather different, since not only do you fail to do this in your own clinic, but also fail to make a distinction between an accurate diagnosis made before treatment has been given elsewhere, and the effect which treatment has had upon that diagnosis. The failure to recognise severe radiation reaction, particularly in the pelvis, a well-known source of error in cancer departments which can cause difficulties even in a hospital fully equipped to carry out investigations, has I am afraid been a major source of confusion in the presentation of your results.

Lastly, may I say that total regressions of multiple metastatic disease in cancer patients today is not at all uncommon. We could find no real evidence of such patients in your clinic who had not had chemotherapy and the number on chemotherapy with regression shown to us was small; with surgery, radiotherapy and chemotherapy used in co-ordination here we could show you many patients in this category where the evidence for metastatic disease would be generally acceptable. I am afraid that it seemed to us that you were not fully acquainted with the present state of cancer treatment for advanced disease in the best centres in many countries.

I am glad that you understood the tone of our report which was concerned only with a publicity situation created in this country by a well-made film of interest which carried a most misleading commentary. I regarded it as no part of our business to attack your clinic or your methods in any way but very much our business to straighten out a misrepresentation that had been made to the British public.

May I say that you have one straight course before you if you wish to convince the medical profession that you have something new to offer in the cure of cancer patients, and that is to publish a new account of your work; it must, however, be in a form that is self-critical and scientifically acceptable; you have so far put forward no evidence that could be so accepted in any serious cancer clinic at the present time.

Josef Issels was not surprised that Smithers responded in such a way. Issels noted:

Sir David's letter took no account of the fact that I had presented his team with 26 properly verified cases *in persona* of incurable cancer which we had cured. Many of them had survived up to 20 years. Further, the team was shown over 30 case histories, with X-rays and precise clinical data.

This presentation had taken place on the two afternoons available in the team's programme. Some of its members had shown they were impressed at what they had seen. Sir David gave no reaction. When I suggested a further presentation for the next afternoon, Sir David suddenly told me, 'I thank you. We have seen enough'. I was astonished, recalling there had been much talk originally of the need for a thorough investigation, one that might even last two or three months. It was not to be. In spite of their brief visit the team concluded the therapy was not effective and that no further investigation was called for. This verdict ultimately closed the door for the only possible treatment of incurables in the whole world.

Nobody, not even an unusually perceptive Josef Issels, could have realised that the Report would become a weapon to attack his beliefs, and that in less than three years he would feel forced to close down his clinic, in October 1973, a decision he would directly trace back to renewed medical opposition engendered by the Report. Nor would Issels have anticipated that Smithers, on the day of his retirement, September 27, 1973 would inform the *Daily Telegraph*, London, that he 'shed no tears' at the closure. Smithers was quoted by the *Telegraph* as saying:

> Patients do not need to be worried about not being able to go to Dr. Issels. He was very good at looking after people who had been abandoned by doctors who should not have abandoned them. But I am not sorry about his cancer treatment at the Ringberg Klinik shutting down.

In Smithers' opinion the level of treatment in Britain was a 'lot better'. Issels dismissed Smithers' statement as:

> Unimportant. Whether Sir David was aware or not does not matter, but the fact is that several patients have come to me for treatment from the Royal Marsden Hospital, where Sir David was a consultant. I am quite sure Sir David did not mean to convey the idea that his colleagues had 'abandoned them'.

By the autumn of 1973, in spite of all his trials and tribulations, Josef Issels felt he had more important things to do than discuss such matters with Smithers. He had aimed at a dialogue with Dr. Robert Good, medical director of New York's Sloan-Kettering Institute for Cancer Research. Good, open-minded and ready to form his own opinion about other methods of treating cancer had earlier in 1973 arranged for Issels to address senior members of the Institute's medical faculty. They had been 'impressed' by what Issels had told them. At the end of the meeting—a marathon talk-in lasting four hours—Robert Good had asked Issels if he had given a similar presentation to Smithers' team. Issels said he had.

The Americans had looked bewildered. Good spoke for them all when he said: 'In that case I simply do not understand how they could have produced the report they did'.

It was a question that Josef Issels could not answer in

1973, just as two years earlier he had been unable to understand how the Department of Health Report could have been allowed to see the light of day.

In the summer following its publication Issels wrote a lengthy critique of the Report.

It took Issels and his staff several weeks to go through the case files the visiting team claimed to have analysed in three days. Issels found serious discrepancies in the Report:

> It stated facts which were completely at variance with the case-notes. For example, the Report referred to a case of cancer of the uterus and stated that the patient had been cured by surgery. Yet the case-notes showed that she had never been operated upon. There was another case in which the Report stated: 'One patient had a brain tumour in which a cyst aspirated seven years after radiotherapy contained what were thought to be tumour cells.' The Report failed to mention that as well as the cyst there was a large, malignant tumour. The Report quoted only part of the operation report. The full sentence read: '. . . first, there is a cyst in the area of the resected parts of the left cerebellum which is evacuated. It fills a large part of the left dorsal cranial fossa. Apart from this there is also a tumour extending mainly to the pons and the foramen occipitale and originating from the wall of the cyst.' There was ample clinical evidence in that patient's case-notes to prove that. Further, the Report failed to make any mention of nine cases which the visiting team had examined. Those cases clearly showed the scope of *ganzheitstherapie* in treating a wide variety of cancers. Most strange of all, the visiting team were given ample proof during the ward rounds to see how the clinic's medical staff repeatedly challenged the original diagnosis. They were shown that in every single case the original diagnosis was either confirmed or modified, or sometimes even rejected. The visiting team almost totally agreed with the diagnosis of cancer they saw in all the patients in the clinic. The same methods of diagnosis had been applied to cured patients. But in those cases they said there had been a wrong diagnosis. Therefore the Report implied that some 600 independent

cancer specialists who had diagnosed the progressive carcinomas in the cases had made a mistake.

He ended with the suggestion that a suitable scientific organisation, British or otherwise, should arrange for properly verified cases of 'incurable' cancer to be treated at the clinic, and: 'This selection should correspond to the accepted criteria for a statistical evaluation. Both the diagnosis and the treatment results should be assessed and published by *the same group of experts.*'

The critique was published in the German medical journal *Das Krebsgeschehen.* Professor John Anderson later cast his expert eye over the contents, and judged the contents to be of real interest to British medical journals. Not one accepted it for publication.

The months following the appearance of the Government-sponsored Report were critical for the Ringberg Klinik. Medical opposition in Germany, and elsewhere, flared anew; the words 'charlatan' and 'false hope' found new voices.

For the first time in many years there was no waiting list for admission to the clinic. By high summer 1971, a third of the 125 beds were empty. But no staff were dismissed. In a few months debts had reached over DM 400,000.

Issels was frequently depressed during that period and would undoubtedly have grown more so but for Isa. She knew better than anybody that he had travelled the road of confidence in full view of everybody for so many years; that alone made it harder for him to accept the crushing verdict of the Report. Yet Isa knew her husband was in no mood to accept consoling advice; equally 'The Task' could not resume if its champion waited upon certainty. So she calmly laid out the inescapable facts. He knew his ideas worked: his patients were living proof of that. He should look upon the Report as no more than another obstacle along the lonely route he had travelled for so many years.

Issels listened to his wife. His confidence and perspective returned. His physical and mental powers became as great, and perhaps even greater, than they had been for some years. Uti and Rolf, both remembered that while his enthusiasm returned, their father mellowed; it seemed too that he had found more time for the children of his second marriage than he had ever been able to spare for his older children.

By the autumn of 1971 Issels completed another draft of a book describing his methods; it was a clear indication of the way he had come. Writing it also had a certain therapeutic value in that it helped to expunge the definitive damnation of the Report.

In November he travelled to Japan to investigate the use of enzymes in treating cancer. He visited various cancer institutes in Tokyo and lectured at the University of Sapporo. He returned home on Christmas Eve to find many of his patients showing signs of improvement. It was, he confided to Isa, the best present he could have.

In February, 1972, he and Isa travelled to the Cancer Conference in Sydney, Australia, with a group of doctors who were members of the German Cancer Society. Issels found the conference had much to offer. Papers were read showing the latest advances in treating that most difficult of all cancers leukaemia and melanoma. He learnt much that was new about immunology. He found an easy relationship with scientists from all over the world who knew his work and appreciated his aims. More than one confided to Issels that his approach, *ganzheitstherapie*, was the most promising of all approaches. But this atmosphere of scientific harmony was disturbed by an unpleasant piece of medical politicking.

They were barred from two official receptions at the direct instigation of Professor C. G. Schmidt, then President of the German Cancer Society. Issels was told by Sir Leslie Herron, Chairman of the Hospitality Committee of the Australian Cancer Society that they had been excluded because Schmidt insisted Issels did not belong to the German group of doctors, and was not a member of any official German Cancer Society. Issels said neither was true. He did belong with the visiting group of German doctors. He was also a member of the Bavarian Cancer Society. Herron was clearly embarrassed by the whole situation, but felt the matter was beyond his control. Issels met Schmidt, and was publicly snubbed before conference delegates. The German

Consul-General in Sydney became involved in the squabble, but he refused Schmidt's request that he cancel Issels' and Isa's invitation to attend an official Consulate reception. Issels looked upon it as yet another example of what he termed 'the power of the medical Mafia'. He returned to Rottach-Egern and began a legal action against Schmidt.

The past twenty-five years of Josef Issels' life have been devoted to discouraging the conclusion cancer was a local disease and that symptomatic treatment was enough. From the time he started treating the disease he remained true to certain fundamental ideas that he restated in July, 1972:

> A healthy body has the capacity to keep all cells functioning properly, and when cancer cells form the body's natural defence mechanism can overcome them. The body's 'resistance' acts as a natural defence against cancer. Once the 'resistance' is lowered to a certain point, and given a certain combination of other factors, the body cannot destroy malignant cells, and the way is clear for a tumour to grow. The breakdown of the body's 'resistance' is the cause of the 'primary' tumour and 'secondaries'. It is equally true for all the theories of the origin of the cancer cells—either by virus, mutation and so on. The 'resistance' should become the core of every cancer treatment. Such a therapy should comprise of two main pillars. A *causal* therapy to improve the body's natural defences; a *symptomatic* treatment directed against the cancer. They cannot replace each other; they must complement one another.
>
> From the beginning, the Ringberg Klinik has not only been a hospital for treating incurable cancer patients. It has also always been a centre for 'research on the sick bed', something repeatedly advocated in medical literature.
>
> The patients the clinic has treated, and still treats, have been the ones who have failed to benefit from conventional treatments. It is these patients who have enabled us to make lengthy observations, and gain new insight into the disease, that is not possible by merely *symptomatically* treating the tumour. Over twenty-five years, we

have come to certain conclusions about new measures to be taken when treating cancer. The most important is that the lowering of the natural bodily defences has not one cause, but is a complex process developing over many years, even sometimes generations. It depends on the poor condition of the 'internal milieu', which in turn depends on the body's capacity to eliminate the waste products of the metabolism, and toxins resulting from chronical infections, such as dead teeth, infected tonsils, degenerated intestinal flora, and inherited factors such as 'masked' tuberculosis and syphilis.

The rules of humoral pathology can explain these correlations, and further explain many of the symptoms discovered in cancer patients, especially in the progressive state. Cellular pathology shows changes in the cells, but not always how those changes occur. Cellular pathology is important for diagnosing, but humoral pathology does not only reveal how cellular changes have occurred, it offers co-ordinated ground rules for treatment. By following those rules it is possible to build up the 'resistance', so providing the basis for active immunotherapy to work. And only then is the optimum benefit from immunotherapy, the third weapon against cancer, open to help the so-called 'incurables', offering a scientific basis for a *real* prophylactic and follow-up treatment of cancer.

This approach is not new. It goes back as far as Hippocrates. He taught that a malcondition of the body liquids, *dyscrasia*, was the bases for all kinds of diseases, which manifested themselves according to the constitution and disposition of the individual person. Thus one patient has chronic rheumatism, another diabetes, a third asthma, and a fourth cancer. So, cancer is not a unique disease. it is not a *disease sui generis*. It is nothing more than another chronic sickness.

We have found that our *ganzheitstherapie* has a beneficial effect on many other chronic diseases, some of which have been termed 'incurable'. By treating cancer, we also found that such illnesses as diabetes, liver cyrrhosis, asthma, rheumatism and a number of other conditions disappeared. *Wholistic* cancer treatment is embodied in *ganzheitstherapie*.

Medicine has made a great progress, but it has now arrived in a *cul-de-sac*, where drugs are used to kill symptoms. Penicillin, however good it may be for many infections, is also more and more being used to destroy a natural fever which the body needs to combat illness. Cortizone, important though it is in many cases, is too often used to destroy the very necessary inflammation which the body uses to fight illness. We forget the consequences the abuse of such drugs could have in the future. The 1970s saw the arrival of computerised medicine. Orthodox medicine thought that was the ultimate in diagnosis. Accurate though the computer is, it can only offer a diagnosis of symptoms. It often misses the cause of an illness.

We must completely re-think our position. We need to go back to the old days when a doctor looked at a patient as a *whole*. We must seek the *cause* of an illness. We must combine humoral pathology with cellular pathology. Both are of equal value. Then we would have found the true way for the future.

The experience and knowledge which we have gained by treating 'incurable' cancer patients can be used by *all* doctors to treat all 'incurable' illnesses. By following the rules of humoral pathology, we could not only remove the symptoms, but also offer real cures for many chronic diseases.

We need to stop training our doctors that cancer is an incurable disease beyond a certain point. The judgment of 'incurable' has been changed by immunotherapy—and only when that does not work can we truly say that a patient is 'incurable'.

But the world at large will not accept that as long as it only puts its faith in surgery and radiotherapy. They have their proper place, and a valuable one it is. But the knife and the deep-ray machine cannot always provide a total cure. Nor can chemotherapy. They are no more than symptomatic tools.

Finally, nobody should be just waiting to find the *cause* of the cancer *cells*. Just as important is to discover the *cause* of why cancer is still treated the way it is. In some ways medicine itself appears to be *incurable* as long as it sticks to a dogma. And daily, people die in their hundreds all over the world from cancer who need not die.

His deep personal convictions were clear in those words. Public opinion had to be aroused over the rigid thinking of conventional medicine. That was the only way to slough off the lethargy, the apathy, and most dangerous of all, the complacency. Cancer research had been in a vacuum too long. In September 1972 he published in Germany his book *More Cures For Cancer,* a restatement of what he believed the disease was and its optimum treatment.

In 1973, in his sixty-fifth year, Josef Issels proposed building a new clinic. But the promise of the drawing board would never be realised. With bewildering speed events overtook his plans, taxing even his furious energy, leaving him embattled and tormented.

The facts are simple. Issels found that staff he had trusted had abused his confidence. Case histories and other medical data had been purloined from the clinic's archives and offered to the Press. A doctor had been filmed by the B.B.C., even though his contract expressly forbade such a thing. Issels' lawyers stopped that caper. But they were unable to halt the flood of publicity which pursued Issels through the summer of 1973. He accepted he was an international figure and fair game for reporters. Some, like Gay Byrne and Des Hickey showed remarkable perception and understanding. Others, he found frankly offensive. He became convinced some journalists, especially those in Germany, were being fed information from the medical establishment. In June, 1973, the publicity reached a new and shriller crescendo when the B.B.C. objected to this book appearing in its original form. The headlines were further fanned by Issels' lecture to the Oxford University Medical Society. He only agreed to appear providing the B.B.C. were barred; he claimed his 'sources' inside the Corporation had warned him he was to 'be set-up for a swingeing attack on my methods'. In the end he received a standing ovation.

The interest abroad only increased the animosity at home. At this critical time Robert Good's parting words at the Sloan Kettering Institute took on a new significance. He said: 'Issels, your problem is that of making your work acceptable to the scientific world. This can only be achieved by double blind trials.' He expressed what Issels had felt for a long time. But how could double blind trials be carried out in a private clinic? Important though the private clinic with its independence had been for the development of the therapy, at this stage it turned out to be an obstacle to acknowledgment and further progress.

Meanwhile, at home, Issels became convinced that the German Cancer Society was planning some possible move against him. Further the clinic's finances had slumped, patient intake had fallen, sacked staff could not easily be replaced. Finally, in tears, Issels announced he was closing down his clinic on October 1. On that day his last patient left. A month later only a handful of maintenance staff remained. Then on November 21, 1973, on his sixty-sixth birthday, Josef Issels showed it is not always easy to disassociate a man from the legend, for the legend is sometimes inextricably woven into his life, and Issels is perfectly aware that he possesses legendary qualities. Responding to a birthday toast, Issels boldly announced he was considering offers to continue his work in various other countries. 'My Task here is finished. But the Task must go on. And I will go on.'

From other men it would have sounded like bravado. From Josef Issels it sounded the most natural of suggestions. By April, 1974, he had already mapped out a world tour which would take him from one medical centre to another, allowing him to evaluate the best possible place for him to continue with what he claims he has done, and will continue to do—helping the incurable.

Acknowledgments

NEARLY FIVE YEARS AND A CONSIDERABLE AMOUNT OF TRAVEL went into the preparation of this book. Many people helped along the way: not a few members of the medical profession asked that their assistance went unrecognised because of a genuine fear of reprisals from more powerfully placed colleagues. That seems to be an alarming situation.

Research fell naturally into two sections. The first was collating all the published material on Josef Issels, the Ringberg Klinik and its patients. By the end of that phase some 4·5 million words had been assembled in a score of languages. There were newspaper stories printed as far apart as Moscow and Buenos Aires; magazine articles from Tokyo and Nairobi, medical journals, official reports and a couple of full-length books.

The second part involved sifting the millions of words in the clinic's archives.

A very special debt must be acknowledged to Ilse Maria Issels. On top of all her other responsibilities she gladly shared with my own wife, Edith, the translation of this material. At times they were driven close to distraction by the frequency of demands for some ancient file or document which might stimulate a reminiscence.

Isa Issels also submitted without complaint to questions about her own life and that of her husband's.

Irmengard Issels received us politely on two separate occasions and gave her version of married life with Josef

Issels. Uti and Rolf talked frankly in the belief it might help their father understand them better. If anything it saddened him.

Margot and Charlotte, two of Issels' sisters, recalled his childhood in Germany nearly sixty years ago in a way that had a haunting quality of its own.

A particular debt is recognised for the contribution of the Ringberg Klinik staff. Anneliese Lipp sketched in a number of small, but important details; Dr. Theodor Weiss, the clinic's statistician, provided useful background material. Professor Franz Gerlach and his wife went to unusual trouble to contribute enough material for a couple of books.

Gisela Ide acted as my secretary and an additional translator, and played her part in ensuring that the finished material was accurately assembled.

There were the patients, too numerous to mention, who answered countless questions; the medical staff were always ready to help.

Above all there was Josef Issels. He was always kind and patient, and conducted nearly all our talks in what he called 'my Ringberg English', a modest assessment for a man fluent enough in the tongue. He provided much material that was precious to him. He allowed totally free access to his private and professional papers. Finally, he gave up all his free time for several months in 1972 to ensure the book would lack for nothing he could offer. No one could ask for more.

Gordon Thomas.

Rottach-Egern,
West Germany,
October, 1974.